IS IT MORAL
to
MODIFY MAN?

IS IT MORAL
to
MODIFY MAN?

Edited by

CLAUDE A. FRAZIER, M.D.
Asheville, North Carolina

With Forewords by

Joseph Fletcher
University of Virginia
School of Medicine
Charlottesville, Virginia

C. A. Hoffman

Cecil E. Sherman

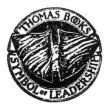

CHARLES C THOMAS · PUBLISHER
Springfield · Illinois · U.S.A.

Published and Distributed Throughout the World by

CHARLES C THOMAS • PUBLISHER

BANNERSTONE HOUSE

301-327 East Lawrence Avenue, Springfield, Illinois, U.S.A.

© *1973 by* CHARLES C THOMAS • PUBLISHER

ISBN 0-398-02632-7

Library of Congress Catalog Card Number: 72-84142

With **THOMAS BOOKS** *careful attention is given to all details of manufacturing and design. It is the Publisher's desire to present books that are satisfactory as to their physical qualities and artistic possibilities and appropriate for their particular use.* **THOMAS BOOKS** *will be true to those laws of quality that assure a good name and good will.*

Printed in the United States of America

HH-11

To
DONALD FRAZIER
my nephew and my friend

CONTRIBUTORS

CHRISTIAAN BARNARD, M.D.

Department of Surgery
University of Cape Town Medical School
Cape Town, South Africa

HAROLD C. BATCHELDER, ACSW

Director of Psychiatric Social Work Services
Assistant Professor of Psychiatry
Virginia Commonwealth University

ERIC BERMANN, Ph.D.

Chief Psychologist, Children's Psychiatric Hospital
Ann Arbor, Michigan
Assistant Professor Department of Psychiatry
Associate Professor Department of Psychology
University of Michigan
Ann Arbor, Michigan

LEWIS PENHALL BIRD, S.T.M. Ph.D.

Eastern Regional Director
Christian Medical Society

JOSEPH E. DAVIS, M.D., F.A.C.S.

President, Association of Voluntary Sterilization
New York, New York

AMITAI ETZIONI, Ph.D.

Professor of Sociology
Director, Center for Policy Research, Inc.
Columbia University
New York, New York

JULIE FULTON, M.A.

National Institute of Mental Health Fellow
Department of Sociology
University of Minnesota
Minneapolis, Minnesota

ROBERT L. GARRARD, M.D.

Chief, Psychiatric Division
Moses H. Cone Memorial Hospital
Clinical Associate Professor
Department of Psychiatry
University of North Carolina School of Medicine
Chapel Hill, North Carolina

BENJAMIN C. HAMMETT, Ph.D.

Senior Psychologist
Assistant Professor of Psychiatry
Virginia Commonwealth University
Richmond, Virginia

ADRIAN C. KANAAR, M.D.
WOLFGANG LEDERER, M.D.

Associate Clinical Professor
Department of Psychiatry
University of California Medical School
San Francisco, California

JAMES L. MATHIS, M.D.

Professor and Chairman
Department of Psychiatry
Medical College of Virginia
Health Sciences Center
Virginia Commonwealth University
Richmond, Virginia

WILLIAM M. PINSON, JR.

Associate Professor, Christian Ethics
Southwestern Baptist Theological Seminary
Fort Worth, Texas

A. HERBERT SCHWARTZ, M.D.

Assistant Professor of Pediatrics and Psychiatry
Child Study Center, Yale University
Assistant Director, Yale University
Children's General Clinical Research Center
Yale-New Haven Hospital
New Haven, Connecticut

ROBERTA G. SIMMONS, Ph.D.

Assistant Professor of Sociology and Psychiatry
University of Minnesota
Minneapolis, Minnesota

JANE S. STURGES, M.S.W.

Social Worker, Department of Pediatrics
Yale-New Haven Hospital
New Haven, Connecticut

MAX J. TRUMMER, M.D.

Associate Clinical Professor of Surgery
University of California
San Diego, California

MERVILLE O. VINCENT, M.D.

Medical Superintendent of Homewood Sanitarium, Ontario

HERBERT WALTZER, M.D.

Assistant Director, Department of Psychiatry
Queens Hospital Center, Hillside Hospital Affiliation
Clinical Assistant Professor, Department of Psychiatry
State University of New York and
Downstate Medical Center
Brooklyn, New York

ARTHUR WINTER, M.D.

Neurological Consultant
Clinical Instructor in Neurosurgery
New Jersey College of Medicine and Dentistry
East Orange, New Jersey

FOREWORD

In a half-century period, breathlessly fast, we have seen a "biological revolution" take shape. Fabulous gains have been won and innovations made all along the biomedical front.

With any imagination at all our minds boggle at what may be entailed in a simple inventory of the changes: contraceptive technologies, transplants, biochemistry and genetics, embryological research and artificial modalities of reproduction, immunizing agents, mind- and mood-changing drugs, computerized diagnosis, psychosurgery, artificial support systems and implants, micrometric instruments, neurological controls, ultrasonics in place of x-rays, intrauterine monitoring. It is an overwhelming record.

This biological revolution is a radical development in man's control of man himself, rushing ahead at an exponential rate of increase. Compared to the shifting forces and factors of his social changes, man's new biological knowledge is truly radical in the exact meaning of the word: It goes to the root of man's condition, to "human nature" itself.

However, every addition to man's knowledge, augmenting his controls over his condition and his situation, is also an added capability for evil as well as for good. Abuse and misuse can take over from use. These radical changes in modern medicine's art and science lead at once to a whole array of problems in biomedical ethics. Many of them are explored by the contributors to this volume. What they have to say to the reader makes it plain that we need to "second guess" these innovations carefully and formulate some policy principles for the life sciences and their application to human beings. Nota bene: guidelines are needed, yes, but I would hope not regulations. This, by the way, is the purpose of Senator Mondale's bill to establish for two years a top level and interprofessional panel (biologists, physicians, ethicists, theologians, sociologists), a National Commission on Health Sciences and Society. (As of March 1972, the Senate has adopted it and House approval is expected soon.)

As I have said several times elsewhere, these questions about human initiatives and our responsibilities for life, health, and death are moral questions, but they are of a *success* kind—not due to failure. "New occasions teach new duties, truth makes ancient good uncouth." Resuscitation and intensive care have brought us, for example, to the place where prolonging some patients' lives (newborns as well as the elderly or terminally ill) is paradoxically only prolonging their dying. Along with the problems of how to save life comes the problem of when to stop it.

When we try to synthesize these frontier problems as they take form along a hundred and one sectors of the front held by the new biology and medicine, it seems to me that the unifying and thematic question, the basic issue running throughout the whole varied complex of right-wrong, good-evil, desirable-undesirable questions, is this: Which do we want, quantity or quality? Are we in favor of a sanctity-of-life etchics or a quality-of-life ethics? This is exactly what is at stake in proposals to replace the classical definition of death in terms of the loss of spontaneous heart function with a "brain death" criterion (loss of cerebral function, to be more precise).

Just here, however, we must be careful and cautious. The biomedical revolution is conceptual or mental, not merely technical. A bill passed by the Kansas legislature in 1971 (Suppl. 1971, 77-202) attempted to adopt a more medically relevant statute favoring "brain death" but did so in such naive terms that the old clinical definition was in fact unaltered. The issue is not whether artificial support is needed, but whether excerebral life (as in "human vegetables") is truly human or *personal*. Is it quantity or quality?

In the chapters that follow we have a galaxy of stellar authors and hardy explorations. This is Dr. Frazier's second symposium and it carries his first one several leagues ahead. All of us in medicine, biology and biomedical ethics are in his debt because of his initiative, and we are also indebted to the experience and learning of the contributors. The readers, each one on his own, will have to sift it all through his own head and heart, but it won't take him long to see that this book is no mere academic or professional treatise.

It touches every one of us where he lives.

JOSEPH FLETCHER

FOREWORD

A generation ago, the French biologist Rostand suggested the predicament physicians face in this age of pyramiding scientific knowledge: "Science has taught us how to become gods before we have learned to be men." The public now looks with alarm as well as awe at what medicine can do. Can medical ethics provide the security individuals need against the impersonal doom of modern medicine?

Hope for the future is found by examining the history of medicine, because this history is one of medicine's efforts to define the ethical conduct of its members in accordance with the spirit of the time, to elevate the dignity of medicine as a profession, to assure proper education and training for all physicians, to resist the imposition upon the public of unscientific cults, to promote harmony within the profession, and to resist exploitation of physician or patient by commercial or political interests. This history extends back more than 5,000 years and its foundation was defined clearly in the fewer than fifty words of classical Greek written by Hippocrates:

> A physician should be an upright man, instructed in the art of healing . . . modest, sober, patient, prompt to do his whole duty without anxiety; pious without going so far as superstition, conducting himself with propriety in his profession and in all the actions of his life.

The value system upon which these words of Hippocrates and the present Principles of Medical Ethics alike are built is respect for the sanctity of human life. This foundation has not changed and cannot change if medicine has a role in society.

Today's Principles of Medical Ethics consists of 500 words, a few more than Hippocrates used, but the basic precepts that guide physicians in their moments of decision are unchanged. The first section of the Principles outlines medicine's aims:

The principal objective of the medical profession is to render service to humanity with full respect for the dignity of man. Physicians should merit the confidence of patients entrusted to their care, rendering to each a full measure of service and devotion.

Ethical problems do not occur until an individual is confronted with a choice. Every choice a physician makes commits him to consequences from which there is no point of return. Medical ethics constitute the physician's continuing search for standards by which choice can be guided and in this sense, ethics are temporal. They represent the interpretation of the eternal moral principles to reflect the choices to be made in a given period of time.

Little, if any, change has occurred in medicine's pattern of morality since Hippocrates first wrote. What has changed is the physician's milieu of practice. The pyramiding fund of scientific knowledge, the vastly increased capability of physicians, the miraculous armamentarium at their disposal, and the economic phenomena we call health care financing create daily problems of choice of which Hippocrates could never have dreamed. Yet, the basic tenets handed down through the centuries are adequate for this and succeeding centuries. The Ethical Guidelines for Clinical Investigation and the Ethical Guidelines for Organ Transplants are two notable examples of the collective conscience of medicine at work in the interpretation of the basic principles to the new phenomenon and resulting problems.

Heart transplants captured the imagination of the public like no other medical advance because of the symbolic significance. The heart has always been the site of life, the source of love and all other emotions and the home of the soul. Tomorrow, heart transplants may be viewed not only as progress resulting in part from the courage with which physicians cross the traditional barrier of harmless treatment but as the spur which renewed public faith in the medical profession's leadership efforts to find solutions to problems made more complex because of social, religious, anthropological and legal interests.

Can we answer yes when we are asked if the basic ethical principles have applicability today and, even more important, will be relevant tomorrow? There is no question in my mind that we can. The evidence is more convincing today than ever before that the best interest of humanity is well served if the self-restraint and the peer-judgment restraint based upon the ethical standards are allowed to govern clinical investigation, experimental medicine, experimental biology and all aspects of the practices of medicine. Hope is lost only if the medical profession fails to rely upon the basic moral principles, values and duties expressed in the ten Principles of Medical Ethics. The prayer of Maimonides can still be heard coming to physicians from across the centuries: "Let me, oh Lord, by my knowledge discover today what I did not know yesterday, because art has no end, and because the spirit of man always presses onwards." The Principles continue to inspire in all physicians an inseparable fusion of conscience, compassion, consecration and experience directed toward a human personality—the patient.

C. A. HOFFMAN

FOREWORD

One of the liveliest themes in medicine or morals is the title of of this book, *Is It Moral to Modify Man?* The possibilities in transplantation and drugs are a bit overwhelming. The best of men is a bit intimidated with the godlike tools that have fallen into his hands. God has not spoken about how we should act in each particular. The responsibility falls upon discerning men to try and try again to find the best ways of coming to terms with the new options that are open to us.

Simple people look upon the modern medical scientist as a magician. He is the wonder worker. He has miracle drugs. Thoughtful people are awed and cast about for the opinions of the wisest of men. This book is a popular effort in a long line of efforts at solutions. Dr. Claude A. Frazier has done us great service compiling essays on these problem areas. We are in his debt for this kind of labor and for making available to us some of today's best thinking.

CECIL E. SHERMAN, D.D.

ACKNOWLEDGMENTS

I would like to extend my sincere appreciation to the contributors of this book.

Also, I wish to thank my former secretary, Miss Sherry Morrow, for the assistance she rendered in making this book a reality. Final clerical preparation of the book for the publisher was made by my present secretary, Mrs. Rosemarie Duda, to whom I am grateful.

C.A.F.

CONTENTS

IS IT MORAL
to
MODIFY MAN?

Chapter 1

TAO PRINCIPLES OF MEDICAL ETHICS

LEWIS PENHALL BIRD, S.T.M. PH.D.

Religion and medicine conferences abound anymore with noted speakers and multidisciplinary panels debating the medico-ethical issues of liberalized abortion, genetic manipulation, humane euthanasia, organ transplantation, human experimentation, and artificial insemination. Whenever *McCall's* magazine[1] commissions a survey or McGill University convenes a symposium on issues of this nature, a ready audience will be found. That a sense of humor is not entirely lacking amidst such solemn assemblies is evidenced by such notable topics as "Through the Umbilical Cord with Bible and Camera"[2] and "Abortion Reform: or Why Labor Under a Misconception?"[3]

University campuses and medical centers have fostered through the decade of the sixties numerous significant conferences where the social and philosophical implications of modern medicine could be examined. The Dartmouth symposium (1961) debated "The Great Issues of Conscience in Modern Medicine." At Ohio Wesleyan (1963), "The Control of Human Heredity and Evolution" was the theme. A symposium on "The Sanctity of Life" was convened at Reed College[4] in Portland, Oregon (1966). A conference at Duke University (1967) discussed "Medical Science and Moral Responsibility." The decade closed with the notable Houston Conference on Ethics in Medicine and Technology[5] (1969). In addition, excellent symposia were variously sponsored in the mid-sixties by the American Medical Association: the First National Congress on Medical Ethics in Chicago (1966); by the CIBA Foundation in England (1963): "Man and His Future";[6] by The United Methodist Church (1967) at the Mayo Clinic, Rochester, Minnesota: A Convocation on Medicine and Theology;[7]

by the Christian Medical Society in New Hampshire (1968): "The Control of Human Reproduction."[8] These deliberations and publications bring fresh perspective to the increasingly complex concerns of the modern medical community. Issues that formerly attracted only physicians and theologians[9] now merit multidisciplinary examination.

The temper of our times demands that every issue of socio-moral ramification must not only authenticate, but also must vindicate its proposed solution. It is not new for the medical profession to apply time-honored principles to the management of difficult cases; what is new is having the larger academic community along with an increasingly sophisticated general public raise pressing questions about recent biomedical innovations, procedures and therapeutics. It was Albert Einstein who reminded us that "we live in an age of perfect means and confused ends.[10] The modern ethical predicament is further complicated and exacerbated by contemporary existential estrangement. Speaking of the latter, Erich Fromm, upon giving the George W. Gay Lecture upon Medical Ethics for 1957 (Harvard Medical School), noted: "We make machines which act like men, and produce men which act like machines. The danger of the 19th Century was that we may become slaves: and the danger of the 20th Century is not that we become slaves, but that we become robots."[11]

The modern medical student, caught in the swirl of the present social revolution,[12] seeks to wed a philosophical perspective with medical procedure. Sociologists have documented the all-too-frequent downhill slide from humanitarian idealism to personal cynicism which the pressures and anxieties of the medical school regimen inflict over the course of four years on incoming freshmen students.[13] Not only medical school curriculum committees,[14] but the students themselves[15] are seeking to reverse this trend through revised curricula[16] or supplementary programming.[17] A long-time advocate of courses in ethics in the nation's medical schools, Dr. Harold E. Jervey, Jr. of Columbia, South Carolina (a former president of the Federation of State Medical Boards), even proposes "that state boards initiate examinations in ethics as a prerequisite to licensure."[18] Needless to say, the debate over programming structure as well as on the specific medico-moral problems themselves will continue well into the decade of the seventies. The real question, given a pluralistic society, is whether or not a value system can be found which will be acceptable to all.[19]

Science, by itself, cannot give us a value system. Karl A. Menninger wrote "biology cannot provide the content of theology. Living by spiritual standards is more valuable than life maintained at the cost of demoralization and depersonalization."[20] Consequently, one must turn from the science of medicine to the art and history of medicine to discover the basic principles of medical ethics which have illuminated the decision-making process for physicians through the centuries. According to *Dorland's Medical Dictionary,* "medical ethics are the rules of principles governing the professional conduct of medical practitioners." From the Babylonian Code of Hammurabi[21] to the Oath of Hippocrates (written in about 50 words of classical Greek) to the writings of Maimonides to the Code of Sir Thomas Percival on through the American Medical Association Code, the Nuremberg Code, the Helsinki Declaration and the Geneva Declaration runs a rich and distinguished history.[22] Carl E. Taylor concludes

> No other group has such a long and consistent tradition of trying to maintain an idealistic view of its function and role; its ethical principles were long ago embodied in the Oath of Hippocrates, the Oath of Maimonides, and in India, the oath prescribed by Susruta from traditional rituals which originated well before the 1st century A.D. The total milieu of medical education specifically provides for the inculcation of these distinctive values.[23]

Anyone who has attended many of the current spate of panels, conferences, and lectures quickly realizes that most are patient oriented or problem oriented. Few are value oriented enough to be able to enunciate definitively the specific principles which stand behind their views. Yet the long tradition of medico-legal and medico-ethical debate has seen a strong interplay between clinical dilemmas and ethical declarations. In the view of Michael E. DeBakey:

> Human values are shaped in social context. Medical ethics, as an expression of that cultural ethos, seeks to reflect the highest humanitarian and benevolent values. Whether the physician

honors the Hippocratic, Nuremberg, or Helsinki formulation, his natural impulse is to alleviate suffering, preserve human life, and enrich man's existence.[24]

Any review of the literature quickly reveals a ready desire to get to the issues, but little effort to sketch out, even briefly, a philosophical prolegomena. One of the prominent Roman Catholic moral theologians who writes frequently on topics of a medical-moral interest, Edwin F. Healy, S.J., does offer at the outset of his study, *Medical Ethics,* ". . . six general principles that will serve as guides in solving the various special problems of medical ethics."[25] They are

1. Every human being has a right to life.
2. Every human being has a right to the truth.
3. Justice is due to every human being.
4. The faculties and powers of man must be used according to the purpose for which they were evidently intended by nature and in the manner evidently intended by nature.
5. If an act is ethically wrong, one is not only obliged to refrain from it himself, but he is also obliged to refrain from formal cooperation with another in the performance of the act.
6. Evil may never be done that good may result from it.[26]

Joseph Fletcher, the "father of 'situation ethics' in America" and an Episcopal theologian, weaves five elementary principles into the fabric of his study on medical ethics:

1. Our right to know the truth.
2. Our right to control parenthood.
3. Our right to overcome childlessness.
4. Our right to foreclose parenthood.
5. Our right to die.[27]

One of the few who also outlines his own basic presuppositions is Leroy G. Augenstein, chairman of the department of biophysics at Michigan State University and a frequent lecturer on these issues. He enumerates "five fundamental beliefs"[28] for resolving difficult problems:

1. There is a basic orderliness in the way things interest throughout our universe.
2. This orderliness was established by a concerned creator.

3. Life has a sanctity which should not be casually violated.
4. There is a "hereafter."
5. Agape must be the most important principle governing the behavior of people toward people.[29]

However valuable these criteria may be to their advocates, they nevertheless frequently evidence philosophical and/or religious presuppositions rather than more strictly medical presuppositions which would emerge from the medical tradition. A careful study must be made, not only of the primary texts on medical ethics but also of the basic studies of medical history in order to distill and refine precisely those principles of medical ethics which have had a hoary history and universal appeal. Only then can the hope emerge of discovering those fundamental principles of medical ethics which have guided physicians through the centuries.

TAO PRINCIPLES OF MEDICAL ETHICS

A very significant clue to the discovery of these ancient, universal principles comes embedded in the writings of the Cambridge Medieval and Renaissance scholar, C. S. Lewis. In his critique of modern education, *The Abolition of Man*,[30] Lewis calls attention to what he calls the concept of "the Tao:"

> It is the doctrine of objective value, the belief that certain attitudes are really true, and others really false, to the kind of thing the universe is and the kind of things we are. . . . [It is] to recognize a quality which *demands* a certain response from us whether we make it or not.[31]

This universal moral sense of mankind Lewis elsewhere calls "the reality beyond all predicates"[32] and "the sole source of all value judgments."[33]

America's principal C. S. Lewis interpreter, Clyde S. Kilby, in his discussion of "the Tao," see Lewis pointing to the law of righteousness at the very core of creation.[34] As Lewis himself pointed out, this universal moral law is called different names in different cultures. For the Hindus, it is the *Rta;*[35] for the ancient Hebrews, the *Law.*[36] For Aristotle, it is the first principles in ethics;[37] for Augustine, the *ordo amoris.*[38] For Roman Catholic moral theologians, it is the concept of Natural Law;[39] for ancient philoso-

phers, it was the "natural metaphysic."[40] Kant spoke of the "cate-
gorical imperative";[41] Brunner of the "divine imperative."[42] J. H.
Newman spoke of society's "common possession":[43] Walter Lipp-
mann called it "public philosophy."[44] Lewis has collected various
citations from both the world's great religions and great philosophers to illustrate the eight Tao principles he adduces from the
universal ethical consensus:

1. The Law of General Beneficence.
2. The Law of Special Beneficence.
3. Duties to Parents, Elders, Ancestors.
4. Duties to Children and Posterity.
5. The Law of Justice.
6. The Law of Good Faith and Veracity.
7. The Law of Mercy.
8. The Law of Magnanimity.[45]

It remains, then, to delineate and to document those *Tao* principles of medical ethics which have arisen in the medical tradition
and which have been the basis of clinical decision for centuries.
These ancient moral insights, perhaps revised and recast, could
form the foundation still of medical-ethical debate. Stumpf sees
no historical hiatus:

> It is rather fascinating that the deployment of a body of medical
> knowledge which has been discovered to a very great extent
> during the last 50 years in an unprecedented burst of discovery
> should be governed by a set of assumptions and insights about
> human nature formulated virtually 2,000 years ago. The great
> disparity in the time sequence of these two bodies of knowledge
> does not necessarily mean that the one is irrelevant to the other.
> It may be that moral insight was gained on the whole swiftly,
> whereas many preliminary steps had to follow before modern
> medicine could consolidate its historic gains and then suddenly
> explode in many directions in the contemporary world.[46]

What follows is an attempt to set in order an irreducible minimum of basic ethical principles, the *Tao* principles of medical
ethics.

I. *Primum, non nocere* (First of all, do no harm)

The origins of this elementary principle are lost in antiquity.[47]
Nevertheless, at least four illustrations of this concept are possible:

1. I will use treatment to help the sick according to my ability and judgment, but never with a view to injury and wrong-doing. —Oath of Hippocrates[48]

2. Do the sick no harm; not even in thought. —Hindus, Ayur-veda[49]

3. Christian morals forbid only one thing, doing ill to one's neighbor. —Claude Bernard[50]

4. Ye shall not cause any man injury by hastening to cut through flesh and blood with an iron instrument or by branding. —Oath of Asaph[51]

II. The Sanctity of Human Life

Numerous illustrations from the various codes of medical ethics bear witness to the centrality of this *Tao* principle:

1. Neither will I administer a poison to anybody when asked to do so, nor will I suggest such a course. Similarly I will not give to a woman a pessary to cause abortion. But I will keep pure and holy both my life and my art. —Oath of Hippocrates[52]

2. Care for the good of all living beings. —Hindus, Ayur-veda[53]

3. Ye shall not dispense a potion to a woman with child by adultery to cause her to miscarry. Nor shall ye reveal which roots be poisonous or give them in the hands of any man. —Oath of Asaph[54]

4. I have given no one a fatal draught. No woman has ever brought about an abortion by my aid. —Private Oath of Amatus Lusitanus[55]

5. Physicians dedicate their lives to the alleviation of suffering, to the enhancement and prolongation of life, and to the destines of humanity.—Principles of Medical Ethics of the American Medical Association[56]

6. I will maintain the utmost respect for human life, from the time of conception. —Declaration of Geneva[57]

7. A doctor must always bear in mind the importance of preserving human life from the time of conception until death. —International Code of Medical Ethics.[58]

8. A man is ethical only when life, as such, is sacred to him, that of plants and animals as that of his fellow men.
—Albert Schweitzer[59]

9. The direct killing of any innocent person, even at his own request, is always morally wrong.—Ethical and Religious Directors for Catholic Hospitals[60]

10. You shall watch verily over the life of man even from his mother's womb, and let his welfare always be your chief concern. —Oath of the Hebrew Physician[61]

III. The Alleviation of Suffering
This core principle of medical ethics finds plentiful support:

1. Here begins the book of the preparation of medicine for all parts of the body of a person. . . . The Lord of All has given me words to drive away the diseases of all the gods and mortal sufferings of every kind.—Prologue, the Egyptian Ebers Medical Papyrus[62]

2. As regards the art of medicine, I should state first of all what I believe to be its scope: to remove the sufferings of the patient, or at least to alleviate these sufferings.
—Hippocrates, *On Art*[63]

3. Not for self, not for the fullfillment of any earthly desire of gain, but solely for the good of suffering humanity should you treat your patients, and so excell all.
—Charaka (Hindu physician) in the Samhita[64]

4. Devote yourself to the healing of the sick even if your life be lost by your work. —Oath of the Hindu Physician[65]

5. The first responsibility of the physician is to prevent disease; if that be impossible, to treat illness; and if that be impossible, to relieve suffering. —ancient aphorism[66]

6. Ye shall not harden your hearts against the poor and needy, but heal them. —Oath of Asaph[67]

7. I have accorded the same care to the poor as to those born in exalted rank. All men have been considered equal by me of whatever religion they were, whether Hebrews, Christians or the followers of the Moslem faith.
—Private Oath of Amatus Lusitanus[68]

8. To cure sometimes, to relieve often, to comfort always.
—Lord Lister[69]

9. You are charged night and day to be custodians at the side of the sick man at all times of his need. You shall help the sick, base or honorable, stranger or alien or citizen, because he is sick.   —Oath of the Hebrew Physician[70]

IV.   The Sanctity of the Doctor-Patient Relationship

1. And whatsoever I shall see or hear in the course of my profession, as well as outside my profession in my intercourse with men, if it be what should not be published abroad, I will never divulge, holding such things to be holy secrets.
                    —Oath of Hippocrates[71]

2. When the physician enters a house accompanied by a man suitable to introduce him there, he must pay attention to all the rules of behavior in dress, deportment, and attitude. Once with his patient, he must in word and thought attend to nothing but his patient's case and what concerns it. What happens in the house must not be mentioned outside.
                    —Oath of the Hindu Physician[72]

3. Ye shall not disclose secrets confided unto you.
                    —Oath of Asaph[73]

4. I have revealed to no one a secret entrusted to me.
                    —Private Oath of Amatus Lusitanus[74]

5. The one rule of practice is to put yourself in the patient's place.   —Lord Lister[75]

6. Confidences concerning individual or domestic life entrusted by patients to a physician and defects in the disposition or character of patients observed during medical attendance should never be revealed unless their revelation is required by the laws of the state.—Principles of Medical Ethics of the American Medical Association[76]

7. I will respect the secrets which are confided in me.
                    —Declaration of Geneva[77]

8. A doctor owes to his patient absolute secrecy on all which has been confided to him or which he knows because of the confidence entrusted to him.—International Code of Medical Ethics[78]

9. Be true to him who puts his trust in you. Reveal not his secret and go not about us a talebearer.
                    —Oath of the Hebraw Physician[79]

V. The Right to Truth

1. You must speak the truth; speak clearly, gently, truly, properly; consider time and place; always seek to grow in knowledge. —Oath of the Hindu Physician[80]

2. Grant me strength, time and opportunity always to correct what I have acquired, always to extend its domain; for knowledge is immense and the spirit of man can extend infinitely to enrich itself daily with new requirements. Today he can discover his errors of yesterday and tomorrow he may obtain a new light on what he thinks himself sure of today —Prayer of Maimonides[81]

3. In diagnosis I have always said what I thought to be true. —Private Oath of Amatus Lusitanus[82]

4. Thou shalt not confess to a belief in occasional lies. —Richard C. Cabot[83]

5. Devotion to the truth does not always require the physician to voice his fears or tell his patient all he knows. But, after he had decided that the process of dying has actually begun, only in exceptional circumstances would a physician be justified in keeping to himself his opinion. In such cases his only question should be whether to tell the patient or the family, and, when both are to be told, which to tell first. —Alfred Worcester[84]

6. The physician should neither exaggerate nor minimize the gravity of a patient's condition. He should assure himself that the patient, his relatives or his responsible friends have such knowledge of the patient's condition as well serve the best interests of the patient and the family.—Principles of Medical Ethics of the Americal Medical Association[85]

VI. The Right to Informed Consent

This last *Tao* principle of medical ethics, while perhaps implicit in the history of clinical practice, has become more carefully articulated in the past several decades. This is due both to the inhumane medical experiments conducted in Germany under Hitler and to the rapidly growing field of research experimentation. "Ethics in research, however, is still rather virgin territory."[92] Illustrations of this *Tao* principle come only from the past century:

1. Among experiments that may be tried on man, those that can only do harm are forbidden, those that are harmless are

permissible, and those that do good are obligatory.
—Claude Bernard[93]

2. The voluntary consent of the human subject is absolutely essential.—Nuremberg Code of Ethics in Medical Research[94]

3. The danger of each experiment must have been investigated previously by means of animal experimentation. —Judicial Council of the American Medical Association[95]

4. The experiment must be performed under proper medical protection and management.—Judical Council of the AMA[96]

5. Under no circumstances is a doctor permitted to do anything that would weaken the physical or mental resistance of a human being, except from strictly therapeutic or prophylactic indications imposed in the interest of the patient.
—International Code of Medical Ethics.[97]

6. Any procedure harmful to the patient is morally justified only insofar as it is designed to produce a proportionate good.   —Ethical and Religious Directives for Catholic Hospitals[98]

7. The human experimental subject must understand and voluntarily consent to the procedure, and must not be selected upon any basis such as race, religion, level of education, or economics status   —Michael B. Shimkin[99]

8. An experiment is ethical or not at its inception. It does not become ethical *post hoc*—ends do not justify means. There is no ethical distinction between ends and means.
—Henry K. Beecher[100]

VII.   The Right to Die With Dignity
1. There is a time to be born, and a time to die.
—Old Testament Wisdom Literature[86]

2. I esteem it the office of a physician not only to restore the health, but to mitigate pains and dolors; and not only when such mitigation may conduce to recovery, but when it may serve to make a fair and easy passage.   —Francis Bacon[87]

3. While one of the physician's functions is to assist at the coming-in, another is to assist at the going-out.
—Oliver Wendell Holmes[88]

4. I hold it to be your duty to smooth as much as possible the pathway to the grave even if life is somewhat shortened.

—S. B. Woodward[89]

5. Everyone has the right and the duty to prepare for the solemn moment of death. —Ethical and Religious Directives for Catholic Hospitals.[90]

6. Our duty to our patients ends only with their death, and in the preceding hours there is much that we can do for their comfort. At the very least we can stand by them.

—Alfred Worcester[91]

IMPLICATIONS FOR THE TAO PRINCIPLES
OF MEDICAL ETHICS

In a certain sense the first three *Tao* principles apply to the physician, the fourth is transitional, and the last three apply to the patient. Reciprocity of integrity between the doctor and the patient is explicitly affirmed in both the fourth and the seventh principles; it is implicitly pledged in both the fifth and the sixth principles. Whether the physician be an advocate of humanism or Hinduism, whether Christian or Jew, whether Oriental or Occidental, the broad stream of the medical tradition carries with it these elementary principles, obligatory upon all. While men of good will and professional competency may debate the essential interpretation and clinical application of these ideals, there can be no escaping their binding moral suasion.

Primum, non nocere has never been intended to be interpreted in so literalistic a fashion as to prohibit the often necessary, short-term discomfort of the patient during therapy. While the scalpel may well be indicated, a hemipelvectomy may not. The Sanctity of Human Life principle, while not advocating a crude biological vitalism,[101] nonetheless does argue for a sense of reverence towards both potential[102] and actual human life. The contemporary social revolution, arguing as it does for elementary human rights,[103] enlarges one's understanding of this principle vis-à-vis the quality of human life. Only a clearer perception of the processes of humanization and socialization will permit a more optimistic prognosis for the quality of human life which incorporates both emotional and spiritual health into the physical dimension of health.

The Alleviation of Suffering has long been the task of both the private practitioner and organized medicine. Of deep concern in the modern world is the present desire to deliver quality health care to the widest reaches of any given population. The right to choose one's own physician and the right to confidentiality in privileged communication undergird the Sanctity of the Doctor-Patient Relationship. While aberrant personalities may jeopardize and/or strain this most unique relationship,[104] nevertheless, for most patients it has been *the* basis for sound diagnosis and rapid recovery, often of healing additional personal, familial, and marital disease.

The physician who is taking a routine medical history has no less a Right to Truth than does the patient upon the completion of the examination. "Speaking the truth in love"[105] adds perspective to the physician's task. Knowing the truth, which sets one free,[106] adds perspective for the patient. The Right to Die with Dignity can restore to the individual a sense of both his own history and his own destiny. Supportive measures which place this last great ritual of life in a family context merit commendation, for the most part.[107] Combining this principle with the Sanctity of Human Life, Thielicke remarks: "For man, unlike the animal, is a being who can suffer ethically. Therefore there can be a *"coup de grace"* for a dog, but not for man."[108] The Right to Informed Consent presupposes that rational volunteers may give a valid and knowledgeable assent to qualified research experimenters in permitting their persons to be the objects of scientific inquiry.

Obviously, these *Tao* principles provide only a starting point in the quest for the solution to modern medico-ethical problems which have, usually, vast personal, social, legal, medical and ethical ramifications. While codes of ethics may well prove to be rigid or absolutist, theoretical or sterile, without legal sanction or unduly restrictive,[109] they have borne witness, nonetheless, to the moral consensus within the medical community at any given point in history. In a sense, to discuss codes of medical ethics or *Tao* principles of medical ethics is to build the cart before securing the proverbial horse. For the motivation (the horsepower?) to consciously, persistently live by these principles, every physician must look within. Says Michael E. DeBakey:

> Ethical decisions in medical science must therefore depend finally on the wisdom, integrity, and compassion of the physician and his peers, because these are the qualities that nourish love and reverence for life in our culture.[110]

Since it is not very difficult to see how most of these *Tao* principles align with the Decalogue and the Judaeo-Christian ethic, a synthesis of their main ideals would prove to be additionally instructive. E. Mansell Pattison[111] and William B. Kiesewetter[112] have done this, essentially, in their studies. Bonhoeffer points to five critical steps in responsible decision-making: (1) to observe, (2) to judge, (3) to weigh up, (4) to decide, and (5) to act.[113] For the responsible Christian physician, clinical data must be joined with the biblical data, when appropriate, for valid results. As Miller has well noted, "a valid Christian decision is compounded always of both faith and facts. It is likely to be valid in the degree to which the faith is rightly apprehended and the facts are rightly measured."[114]

A final insight comes from the wisdom of Coach Vince Lombardi: "Coaches who can outline plays on a blackboard are a dime a dozen. The ones who win get inside their players and motivate them."[115] Given the *Tao* principles of any profession, the winning "plus" will always be an internalized, meaningful value system which calls forth sound judgment and personal compassion. Certainly the Christian faith offers such a philosophy of life—and an incarnate ethical model in the figure of the Great Physician.

NOTES AND REFERENCES

1. E. Fuller Torrey discovered that ". . . in the *Readers' Guide to Periodical Literature* between 1951 and 1953 there were 18 articles on birth control, whereas between 1963 and 1965 there were 120. Headings such as enthuansia, vasectomy, and artificial insemination were not even listed in the early period but are included in the latter." From Toward solutions. In Torrey, E. Fuller (Ed.): *Ethical Issues in Medicine*. Boston, Little, Brown 1968, p. 417f.

2. Montgomery, John Warwick: Original manuscript: The Christian view of the fetus. Read at the Christian Medical Society Symposium on the Control of Human Reproduction, Wentworth-by-the-Sea, New Hampshire, August 1968.

3. The title of the program topic at a luncheon of the Woman's Alliance of the University Unitarian Church of Seattle; cited in the *Emko Newsletter,* August 1970, p. 1.

4. The major papers were published. Daniel H. Labby (Ed.): *Life or Death: Ethics and Options.* Seattle, University of Washington Press, 1968.

5. The published proceedings have appeared. Kenneth Vaux (Ed.): *Who Shall Live?* Philadelphia, Fortress Press, 1970.

6. Wolstenholme, G. (Ed.): *Man and His Future.* Boston, Little, Brown, 1963.

7. White, Dale (Ed.): *Dialogue in Medicine and Theology.* New York, Abingdon Press, 1967.

8. Spitzer, Walter O. and Saylor, Carlyle L. (Eds.): *Birth Control and the Christian.* Wheaton, Tyndale House, 1969).

9. Cf. Some professional views on the role and relevancy of medical ethics. In the *American Medical News,* September 22, 1969, pp. 8, 9. For the standard studies on medical ethics, cf. O. Garceau, Morals of medicine bibliography. *Ann. Am. Acad. Med.,* vol. 363, pp. 60-69, January 1966. Also the competent bibliography in Vaux, *Op. Cit.,* pp. 197-199. Also the bibliography compiled by Lewis P. Bird in Spitzer and Saylor, *Op. Cit.,* pp. 501-521.

10. Cf. Infeld, Leopold: *Albert Einstein: His Work and Its Influence on Our World,* Revised ed. New York, Charles Scribner's Sons, 1950, pp. 120ff.

11 Fromm, Erich: The ethical problem of modern man. At *The George W. Gay Lecture upon Medical Ethics,* Harvard Medical School, April 25, 1957, mimeographed copy, p. 11.

12. Cf. The surprising views of tomorrow's doctors. In *Redbook,* October 1968 and Doctors in the streets. In *Newsweek,* October 14, 1968, p. 63.

13. Cf. the data of Fox and Eron, cited in The medical student mind by David Durica. *Christian Medical Society Journal,* Autumn 1969, pp. 1-7. Also cf. The professional, ethical and intellectual attitudes of medical students. *J. Med. Educ.,* December 1963, pp. 1016ff.

14. Cf. Kepler, Milton O.: Ethico-religious instruction in medical schools of the United States and Canada. *J. Religion Health,* 7:242-253, 1968. Also his article: Religious values in medical

education. In the *Christian Medical Society Journal* pp. 10-15, September-October, 1969.

15. Cf. The medical curriculum and human values. *J.A.M.A.*, 209(9): 1341-1353, 1969.

16. Cf. Should teaching about human value systems be included in medical education? If so, how? In *The Place of Value Systems in Medical Education,* New York, Academy of Religion and Mental Health, 1961. Two significant facts emerged from this symposium: "In the first place, all medical schools have traditionally given *pro forma* recognition to the importance of ethical values in medical education. Second, few if any medical schools have gone any further than this in the effort to educate their students. . . ." p. i. Cf. also the papers by William B. Kiesewetter, Gosta Birath, and Gerrit A. Lindeboom in the symposium, Introducing ethics into the medical curriculum. In *The Responsibility of the Christian Physician in the Modern World,* The Third International Congress of Christian Physicians, Oslo, July, 1969, Oak Park, Christian Medical Society, 1969, pp.11-31.

17. Cf. the Philadelphia series, A conversation in medical ethics, sponsored by Smith Kline & French Laboratories and by the Academy of Religion and Mental Health for the medical students of Philadelphia's medical schools.

18. Quoted in Medical ethics in a changing world. *Med. World News,* May 20, 1966, p. 70.

19. In a widely discussed editorial, the *Br. Med. J.* questioned whether any code or value system could be drawn up that would satisfy all groups. It referred to "the prevalent anxiety among investigators that a guide drawn up by doctors for themselves will have the force of law. We suggest that their real fear is of interference with the freedom of the investigator to decide for himself what is ethical or not." Cited in *Med. World News,* May 20, 1966, p. 68.

20. Menninger, Karl A.: In the foreword to Joseph Fletcher's *Morals and Medicine.* Boston, Beacon Press, 1960, p. xii.

21. Of the 282 sections of the Code of Hammurabi, eight refer to matters of medical practice. Cf. Samuel X. Radbill, A history of medical ethics. *AMA Medical Ethics and Discipline Manual,* Chicago, American Medical Association, n.d.

22. Cf. Richard Thomas Barton, Sources of medical morals. *J.A.M.,* 193(2):127-132, 1965. Also cf. The medical oath: empty ritual or wellspring of dedication? *Spectrum,* Winter 1965-1966.

23. Taylor, Carl E.: Ethics for an international health profession. *Science, 153* (3737):716, 1966.

24. DeBakey, Michael E.: In the foreword to Vaux *Op. Cit.*, p. vii.
25. Healy, Edwin F.: *Medical Ethics*. Chicago, Loyola University Press, 1956, p. 10.
26. Healy, Edwin F.: *Medical Ethics*. Chicago, Loyola University Press, 1956.
27. Fletcher, Joseph.: *Op. Cit.*
28. Augenstein, Leroy G.: *Come, Let Us Play God*. New York, Harper & Row, 1969, p. 135. He speaks of himself as "a practicing Protestant," pp. 6, 72.
29. Augenstein, Leroy G.: *Come, Let Us Play God*. New York, Harper & Row, 1969, pp. 135-139.
30. Lewis, C. S.: *The Abolition of Man*. New York, Macmillan, 1947.
31. Lewis, C. S.: *The Abolition of Man*. New York, Macmillan, 1947, p. 29.
32. Lewis, C. S.: *The Abolition of Man*. New York, Macmillan, 1947, p. 28.
33. Lewis, C. S.: *The Abolition of Man*. New York, Macmillan, 1947, p. 56.
34. Kilby, Clyde S.: *The Christian World of C. S. Lewis*. Grand Rapids, Wm. B. Eerdmans, 1964, p. 190.
35. Lewis, C. S.: *The Abolition of Man*. New York, Macmillan, 1947, p. 27f.
36. Lewis, C. S.: *The Abolition of Man*. New York, Macmillan, 1947, p. 28.
37. Lewis, C. S.: *The Abolition of Man*. New York, Macmillan, 1947, p. 26.
38. Lewis, C. S.: *The Abolition of Man*. New York, Macmillan, 1947, p. 26.
39. But Fletcher, in his disaffection for the classical concept of Natural Law, suggests "moral order." *Op. Cit.*, p. 223.
40. Cited in Labby, *Op. Cit.*, pp. 12, 38.
41. Kant, Immanuel: In Lewis White Beck (Ed.) *Critique of Practical Reason*. Chicago, University of Chicago Press, 1949.
42. Brunner, Emil: *The Divine Imperative,* Trans. Olive Wyon. Philadelphia, Westminster Press, 1947.
43. Newman, J. H.: *Historical Sketches*. London, 1872, I, p. 161.
44. Cited in Norman St. John-Stevas' article, Law and the moral consensus. In Labby, *Op. Cit.*, p. 42.
45. Cf. the Appendix, Illustrations of the *Tao*. In Lewis, *Op. Cit.*, pp. 95-121.
46. Stumpf, Samuel Enoch: Some moral dimensions of medicine. *Ann. Int. Med., 64*(2):467, 1966.
47. Cf. Chavez, Ignacio: Professional ethics in medicine in our time. *J.A.M.A., 190*(3):226-231, 1964.

48. Cited in Will Durant: The life of Greece. *The Story of Civilization, vol. II.* New York, Simon and Schuster, 1939, p. 347.
49. Cited in Benjamin Lee Gordon, *Medicine Throughout Antiquity.* Philadelphia, F. A. Davis, 1949, p. 348.
50. Cited by Henry K. Beecher, Medical research and the individual. Labby, *Op. Cit.,* p. 122, ftn. 7.
51. Quoted in *Spectrum,* p. 7.
52. Cited in Durant, *Op. Cit.,* p. 347.
53. Cited in Gordon, *Op. Cit.,* p. 348.
54. Cited in *Spectrum, Loc. Cit.*
55. *Spectrum,* p. 9.
56. Quoted in McFadden, Charles J.: *Medical Ethics,* edition 5. Philadelphia, F. A. Davis, 1961, p. 417.
57. Quoted in McFadden, Charles J.: *Medical Ethics.* Philadelphia, F. A. Davis, 1961, p. 430.
58. Quoted in McFadden, Charles J.: *Medical Ethics.* Philadelphia, F. A. Davis, 1961, p. 431.
59. Schweitzer, Albert: *Out of My Life and Thought.* New York, Henry Holt and Co., 1933, 1949, p. 126.
60. Quoted in McFadden, *Op. Cit.,* p. 411.
61. Cited in *Spectrum,* p. 8.
62. Cited in Gordon, *Op. Cit.,* p. 208.
63. Cited in Arturo Castiglioni: *A History of Medicine,* 2nd ed. Trans. and Ed. E. B. Krumbhaar. New York, Alfred A. Knopf, 1958, p. 156.
64. Cited in Durant, *Op. Cit.,* vol. I, Our oriental heritage, p. 530.
65. Cited in *Spectrum,* back cover.
66. Quoted in Taylor, *Op. Cit.,* p. 717.
67. Cited in *Spectrum,* p. 7.
68. *Spectrum,* p. 7.
69. Quoted in Maurice Davidson: *Medical Ethics.* London, Lloyd-Luke Ltd., 1957, p. 154.
70. Cited in *Spectrum,* p. 8.
71. Cited in Durant, *Op. Cit.,* II, p. 347.
72. Cited in *Spectrum,* back cover.
73. *Spectrum,* p. 7.
74. *Spectrum,* p. 9.
75. Quoted in Short, David S.: Ultimate loyalties. In Vincent Edmunds and C. Gordon Scorer, (Eds.): *Ideals in Medicine.* London, Tyndale Press, 1958, p. 157.
76. Quoted in McFadden, *Op. Cit.,* p. 421.
77. McFadden, *Op. Cit.,* p. 430.
78. Quoted in McFadden, *Op. Cit.,* p. 431.
79. Cited in *Spectrum,* p. 8.

80. *Spectrum,* back cover.
81. Cited in Rogers, Fred B.: *A Syllabus of Medical History.* Boston, Little, Brown, 1962, p. 22.
82. Cited in *Spectrum,* p. 9.
83. Cited in Fletcher, *Op. Cit.,* p. 48.
84. Fletcher, *Op. Cit.,* p. 53.
85. Quoted in McFadden, *Op. Cit.,* p. 421.
86. Old Testament, Eccl. 3:2.
87. Quoted in Fletcher, *Op. Cit.,* p. 179.
88. Cited in J. Clifford Hoyle, The care of the dying. In Davidson, *Op. Cit.,* p. 139.
89. Quoted in Fletcher, *Op. Cit.,* p. 204.
90. Cited in McFadden, *Op. Cit.,* p. 410.
91. Cited in Hoyle, *Op. Cit.,* p. 139.
92. Wolfensberger, Wolf: Ethical issues in research with human subjects. *Science, 155*(3758):47, 1967.
93. Cited in Henry K. Beecher, Medical research and the individual. In Labby, *Op. Cit.,* p. 122, ftn. 7.
94. The Nuremberg Code of Ethics in Medical Research is given in full in Otto E. Guttentag, Ethical problems in human experimentation. In Torrey, *Op. Cit.,* pp. 214f.
95. Cited in Pappworth, M. H.: *Human Guinea Pigs: Experimentation on Man.* Boston, Beacon Press, 1968, p. 189.
96. Pappworth, M. H.: *Human Guiena Pigs: Experimentation on Man.* Boston, Beason Press, 1968, p. 189.
97. Cited in McFadden, *Op. Cit.,* p. 430.
98. McFadden, *Op. Cit.,* p. 414.
99. Quoted in Gerald Kelly: *Medico-Moral Problems.* St. Louis, The Catholic Hospital Association, 1958, p. 264.
100. Cited in Pappworth, *Op. Cit.,* p. 185.
101. Cf. The discussion of this point by Fletcher, *Op. Cit.,* pp. 193, 215.
102. The current debate over the liberalization of America's abortion laws centers on this point. It is interesting to note, in passing, that most of the codes of medical ethics, from a historical viewpoint, emphasize the sanctity of human life *from the moment of conception.*
103. Cf. Iago Galdston, The third revolution: prelude and polemic. In Torrey, *Op. Cit.,* pp. 1-23.
104. Cf. Lois G. Forer, professional ethics and aberrant personalities. *Medical Opinion & Review, 5*(10):176-191, 1969.
105. New Testament, Eph. 4:15.
106. A free rendition of the New Testament, John 8:32.
107. Cf. Elisabeth Kubler-Ross: *On Death and Dying.* New York, Macmillan, 1969.

108. Thielicke, Helmut: *The Ethics of Sex.* Trans. John W. Doberstein. New York, Harper & Row, 1964, p. 266.
109. Cf. Pappworth's discussion, *Op. Cit.,* pp. 199f.
110. DeBakey in Vaux, *Loc. Cit.*
111. Pattison, E. Mansell: Medical ethics and christian values. *Christian Medical Society Journal, 15*(4):12-16, 1963.
112. Kiesewetter, William B.: Medical ethics—Can they be distinctively Christian? *The Responsibility of the Christian Physician in the Modern World* Proceedings, pp. 11-19.
113. Bonhoeffer, Dietrich: *Ethics.* Ed. by Eberhard Bethge, Trans. Neville Horton Smith. New York, Macmillan, 1955, p. 217.
114. Miller, Alexander: *The Renewal of Man: A Twentieth Century Essay on Justification by Faith.* Garden City, Doubleday, 1955.
115. Cited in *The New York Times,* Vol. CXIX, No. 41, 131, September 4, 1970, p. 24.

Chapter 2

CHAOS, ORDER, AND PSYCHOTHERAPY

Wolfgang Lederer, M.D.

W hen Freud began the studies of hysteria which were to become the foundations of a vast edifice of psychoanalytic theory and practice, Queen Victoria ruled in England. The age which bore her imprint and her name took pride and comfort—at least on the surface, at least officially—in the clarity and orderlines of its morals, in the simple, self-evident, God-given and rock-based ethics of its society. Individually, Victorians the world over did their consciencious best to *be* as they would *seem*. When feelings and thoughts just would not be contained within the forbidding rules and limits of custom and upbringing, they would develop symptoms: paralyses, faints, fits and fears, compulsive actions and obsessive thoughts—the whole gamut of the neuroses which were, according to Freud, nothing more nor less than primitive, chaotic instincts running afoul of a petrified social order and turning their frustrated vehemence against themselves, against the body and soul, against the person whose damned but civilized destiny it was somehow to contain them. It was, according to Freud, the purpose of therapy to soften the severity of conscience, to render more reasonable the demands of society as represented within the psyche by the superego. Reasonable—indeed, the age of reason would plausibly dream of a reasonable compromise between the wild horses of instinct and the orderly demands of society visualized as the rider: an immaculately clad, a purposeful and strong-willed rider, to be sure, who would give his mount all the exercise needed provided, of course, that it prance and lope and gallop within the well-established bridle paths in the park: provided it give due precedence to rank, due courtesy to ladies, due respect to officers and due caution to babies in perambulators. Restraint was the guiding principle—reason and re-straint, restraint and reason, and balance in every way, balance —and order.

Today the shoe is on the other foot: we no longer need to quote Heraklitos to maintain that everything is in flux; we know it by the testimony of our own senses: nothing stays still, nothing stays the same—no street and no city, no custom and no technique, no friend and no enemy, the very oceans and the very continents do not stay the same. Obviously, rules and guidelines are obsolete; there is no moral rock on which to base a sure-footed stand, no rank or caste, no guild or precedent to help define ourselves, our conduct and our identity. As a consequence, the neuroses are obsolete—we rarely see them any more, and if we do, then in old-fashioned people, who still plague themselves with notions of duty and decency and responsibility. But that is not where it's at: today the thing is not knowing who you are, man, the thing is identity confusion and diffusion.[1] The thing is to do your own thing or whatever you think your own thing may be today, for tomorrow it will be something else again be-cause the thing is to be protean, man, to be a protean man[2] and change all the time with the changing time, to hang loose and to let go. Oh, today, the rider and the horse, they are having a jolly time, dashing off the bridle path and through the flower beds and fish ponds and through the trash left from the picnic on the green, riding bareback and bare ass and without a bridle. Oh, it is great fun until, suddenly, it becomes a great panic and a horror not knowing where to go or how to stop going there, what with the horses all out of control and the riders just hang-ing on for dear life. So today, a growing number of therapists feel that the much-maligned and once so dictatorial superego has been too powerfully exorcized and has been excessively soft-ened and diminished.[3] It would seem today that conscience and morality, not in the shape of a rigid ethic but in their more adapt-able form of moral concern,[4] could stand a therapeutic helping hand.

However that may be, the phenomenological polarities of order (such as it stifled the Victorians) and of chaos (such as it threatens to drown us today) impress themselves on the observing mind. Those of us for whom it is a need and a joy to strive for some sort of order, at least in our own thinking, will wish to put the matter into a scheme, a patterning, no matter how provisional, that gives us at least a semblance of understanding, one that seems reasonable. In the following, I have attempted to do just that: I have tried to show that this polarity of chaos and order, which both history and psychology have so recently impressed on us, actually constitutes a principle so basic that it underlies all natural, social and psychological processes. I will also try to claim that the phenomenon of *life* can occur only somewhere *between* the extremes of chaos and order, that certain modalities of our *feeling* and *perception* belong more to one extreme than to the other; and that, in a primarily symbolic but nevertheless deeply meaningful way, the polarities of *male* and *female* are intertwined and interdependent with those of chaos and order. If correct, even if only within the broadest outlines, these reflexions should cast some light on the current social and psychological scene.

THE ATOMIC LEVEL

Let us contemplate, to begin with, Chaos: that murky, steaming, bubbling, largely undifferentiated mush of gas and liquid and a little solid which presumably existed before the Lord separated the heavens and the earth, or before the earth cooled sufficiently to permit the beginnings of life. Even in this chaos there already existed some order—the order first divined by the Russian chemist Mendeleyev in 1869, when he began to present succesive refinements of what came to be known as the *Periodic Table of Elements.*

For while the elements in chaos were wiledly intermingled, they were already, in themselves, structured, and after a very orderly pattern: each had a nucleus and around it one or more layers of electrons. Each layer of electrons is "satisfied," so long as it is granted its favorite number of negatively charged particles. And once it is satisfied, it refuses to budge any further or, as we say, it becomes inert. In consequence, as each layer of electrons is completed, we periodically encounter in the table of elements the inert gases, such as helium, neon, crypton, which being non-reactive* combine with no other element. Hence, they cannot take any active part in the formation of the world or, in particular, of life. They exist; they are perfect in themselves, perfectly ordered within themselves and perfectly dead, from eternity to eternity.

Between the dead perfection of helium, which stands in second place, and the equally dead perfection of neon, which stands in the tenth place of the periodic table, there is room for seven elements. And between the inertness of the two extremes, the elements of the first row become, from either end, more reactive toward the middle: they become increasingly dissatisfied the farther they depart the perfection of helium, until, having reached the midpoint and greatest dissatisfaction with carbon, they become gradually less reactive as they approach neon at the end of that line. Hence lithium has one free valence with which to attach to other elements; beryllium has two, borium has three, and carbon has four. And it is upon the latter, this most imperfect, most dissatisfied, hence most available and gregarious element halfway between the perfect ones, that organic compounds —that Life—was to be built.

After neon, the process starts all over again: a new layer of electrons is added. Layer by layer, the atoms become more complexly organized, more intricate, more bulky. By the time the ninety second element, uranium, is reached, the ordering and organizing genius of nature seems to have overextended itself: too large, too heavy, too clumsy, the trans-uranium elements are no longer stable; the last in line are too precariously short-lived to exist in nature and some, such as plutonium, appear so loaded with a rage at their own complexity that they may quite willingly blow all our created order back into primeval chaos. All of which we may take as a first hint that both *perfection* and *complexity* are, like chaos, inimical to life.

THE MOLECULAR LEVEL

But life did form: the carbon picked up oxygen and hydrogen and nitrogen, and the new tentative order of the organic com-

*With a few recently discovered exceptions.

pounds came into being. Their formation required heat and ample moisture and probably near darkness, for life withstood neither freezing nor drying out: exposed to either, the tender, evolving organic substances were likely to compose themselves into a deadly order of their very own they would likely, each in its own specific way, *crystallize*. There is no more perfect example of perfection than a crystal, but crystals are incompatible with life.

To be of use to life, the organic substances must be loose and free, free in a moist medium to combine and split, to oxygenate and hydrogenate, to link with sulfur and iron and magnesium, to form amines and acids and alcohols, and to build up and up into the slimy substance of life, protoplasm. Once formed, protoplasm has its brief moment of glorious complexity, its teetering instant of more-than-matter, only to promptly break down again by oxidation, fermentation, decomposition and decay into the simple rudiments of chaos—water, salts, carbon dioxide, ammonia, methane—all simple, and chaotic, and again less than life. So that once again we see on the biochemical level life existing only between the crystalline death of ordered perfection, on the one hand, and the putrid chaos of biologic death on the other.

The smelly chaos remains, of course, our ultimate destination: when out time comes we must all return the borrowed carbon compounds to the general biochemical pool; chaos is always waiting to retrieve its own. But while life lasts, is the organism as such, quite like the elements and the compounds, threatened not only by decay but also by a too-much of order?

THE ORGANISMIC LEVEL

Why yes, it is. Biology evolved flexibly, with a marvelous knack for adaptation. But only those species which remained flexible could adapt further. All along the line, species of vegetal or animal life drove adaptation beyond flexibility, developed the complexity of *specialization*. Such specialization, once achieved, can never be taken back, can never be undone. Specialization, whether in physical structure or by way of instinctive behavior patterns, increasingly limits the organism to a special environment. Together with its environment, which never really stands still, it must sooner or later perish.

Or again, the "too much" of organization may express itself as *gigantism:* not excessive complexity, but excessive mass; an order so unwieldy as to become a burden. The species of giant animals, like the giant atoms, were destined to have a relatively short life. In other words, on the organismic level both the rigidity of specialization (somewhat comparable to the crystal) and the bulk of hypertrophy (comparable to the trans uranium elements) are inimical to the survival of the species.

THE HUMAN LEVEL

It is lucky for us that man, like the carbon atom, takes a middle stand, in biological terms remarkably unspecialized—what with an as yet largely unassigned brain and few inherited, unalterable behavior patterns therefore highly adaptable; and in size, of conveniently medium build.

If man were five times bigger, he would, by virtue of the laws which govern relationships between size, surface, and volume, weight 125 times more than he does now, i.e. about twenve tons or as much as the biggest elephant. To support such a weight he would, like the elephant, have to walk on four stubby and pillar-like extremities. If man were five times smaller, he would have to eat twenty-five times more per pound of body weight to maintain his temperature, and this would keep him as busy eating all day as a mouse. If man were bigger, then, he would lack the use of his hands; if smaller, he would lack the time to develop his brain; in either case, he would not have become Man.

The hands and the brain—how are they informed?

In the primordial chaos, in that moist, warm, dark and continuous womb, life had at first neither brain nor hands. When, little by little, a nervous system developed and sense organs formed, they were adapted to their environment. The skin senses came first—touch, temperature, pain, vibration, then the chemical sense of smell, and then hearing. To this day, almost everything that grows, grows first in darkness before it emerges into light. In the marsh, in watered soil, in the egg, and in the womb, we have brought the moisture and darkness and the tactile continuity of the chaos along through evolution. The human infant, following birth, first perceives his mother by touch and smell (of which sucking and tasting are combinations) and is largely so perceived: the warmth and softness and fragrance of mother and infant, registered by the phylogenetically oldest parts of the brain, become and remain the basis of experience and well-being.

Only when life emerges from darkness into light, and further from wet to dry, from the continuity of the internal symbiotic environment to the discontinuity of external space does it need eyes. To serve the eyes, a new brain had to be developed; through the eyes, a new order began to be perceived.

In place of the uterine enclosure, so unified and in its brooding fertility so static, ripe with feeling and urge but lacking in discernement, there is now the intermittency and strangeness of objects, the separating distance, the identifiable goal requiring for its attainment not merely growth but purposive struggle. Hence, with vision and with distinction comes the recognition of sequence in space and time; hence the ordering of cause and effect; hence the essentially male (a-biologic) persuits of ordering by logic, of naming by categories and, abstracted from reality, of numbering and calculating—mathematics, a most perfect order sensed as underlying the imperfection of the created world. There is a new air to breathe in, clear and sharp and thin, whither man must go, no longer as family or tribe or clan, but for the first time, alone, as an isolate, as an individual.

Man—and not woman?

Woman had her age, yes, her vast ages, all but the last seconds of humanity, when she ruled as a goddess. Throughout the Paleolithic, under her nurturing care, mankind gathered and hunted in small bands, and planted in small patches, and lived at the most in small villages subject to a sort of localized mini-order, submerged in dark forests and ignorant of the world beyond. Inwardness was the guiding direction, inward and downward into the earth, whence came the food, where lived the earth goddess in darkness and death. Worship and sacrifice was down to the powers below in the darkness of cave and hollow temple, except it be to the darkness of night and to the moon, goddess of the night and of changeable womanhood. Fertility was the goddess, receiving the dead and perhaps granting rebirth to corn and man, chaotically scattering her seeds of plants and animals and frightened men without rhyme or reason over the empty earth. During the millennia of feminine chaos, man was a herd animal, a part of nature, not yet building up, not yet man.

Then came an explosion.

THE SOCIETAL LEVEL

Perhaps it came with the perfection of speech, which enabled man to share what he knew and to report on what was distant or past. At any rate, when the day breaks on the Neolithic, on that inspired youth of mankind, suddenly everything changes. Over a scant two to three thousand years hunting becomes herding, planting becomes agriculture, villages become cities, and cities grow into states. Suddenly, man has mastered space, and he throws over the compliant earth boundaries and canals, roads and road stations, accomplished and run by administrations and guarded or conquered by armies. Suddenly, man has learned to organize and to work together, to parcel out skills and duties and, above all, to plan ahead. The eye of man, having measured space and distance, has learned to gaze into the future.

The man who accomplished this is the hero with a thousand faces. He worships and often joins the new gods who no longer live below or in darkness where one cannot see, but up above, in the heavens, among the stars. First among them is the sun, god of vision. The measuring eye reaches for the stars and returns with new measurements for man—measures of time, of the hour and the calendar, of dizzying pasts and futures. To better reach his stars and to be closer to heaven, man now worships, no longer from mountain caves but from mountaintops, and builds his own mountains where natural ones are lacking, i.e. the ziggurats, to stand upon, similar in shape but distinct in essence from the pyramid, that tomb-and-womb structure which was the new man's last obeisance to the goddess.

What a heroic age when civilization was first born, when man created, for the first time anywhere, a reality truly supernatural: human society—nature now subject to a new kind of order.[5]

We have ever since—for the last five thousand years or so—tried to make it work.

From the start, we fell into hyperorganization. Priestly order and royal administration were no sooner set up than they became oppressive tyrannies, devouring in luxury the wealth they were to govern, draining on altar and battlefield the lifeblood of their own populations. From the dawn of history to that belated neolithic spurt of the Mayan and Toltect people., complicated hierarchical states collapsed under the load of their own secular and priestly administrations.

Out of the repeated rise to order and decline into chaos of which only archeology informs us, there eventually emerged within recorded history three great systems of distinctly different kind.

THE CLASSICAL ORDERS

Out of Mesopotamia and the Fertile Crescent, still strewn with statues of the goddess and the bones of her sacrificial victims, there arose Yahveh, the single, male God, and Abraham, who proclaimed Him the One and Only, and Moses, who obtained from Him *The Law,* which, derived from the one and only God, could claim to be the one and only law; for the first time in history not a local and national but a *universal moral law,* claiming to be equally valid for everybody any time and anywhere. A new order of right and wrong (a justice without emotion to replace the customary vengeance of the goddess) now set out with many a false start to spread itself over the face of the earth, promising to bring with it the secure freedom man can only enjoy within the limits of the law.

About a thousand years later, a brilliant light began to shine from Greece. Within the walls of their confined city states, in the limited freedom of their limited democracies, Greek philosophers began to look at nature in a new way. By the clear, unclouded and unbefogged radiance of Phoebus Apollo they began to see things as they are, unembroidered by the demons and goblins of the goddess. They strove to tell true from false, and nature, studied thus without emotions, surrendered to man the rudiments of *a universal natural law*. It too, like the universal moral law of Moses, had a fitful and uncertain start and went through many a decline, but how effectively, under the name of Science, it eventually imposed its own brand of order upon the whole world we know well enough.

A little later still (perhaps 300 years) a third order spread from Rome to conquer the world. What Rome had to offer was neither moral nor particularly scientific. What Rome had to offer was the *Pax Romana,* the rule by universal subjugation which, thanks to the spears and swords of Roman legions, could claim to settle *a universal administrative law* over the known earth—a law on the whole so shrewd and fair that it effected one of the longest periods of relative peace and prosperity in the history of mankind.

These three classical orders represent, each in their own way, peaks of human thought and organization. Not one of them was to last.

THE DECLINE AND FALL

The Hebrew law, with its claim to worldwide morality, lost its grand scope and became more and more concerned with technicalities of conduct and worship. A fanatical hyperspecialization made the law oppressive to the Jews and inacceptable to the Gentiles. Christ came, He said, to fulfill the Law, not to break it; but Paul broke the law in pieces, thus freeing some of its legally encrusted principles for the use of all mankind. In the following centuries, a considerable part of Christendom drifted away from the last remnants of paternal law; the simple people increasingly sought the all-forgiving, basically a-moral protection of the Virgin Mary. A few inspired individuals steeped themselves in a mystic inwardness which, by emphasis on a personal ecstatic experience of God and on a sensual at-oneness with Christ or the Virgin Mary, as well as by a sometimes vehement rejection of ecclesiastic authority and organization, equally tended toward the realm of emotion and chaos.

Nor did Greek natural law fare any better. The people, never really quite with it, found Euclidean geometry too precise, Praxitelean statues too static and calm, and the gods of Olympus too deficient in spiritual values. First Dionysos then Orpheus seduced them back into the night of the goddess, with midnight revels on hilltops and obscene mysteries in the underground sanctuary at Eleusis.

As to the Romans, their virtues did not in the long run equal the demands of empire. A true Roman senator or consul had to be a man of incorruptible integrity, indomitable courage and ascetic habits; a man reserved and jealous of his privacy, detached and superior to the politics and wars of the moment, yet ruthless in their prosecution; a man ruling his passions and ruled by reason. There were few such men, and their example, with the increasing wealth of empire, became more reproach than inspiration. The Romans, living well, deserted virtue (*virtus*, the conduct becoming a man, a *vir*) and fell into sexual excesses, group orgies, the use of ecstatic drugs imported from the Orient, and debauche to satiation and exhaustion.

Thus the three orders ended, at least for the time being, much the same way: emotional frenzy, touching, tasting, physical closeness and the uncritical mutual acceptance of carnality, or mystical union and oceanic continuity. In either case it was a victory for the goddess, resurging from her Eastern strongholds, and a victory for chaos; and yet, at the same time, an escape from the stifling rigidity of excessive order.

THE CHURCH

The first 500 years of our era saw chaos indeed: the Roman empire torn and shredded by invaders, the Christian churches rent by savage and passionate schisms. But eventually there emerged a new order with a new claim: to be a religion for the whole world (*kat-holon*), a *universal faith:* The Roman Catholic Church. It was a very male and very orderly effort. Building on the ruins of empire, the Church grew and extended a carefully structured, centrally controlled ecclesiastic hierarchy, from village priest to pope, composed entirely of men. It salvaged from the hunger and disease of the early Middle Ages an army of monks, regimented in "orders" and cared for in cloisters (and a lesser troup of nuns, equally regimented). The better ones observed strict and ascetic rituals, and while serving their church and the Spirit, also furthered the cause of learning by reading and copying whatever ancient volume they could find. Where earlier Roman consuls had gone to seed in North Africa, now Augustine escaped the debauch of the same shores to find a life of disciplined purity in the Church.

Indeed, a worthy prior commanding a monastery would have had much in common with a good Roman provincial governor, and it was not to be long before the monks were actually armed, and their leaders called generals. Nor did the Church militant lack heavy armor: the Templars, the Knights Hospitallers, the Teutonic Knights and other such more or less ecclesiastic armies offered military structure and security (and often homosexuality) to a society of males disenchanted with women. The goal of life was, after all, no longer the propagation of life on earth, but individual life eternal—a reach of the spiritual eye for vision without end, for an ultimate deliverance from darkness.

Again, however, organization overreached itself: the people, already poor, groaned to build more altars or fatten more prelates for the sake of salvation. The monasteries took their young men, and the priests castigated and reviled their women. Oppression forced revolt, and it came in three ways.

THE DECLINE OF THE CHURCH

On the one hand, starting about the twelveth century but culminating during the sixteenth, there occurred a regular underground rebellion of women, the conspiracy of witches.

Some have questioned whether witches ever existed. Of course the spectacular aspects of popular witch-lore, the levitation on broomsticks and metamorphoses into animal shapes are pure invention. But evidence does seem to support that witches did indeed exist, that they met in the dark of night, sometimes in great numbers; that they made a mockery of the Church in the upside-down ritual of the black mass; that they practiced sexual license, were experts both in contraception and fertility, and made ample use of halucinogenic drugs; and that they sometimes served and worship Satan, but more generally Satan's wife or one of the old heathen goddesses. It is also likely, though no doubt much less frequent than their accusers claimed, that they revived that old terror of goddess worship, the sacrifice of children. On the other hand, it is quite certain that they were able to bestow upon their times not only some rather questionable curses and bewitchments but the very real benefits of herbs and brews and the whole paraphernalia of folk medicine. The Church considered the witch movement not merely heretical but subversive of the social order and decimated Europe to stamp it out.[6]

The second rebellion against ecclesiastic order was more open, has been much better documented, and fits less clearly into our scheme of things. True enough, the Reformation was destructive of Roman order by pointing out its abuses and by effecting a decentralization of at least some of Christendom. On the other hand, it did not swing over to the side of femininity and chaos. In fact, it abolished the worship of Mary and quickly gave rise to teachings, such as those of Calvin and Knox, which commanded a more severe and sombre ordering of life than anything ever ordained by Rome. However, in the course of time the antiauthoritarian, antinomian spirit which gave birth to Protestantism did assert itself and brought about a splintering of its adherents into hundreds of independent factions and churches. Some of these, such as the Holy Roller fundamentalist sects and the snake handlers of the American South, converted their services, frequently presided over by women, into rites so inspirational, so ecstatic, so entirely and wildly emotional, as to cede in nothing to the spirit possession of a voodoo cult or the orgiastic rites of the Phrygian goddess of old.

The third rebellion against Rome was of a different order entirely, as witnessed by the fact that it was, in part, supported by the popes themselves. It was the Renaissance, occurring contemporaneously with the Reformation in the fifteenth to seventeenth centuries, which took issue with the moralistic dogmatism and materialistic sordidness of the Church by reaching back to an older and infinitely more esthetic and joyful order, that of classical Greece. Under the influence of Renaissance spirit the real world, for the first time in centuries, was once again looked at with a clear and loving eye. Paintings lost their flat, mainly ornamental and didactic sameness and acquired depth, perspective, and realism. The nude body once again emerged, an object of joy and wonderment. Statues once again expressed not merely gothic sadness, grief and decay but physical vigor and sensuality. An inquisitive gaze at the world took medicine, once again, out of the hands of wise women and placed it into the experimental study of the physician. A new light, a new vision, a new insight went below the surface and dissected for the first time the human body; measured once again the firmament; reached with telescope as well as with the imagination further than God in heaven.

The yearning for a universal reasonable ordering of the world, for an all-encompassing, rational understanding resembled in scope and spirit the far-ranging exploits of the neolithic. But it went beyond: reason claimed that the earth was finite and could be totally comprehended; courage demanded such reaching out, such looking for what had not yet been seen; the inherent expansiveness of order and of ordered thinking, as against the statism of chaos, led to the age of exploration, the discovery of the Americas, the first circumnavigation of the globe. This was followed in the seventeenth and eighteenth centuries by the aggressive euphoria of the mind known as *the Enlightenment.* Surely, it was thought, *everything* could be understood, classified, ordered. Worshiped were reason and learning, idealized were poise and balance, serenity, proportion, and health. Woman had status as man's muse, his inspiration, the basis—but never the pinnacle—of his existence.

From then on, the forces and enticements of chaos and order no longer succeeded each other in time, but intermingled and opposed each other like dancers in a ballet.

THE MODERN AGE

The material reflection of the enlightenment was the growth of industry and commerce. Both exploration and science furthered the new economic order of capitalism which, guided by new arrangements of international finance, created from factories, mines and plantations an iron order of deprivation and death for some and luxury for others. Shipping lines, steel rails, and eventually the invisible flight lanes of aviation were to lay down a dense, utilitarian grid over the globe, trussing it like a giant Gulliver.

Against the clamor of these developments, as against the entire spirit of the enlightenment, there protested in the eighteenth and nineteenth centuries a new literary and popular movement: *the Romantic.*

Romanticism and yearning are near synonymous: a yearning for nature, for simplicity, for the ways of the simple people; a yearning for fairylands and for the folktales and folksongs that tell of them; a yearning for pure love, for pure beauty, uncontaminated by necessities. And yet, at the same time, Romanticism wallows in the excesses of the East and the agonies of turmoil and disease, it seeks the dark of night and the drug-induced dream, it thrives on steaming blood and pain and the sweet smoke of opium dens, and it looks to woman as ultimate temptress, despair and death.[7] Romanticism itself became, in time, a heady intoxicant for dizzy minds and helped produce one of the worst nightmares of history. For among its direct and linear descendants there arose, midwived however innocently by Wagner and Nietzsche, the blood-and soil mythology, the apocalyptic blood orgy of Hitler and the Third Reich.

But long before history arrived at that particular climax of chaos, the march of order had, in its turn, gained new ground and new forms. Moving with incredible speed into every power vacuum, the economic and military forces of the Western nations were busily erecting a system of colonial empires and between them divided up the globe. Against such horizontal apportionment of the world a new order now proclaimed itself, bent on ignoring national boundaries but visualizing a world structured vertically, with the exploited proletariat below and the exploiting, colonalist capitalists above. Counterpart to previous laws and religions with claim to universality, socialism now presented itself as *a universal economic doctrine* or dogma. Its appeal and strength, apart from the obvious humanitarian concern, lay in the emphasis on a new kind of vision: the foresight of economic planning. A blind interplay of economic and social forces and balances was to be replaced by a reasoned, goal-directed, consciously progressive scheme. The future, last realm of darkness, was to be taken out of the laps of the gods. Where chance had been, there planning was to be.

While socialism and communism began to subvert the establishment by organizing the minds of men, a more subtly revolutionary new order undertook to organize the mind of man. Moving not outward but in, seeking not foresight but insight, integrating not the future but the past, psychoanalysis attempted by reason to order unreason itself. Freud invaded a darkness only poets had ever visited: where chaotic *id* had been, there ordered *ego* was now to be. One of the last great figures of the enlightenment, he believed that reason could even cure the soul.

We know today how all the various ambitious systems and orders of the late nineteenth and early twentieth centuries were doomed to fail.

THE DECLINE OF SYSTEMS

The empires, with their colossal expanse, their colossal administrative buildings and appartuses, their colossal wealth and colossal exploitation, fell apart after WW II. National, local, separatist enthusiasm and obstinacy everywhere encountered and defeated the mighty armies and the lofty purposes of empire. Nationalists repeatedly rose or at least tried to rise against the alliances of political dogma, and separatists threatened, if they did not destroy, the integrity of long-established countries. The United Nations, created like the League of Nations twenty-five years earlier to attempt a global order, found this globe more splintered, more disjointed than anyone could have predicted before the war.

But even before the empires fell, those doctrines which had so surely meant to supplant them ran into turbulence and faltered and, in their grand design, failed. While communism with its five-year plans, its dictatorship of the proletariat and its collectivization of the individual churned on in Russia, former adherents and sympathetic onlookers increasingly reckoned the price too high, the cost in terms of freedoms surrendered incommensurate with the gains. Little by little, leading thinkers in the West became disenchanted with political systems and ideologies. For a few grim years during the thirties and early forties, that odious bastard between systematic socialism and romantic nationalism, the National Socialism of Germany, furnished the world a negative pole against which to orient itself. But after the Nazi defeat the victors found that, like the vanquished, they had lost their convictions. As empires crumbled into mini-countries, so ideologies splintered into dissident factions and in the end right down to the individual who, deceived by all previous attempts at order, now proclaimed himself both unattached and lost. Estrangement became the catchword, and existentialism preached the accidental, the thrownness of each and every life, the obligation of every individual to create, alone and on his own and incomprehensibly to everyone else, his own particular world.

It had been the anarchists of the nineteenth century who first stated the extreme antinomian position. Thus Proudhon: "The government of man by man, under whatever name it is disguised, is oppression"; and Bakunin: "All exercise of authority perverts, and all submission to authority humiliates."[8] Turgenev, in his novel *Fathers and Sons,* which appeared 1862, puts the matter as follows:

Pavel Kirsanov flung up his hands. "I don't understand—how is it possible not to acknowledge principles, rules? By virtue of what do you act, then?"

"I've already told you that we dont acknowledge authorities," Arcadii broke in.

"We act by virtue of that which we acknowledge to be useful. At the present time repudiation is the most useful of all. We repudiate."

"Everything?"

"Everything."

"What! Not only art, poetry . . . but also—one dreads to say it—"

"Everything," Bazarov repeated with inexpressible calm.

Pavel Petrovich stared at him. "You're repudiating everything or, to put it more exactly, you're demolishing everything. But then, it is necessary to be constructive as well.

"That, now, is no business of ours. The ground must be cleared, first of all. That's what the present state of the people

demands. We are obligated to fulfill these demands; we haven't
the right to indulge in personal egoism."

In our day such extreme aversion to order (Proudhon even
disapproved of symphonic music because of its cooperative aspect)
has found expression in two distinct, basically similar but in some
regards opposite youth movements.

The first of these consists of activist university students, of
whom by far the most successful and the most vocal to date is
the French-German-Jewish firebrand and genius, Daniel Cohn-
Bendit. In his book about the French uprising of May, 1968, he
goes to great pains to deny for himself and all similar-minded
revoultionists every intent of forming a party or organization and
any aspiration to leadership:[9] (p. 58): "What was remarkable
about the events of 3 May was the spontaneity of the resistance—a
clear sign that our movement does not need leaders to direct it;
that it can perfectly well express itself without the help of a
'vanguard' . . . (p. 67) simply as a natural response to a concrete
situation." Or again (p. 250): "Democracy is not suborned by
bad leadership, but by the very existence of leadership . . . (p. 256)
Every group must find its own form, take its own action, and
speak its own language. When all have learned to express themselves, in harmony with the rest, we shall have a free society."

Cohn-Bendit is quite explicit in stating that his chief enemy
must be, not the tottering bourgeois state but the iron organi-
zaion of the Community Party. He is concerned lest, as it happened in Russia, a managerial class should once again take over
in the wake of a successful revolution (p. 104) and deprive the
workers of what would otherwise quite naturally come about,
i.e. a society of equals cooperating without constraint, in perfect
harmony, sharing fairly between one and all (p. 106). Brilliant
though he is, he apparently fails to perceive his own repeated
assertions that his movement collapsed in most instances simply
because the enemy, i.e. the government and the unions, were
better organized (pp. 60, 68, 70); he does not notice what he is
saying because, like the Populists in Tsarist Russia, he profoundly
believes that all good comes from the people, that the people will
naturally achieve heaven on earth if only they are left to them-

selves, to their own kindhearted, innocuous, unambitious simplicity. Like Rousseau, he seems to be calling for a return to nature, and to him, this means above all a rulerless, lawless, anarchic condition.

What is true for Cohn-Bendit appears to be characteristic of most student radicals as well in this or any other country in our day, in that they expect a miraculous improvement of their world to result from the mere removal of the present order. There is little consideration given as to what sort of order, if any, should replace it.

The second relevant youth movement is, of course, that of our hippies: it resembles the first in its repugnance for order, but differs by being not in the least political. As Leonard Wolf explains,[10] the hippie lives by the code of his own small and compact tribe or group, "making it" in the midst of an indifferent or hostile environment which he seeks not to conquer or to destroy, but to elude (p. XXI). The emphasis is all away from organization, away from reason and logic, and toward feelings and mystic-orgiastic sensations, toward dissolution in "the germ plasm of the race" (p. XXIII) and "cellular consciousness," toward "that constant feeling of abandon . . . that cool, damp breast-milk feeling of satisfaction." To "do one's own thing" acquires an almost tabu quality, is considered self-justifying, beyond interference, unquestionably good and therefore morally superior to any societal demand or code. Accordingly, the emphasis is entirely on the unplanned, on the "happening:" on nature, on now, on kicks, on inspiration through oriental mysticism or through drugs, on improvisation. Thus, rock-music is said to be "participational and non-typographic" (p. XXXIII)—it would die in the process of transcription for it would become lasting and historical—and the hippie world is totally a-historic.

It is a feminine world, with uncritical, maternal acceptance of every flower child, of everyone who quietly "turns on" to whatever his particular "bag" may be, like a toddler in the corner of a nursery. It is an undemanding world of smelling and touching, a world, in short, of chaos, and of the characteristic sensory and emotional modalities of chaos as we have described them. And if, as the Durants stated in their *Lessons of History*,[11] the replacement of chaos with order is the essence of art and civilization, then the dazzling light shows and deafening commingled noises of hippieland constitute a sort of anti-art, clearly aiming at replacing order, and with it civilization, by chaos.

No doubt the psychedelic drugs serve the same purpose: they dissolve, or at least distort, the natural and familiar order of things and place the subject into a dream world uniquely his own. Throughout history—from the ecstatic services of the goddess to the mystery cults, from the midnight rites of the witches to the trances of seers, from the poets of nineteenth century romanticism to the escapists of our day—drugs have been used in just this manner: to breach the hard boundaries of ordering reason and to return to at least a semblance of infantile security and uniqueness.

It should be pointed out, however, that long before the blossoming forth of psychedelia the establishment itself had fondly fostered the rudiments of that which the hippies lead to conclusion: a-melodic, cacophonous music produced on noninstruments; nonrepresentational paintings varying from random dribbles to canvasses of a single, solid color, and therefore void of content: these have long been applauded by esoteric connoisseurs. One must admit that such experiments, like hippie art and music, have their engaging impudence and confer, at least until boredom supervenes, a sense of liberation from form. No doubt it is a surfeit with such contentless liberty which, on the other hand, has brought about today's unprecedented popularity of baroque composers, with their mathematical precision and elegance of form, and which in Europe is spawning new schools of imaginative, often surrealist but always clear and representational painting.

Finally, beside the far-flung empires and the all-embracing political doctrines, there is one more universal system of orderly understanding which has been abandoned by all but the old guard: the system of psychoanalysis.

Even in Freud's day, the orthodoxy splintered into many protestant sects; but increasingly the very goals of understanding and insight are now being abandoned. The painstaking cooperative research once conducted by the exclusive team of patient and analyst is increasingly replaced by the free-for-all of encounter and sensitivity groups.[12] And where some years ago such groups still had a group leader, the newer ones tolerate no more authority figures: like the nihilistic factory workers of Cohn-Bendit, like the hippies in their Haight-Ashbury pad, these latest children of psychology do not wish to understand, or even to think, much less to plan. What they want is to feel, to emote, to react, and to erase individuality and personal boundaries in the sensuous chaos of communality. Hence, space and distance must vanish; the original continuity of the primeval ocean must be reestablished; hence feeling and caressing, preferably naked, preferably in the dark, and if possible in warm water. And so, in the expensive swimming pools of Beverly Hills and in the hot springs of the California coast, the Great Mother, now in the guise of group therapist, once again opens wide her arms to receive her bruised and aching children, disillusioned as they are with all efforts at manly order, to receive them back into her warm, dark, moist, sheltering womb.

THE PERSONAL LEVEL

But when all is said and done we deal, as therapists, not with historical or social development nor even with groups but always with the individual. Does the dialectic apply here, too?

The child is, indeed, not only a child of mother but a child of chaos. Its earliest impressions, largely enteroceptive, are of necessity unstructured; its earliest world is one of feelings and random percepts void of meaning or regularity. It takes many years, as Piaget has demonstrated, before the mind of the child relinquishes the syncretistic fusion and confusion of infancy and masters the skills of category and logic.[13]

As it grows, it is introduced to the world: the world of rules and regulations, of bedtime and mealtime, of worktime and resttime, of making messes and cleaning them up, of taking things out and putting things away. It resists as best it can. It tries to claim that at least the nursery is child territory and proves the point by scattering toys, pencils, clothing, beeds and chocolate helter-skelter over and under bed and rug and table and chair.

Into this cozy chaos enters Mother, this time not to nurture or comfort but to instruct on the most basic level. "You must learn some order, you must learn to clean up your room." And the child thinks, "Must I?"

But he catches on, gradually. Next comes school, with the precision of the school bell, and of math, and of assignments to be completed within a given time; with the gradual extension of the awareness that this is a world of graduated authorities—parents, teachers, principals and God knows what else: policemen, judges, presidents—no end of structure, no end of what is done and what is not to be done.

The commandments present themselves, on one level, in the mundane form of manners and dress, and these constitute the first battlegrounds and serve the first testing of society. How short the skirt, how long the hair, barefoot or shod, the language polite or profane—these are experiments probing leeway and elbowroom, testing softness within the order, alternating rebellion and accommodation.

On a larger scale outright delinquency, on the one hand, or adolescent depression and despair, on the other, are still part and parcel of a general reluctance to emerge from the soft warmth and irresponsibility of childhood, i.e. the realm of the Mother, into the hard demandingness of society and of work, of politics and economics and war, the complex, responsibility-laden, terribly consequential organizations of men.

Most of us eventually "make it" and find our particular individual place and mesh more or less smoothly, a gear among gears, into the apparatus of society. But still the balance between chaos and order remains, for each individual, of the essence. Good health demands, in fact, that we partake of each in rapid alternation: day and night; the order of activity, the dissolution of sleep; the effort of work, the dissipation of rest; the intense mobilization for a creative effort, the depressive aimlessness of lying fallow. If we disrespect either, we are likely to fall short of our potential.

Or again, as a matter of balance, if only in fantasy: in the midst of disciplined and wearisome effort, the hope for a swim in a warm ocean; in the midst of the chaos and smoke of battle, the recitation of a sonnet, the solution of an algebraic problem, both so sane and orderly—these may bring comfort. It is all so obvious, it should not need saying. Yet many, especially among the young, do not know it and need to be taught that we must be able to take hold and to let go, that we must remain related both to the Mother and to the Father, if we are, as individuals, to last and to accomplish.

As to outright psychopathology, I have already said that the neuroses of Freud's time, products of societal repression, have vanished. Today, as one would expect, the danger comes from the other side—from the side of chaos. Those who do not "make it" today are not immobilized by formality, they are rendered ineffective by lack of form, by lack of identity. Characteristic of our day is the "identity crisis," the "young man sans identity,"[14] the need of the young for educational "moratoria" indicative of their unreadiness to assume identity. In precarious proximity to these still normal developmental hang-up there are the "border-line personalities," individuals whose lack of inner structure and of integration into societal order renders them forever susceptible to the seductions of that outright chaos which we call psychosis. It is one of the objectionable aspects of psychedelic drugs that they offer to such ill-defined individuals what they least need, a further dissolution of structured reality. Similarly, the intentional unstructuring inherent in some varieties of group therapy, if not handled with skill and care, may lead to decompensation into psychosis. We need to be reminded today that emotional chaos, like emotional rigidity, is deadly.

We need to be reminded? No. We, the therapists, need to remind ourselves that our function is compensatory: the popular pendulum has swung far to the side of chaos, so it is now our task to teach order—no longer merely to analyze, to take apart, but on the contrary, to build, to structure. The need today is for the therapist to be "square."

The young, in so far as they seek us at all, do not ask for us to join them in their pad; they despise the adult who craves to act young; what they come to us for are precisely points of orientation, the reaffirmation that values and standards of conduct may be chosen and adhered to. By the time the young hippie consults us, he is at the point of drowning in chaos; whether he admits it or not, he is tired of swimming, he wishes to come aboard and to dry out and to find the support of those solid purposes and responsibilities which society has, after all, to offer. To accomplish such a transition without the sacrifice of moral and individual essentials, to help build the sense of integrity which comes from the adoption of consistent, self-chosen and self-tested values—this should be the proper task of therapy today.[15]

The concept of a dynamic balance between chaos and order is, of course, not new. Many philosophers of history, such as the Comte de Saint-Simon or Oswald Spengler,[16] have advanced it and have stressed the dangers of either extreme. The founding fathers of these United States had the matter much in mind. Perhaps the constitution they shaped, with its checks and balances, is one of the finest examples of chaos ordered and order mitigated. Science, today, is increasingly aware that not everything that *could* be ordered and structured and built (freeways, interstellar rockets, H-bombs, automated hospitals, artificial organs and what not else) *should* be built. Suddenly we realize that we must not, that we cannot continue to violate Mother Nature with our clever gimmicks and contrivances, lest she reassert herself and, one way or another, return this world to the lifeless chaotic conditions of its beginnings.

Even more, of course, is the concept of male-female polarity an old familiar notion. The Jungians, in particular, have written voluminously and well of the struggle and balance within each psyche between the masculine and feminine elements. But it is the pairing off of these antagonistic couplets which seems to me of phenomenologic and diagnostic interest.

Whenever order is in the ascendant, things move in the direction of what is predominantly male, i.e. toward systems and ideologies and abstractions, toward the mastery of great distances in space and time, toward the visual values of clarity and light in the sciences and in art. Chaos resurgent always moves toward the essentially feminine, i.e. toward feelings and primary sensations, away from society and toward nature and anarchic separateness. This, I believe, is just as true of individuals as of whole societies, and since I apply the terms male-female in this fashion, I clearly do not equate them with the terms man or woman, but mean to designate by them a behavior pattern which is by now independent of and sometimes opposite morphologic or genetic sexual identity. Nor do I attach blame or praise to either, but I wish to stress precisely the necessity of both and the need for a balance between them.

In the overall, the dialectic of chaos and order, as it is carried on throughout all nature and society, seems to suggest an inherent tendency toward ever more structure with repetitive regressions into chaos whenever structure becomes unworkable. Human development, paradoxically, seems to aim both toward greater awareness and separateness of the individual, and toward integration of the individual into ever more complex orders of society. Despite the repeated appearance of isolated communes and utopian experiments, despite ever renewed nationalistic splintering, we seem surely headed for a world order.

Inevitably, in such a complex attempt there must be many false starts that need to be undone. It is here that the chaotic modes, be they anarchist, activist, hippie, or encounter-sensitivist, have their important destructive, ground-clearing role to play. They correspond in the individual to periods of depression or dissocial behavior or some such decompensation and disorganization as alcoholism or psychosis, following which the self can reconstitute on a different and possibly higher level.[17]

But the main march of history is toward more organization. Working towards it, men may fear and shun the seductions of feminine chaos[18] or may give in to it; they may build systems and structures or be imprisoned by them. The therapists role in this conception would be that of exerting, over the fluctuating decennia, a corrective influence either way: helping to keep man and mankind both alive—and human.

NOTES AND REFERENCES

1. The great identity crisis started officially in the late 1950s, with Allan B. Wheelis's *The Quest for Identity*, New York, Norton, 1958, and Erik H. Erikson's *Identity and the Life Cycle: Psychological Issues*, New York, International Universities Press, 1959, vol. 1, No. 1, and was then fully instrumentated by many writers, notably again Erikson in his *Identity: Youth and Crisis*, New York, Norton, 1968.

2. Lifton, Robert J.: Protean man. *Arch. Gen. Psychiatr. 24*:298, 1971.

3. I expounded the positive function of the superego in the monograph: *Dragons, Delinquents and Destiny, Psychological Issues,* New York, Int. Universities Press, 1965, vol 4, no. 3; and in the fat volume O. Hobart Mower, (Ed.): *Morality and Mental Health,* Chicago, Rand McNally, 1967. numerous authorities from various professional disciplines (Dr. Benjamin Spock among them) reassert the importance of morality in life and therapy.

4. Lederer, W.: Some moral dilemmas encountered in psychotherapy. *Psychiatry, 34*:75, 1971.

5. In *The Fear of Women,* New York, Grune & Stratton, 1968, I have attempted to show at much greater length how the woman-nature, man-civilization dichotomy persists psychologically to this day and causes stresses between the sexes.

6. For documentation of the witches' rebellion see the Chapter 22, Broomsticks and acts of faith, in *The Fear of Women* cited above.

7. Praz, Mario: *The Romantic Agony.* London, Oxford United Press, 1951.

8. Both quotes from Burrow, J. W.: The anarchists. *Horizon, 11*(3): 32-42, 1969.

9. Cohn-Bendit, Daniel: *Obsolete Communism—The Left Wing Alternative.* New York, McGraw-Hill, 1968.

10. Wolf, Leonard: *Voices from the Love Generation.* New York, Little, Brown, 1968.

11. Durant, Will and Ariel: *The Lessons of History.* New York, Simon & Schuster, 1968.

12. Kubie, L. S.: The retreat from patients. *Arch. Gen. Psychiatr. 24*: 98, 1971.

13. Piaget, Jean: *The Construction of Reality in the Child* and *The Growth of Logical Thinking* (both N. Y., Basic Books).

14. See notes under 1 and 3 above.

15. See reference 4 above.

16. Discussions of both are to be found, briefly, in Durant, *op. cit.*

17. Sarbin, Theodore R., and Adler, Nathan: Self Reconstitution Processes: A Preliminary Report. *Psychoanal. Rev., 57*:599, 1971.

18. For a discussion of man's fear of seduction by feminine chaos— a fear which includes far more components and dimensions than the well-advertised "castration anxiety," see again *The Fear of Women,* quoted above.

Chapter 3

POPULATION PROBLEMS

WILLIAM M. PINSON, JR.

A cancer is an uncontrolled multiplication of cells; the population explosion is an uncontrolled multiplication of people. Treating only the symptoms of cancer may make the victim more comfortable at first, but eventually he dies—often horribly. A similar fate awaits the world with a population explosion if only the symptoms are treated. We must shift our efforts from treatment of the symptoms to the cutting out of the cancer. . . . The disease is so far advanced that only with radical surgery does the patient have a chance of survival.[1]

The words of a crank? Hardly. They came from Paul R. Ehrlich, Professor of Biology and Director of Graduate Study for the Department of Biological Sciences, Stanford University. His specialty is population biology. He along with many other experts insist that the population explosion is the world's number one problem.

POPULATION TRENDS

The increase in the world's population is rapid enough to be labeled an explosion. Only about 250 million persons lived in the world when Jesus Christ was born. Sixteen hundred years later the population had doubled. It doubled again in only two-and-one-half centuries. By 1850 approximately a billion people were living on the earth.[2] Within the past hundred years the population has soared like a skyrocket. The 2 billion mark was passed around 1930. Now over 3 billion people crowd our planet.

Professor Clyde E. Fant, Jr., and Dr. Donald Hammer were closely associated with me in the research. The chapter "Population Problems" is a revision of a resource paper done for the Christian Life Commission of the Southern Baptist Convention and is used with their permission.

49

At present growth rates it will take only thirty-seven years to double the human population. The fastest rate of growth is in Latin America: 2.9 percent per year as compared to 2.0 in Asia, 2.4 in Africa, .8 in Europe, and 1.1 in North America. It will take the population of Latin America only twenty-four years to double if present trends continue.

The areas which can least afford an increase in population are the ones experiencing the highest rate of growth. The United States and Sweden, two of the highest per capita income nations ($2893 and $2204), rank among the lowest in terms of the rate of population growth. Nations such as the United Arab Republic, Iran, Thailand, El Salvador, Paraguay, and Nicaragua have population growth almost three times as high with incomes only about one-tenth as great.

Has the upward trend slowed down? No. The population boom is in the beginning stage. The major causes of population increase are just being felt in many parts of the world. And the number of persons who will reach the age to start families in the next ten to fifteen years in staggering. Over one third of the world's population is under fifteen. But in many of the poorer, rapidly growing nations, 40 to 50 percent of the population is under fifteen.*

The United States has a rapidly increasing population, though not as rapid as most of the world. It took approximately 300 years for America to reach 100 million in population. That was in 1918. It took less than fifty years to add the second 100 million. By the year 2000 at least another 100 million will be added, maybe many more. Some estimate that the population of the United States will be 400 million by the turn of the century.

CAUSES OF INCREASE

The change which triggered the population explosion was not an increase in the birth rate but a decrease in the death rate.**

*Some samples: Honduras, 51 percent; Mali, 49 percent; Costa Rica, 48 percent; Colombia, Dominican Republic, Philippines, Sudan—47 percent; Niger, Kenya, Jordan, Syria, Iran, Guatemala, Mexico, Venezuela—46 percent.

**Some examples:[3] Mexico's crude death rate from 1940 to 1960 fell from 23.2 to 11.4; Venezuela from 16.6 to 8; Singapore from 20.9 to 6.3.

A decreasing death rate without a corresponding decrease in the birth rate has resulted in rapid population growth.

At the time of Christ the life expectancy at birth in Egypt, Greece, and Rome was probably not more than thirty years. By the eighteenth century life expectancy had increased to about thirty-three years in North America and Europe. By 1900 life expectancy had increased to forty-five or fifty years. By 1960 it had reached seventy years. Today in Sweden and the Netherlands it is seventy-four years and in the United States seventy-one years.[4] Within the past seventy years the drop in infant mortality has been dramatic.[5] With more children surviving infancy and people in general living longer the total population has soared.[6]

The death rate has declined dramatically for several reasons. Most are related to advances in technology and modern medicine. When man discovered the basic causes of disease and as a result improved his personal hygiene and public sanitation the death rate plummeted. The improvements in medical technique have also saved millions of lives. Technology has enabled man to control disease-carrying animals and insects, raise more food to avert starvation, and to spread the healing effect of modern medical care.

Europe and North America enjoyed these benefits first. While the rest of the world marked time the West forged ahead in technology, sanitation, and medical care. As a result the death rate declined in Europe and the population boomed.

But the birth rate also declined in Europe and North America because of the impact of technology. At one time a large family was an economic asset. The children helped with farming, the dominant economic activity. But mechanized farming and automated industry made children an economic liability. Families wanted fewer children. Improved birth control techniques made it possible for a couple to keep down the number of children. Birth rates declined. The rest of the world is now experiencing the impact of medical, agricultural, and industrial technology. Death rates are declining. But birth rates are still high. The result is a rapid increase in population.

EFFECTS OF THE POPULATION EXPLOSION

The real problem is not too many people. It is too many people for the limited room and resources of spaceship Earth. Birth rates cannot indefinitely outpace death rates. Sooner or later we humans will run out of something necessary for life—either food, clean air, pure water, or room. Then death rates will soar, billions will die, and hordes of others will suffer intensely.

Already we are straining our planet's capacity to maintain human life. The chief evidences of this fact are widespread malnutrition, starvation, poverty, and pollution. With the big boom still to come, the misery has only begun.

One half of the persons on earth suffer outright hunger. As many as two thirds are probably undernourished. Millions starve to death each year* and the world's food situation is growing worse, not better. Recent breakthroughs in food production only serve to delay massive starvation unless the population growth is checked. In areas where the greatest numbers are crowded, food is scarcest. The Far East contains over 53 percent of the world's people but produces only about 28 percent of the world's food. In contrast, North America has 7 percent of the people and 21 percent of the food.

Hunger is only one aspect of the poverty created by overpopulation. In many nations housing, education, clothing, and medical care cannot keep pace with galloping population increases. These problems are compounded by the current mass movement to urban areas. Sprawling slums mar most cities. Dirt floors, rats, vermin, foul air, poor sanitation, and lack of privacy are common household items for millions. Many can afford no house at all. They sleep, and often die, in the streets. Others set up living quarters in alleys and under stairways.

For multitudes, adequate clothing is rare. Education is a

---

*No one knows how many starve. Starving people often fall victim to disease as they weaken and their deaths are not recorded as due to starvation. In some crowded places the deaths go unnoticed; corpses are loaded on carts like so much firewood and dumped outside the city. A minimum of 3 to 4 million persons, mostly children, starve to death annually under present world conditions. Ehrlich, p. 17.

novelty. Rotting teeth and festering sores are daily companions. Brains and bodies are permanently damaged by lack of proper food. Sapped by disease, gnawed by hunger, devoid of hope, with pain as a daily companion, life itself is torment. Often they resemble walking skeletons. They are the living dead of the earth.

Another effect of runaway population increase is pollution. Man has been called the "dirty animal." A look at the mess he has made of the world shows that the label is appropriate. As the number of dirty animals increases so does the amount of pollution. Technology is at the root of the pollution problem. Technology has triggered the population explosion, made modern urban life possible, and polluted the environment. Man has used technology to try to remedy the effects of overpopulation. He has mainly succeeded only in further corrupting his environment.

For example, pesticides have been used to increase crop production and reduce hunger. A side effect has been the pollution of the soil and water and the poisoning of fish, animals and men. Huge industries produce items necessary to care for vast populations. They also vomit corrupting wastes into the waterways and belch harmful substances into the air. Massive transportation systems shuttle the world's growing hordes from place to place. But they also produce destructive noises and poisonous gases.

Other effects of crowding are not as easy to document. War, for example, is often cited as a result of overpopulation. Poverty and hunger have contributed to most major revolutions.

The crowding brought on by population increase may be contributing to the widespread crime, rioting, and unrest in the world. After a careful study of available evidence, Congressman Morris Udall wrote, "Most of our tensions and our failures are directly due to an unrestrained, spiraling population growth."[7] Man may simply not be equipped to function well in a crowded, noisy dirty setting.[8]

RESPONSE TO THE PROBLEM

A few nations, most notably Japan and India, have put forth extensive efforts to stem the population flood. In India governmental and private forces have united in a widespread birth control campaign. Information on the advantages and techniques of birth control has been widely distributed. Free materials to prevent conception are made available. Special teams have been sent from village to village. Financial inducements have been offered for sterilization and use of contraceptives. The results have been disappointing. At the start of the program the growth rate was about 1.3 percent per year. After sixteen years of family planning effort, the growth rate was over 2.5 percent per year and the population had increased over 150 million.[9]

Japan has had better results. After World War II the Japanese were confined to the islands of Japan. It was obvious that the population had to be limited. Government, industry, mass media —in fact almost all phases of Japanese life—joined together to hold the population down. Most types of birth control were encouraged and made available, including abortion. The result was a rapid decline in the birth rate. It is now one of the lowest in the world.[10]

The United Nations has sponsored birth control efforts on a rather limited basis.[11] Some communist nations have stressed limitation of the number of children. Generally speaking, the communist countries have a much smaller rate of population growth than the rest of the world.[12] But on the whole, serious efforts at reducing the population growth have been few.[13]

The United States has no extensive official program of population control. The Federal government has done little. Less than 1 percent of the Department of Health, Education, and Welfare's budget goes for population control. The population budget of all government agencies would not buy more than a dozen modern military jet planes. On the other hand, the Federal government spends billions for death control programs. But unless birth control matches death control the end result can only be catastrophe. In July, 1969, President Nixon delivered an address dealing with the population problem. He called for the establishment by Congress of a Commission on Population Growth and the American Future.[14] Hopefully, government action will increase.

Private agencies in the United States have sponsored widespread education programs on population problems and birth control. (A list of these can be found at the end of this chapter.) The Ford Foundation and Rockefeller Foundation have made large contributions for research in population control. Medical science has produced effective birth control methods which have been widely used. But many people evidently don't know about birth control methods, or they can't afford them, or they are not adequately motivated to use them. Certain religious groups, particularly the Roman Catholic Church, oppose many birth control programs.

SUGGESTED REMEDIES

Faced with the fact of the world's population trend, it is clear that the options are limited if we are to avert widespread disaster. Basically we must provide either more space and food or reduce the growth of population.

Some believe that we should concentrate on adding space and increasing food production. The prospects for significantly increasing food supplies are dim. Bringing much more land into cultivation is unlikely. Population growth is actually reducing the number of acres per person available for growing food.

Proposals have been made to gain food in new ways: harvest the sea, culture microbes on petroleum, produce new high-protein grains and foods, culture the algae in the fecal slime of our sewerage treatment plants. Some of these may eventually be helpful, but many have been dismissed as unworkable, and none are much more than at the drawing board stage presently.[15] The only real immediate hope of increasing food production is to use new, high-yield grains and modernize ancient farming techniques in many of the underdeveloped nations. This is not easily accomplished. It requires a degree of capital and technical know-how which most underdeveloped nations lack.

Even if food production is increased, it cannot indefinitely keep up with the current population increase. In light of this fact, proposals have been offered to export the excess people to other planets. The earth would use other planets in this scheme much as seventeenth and eighteenth century Europe used the New World to absorb a booming population. In this way we could, in a sense, create more room. But this approach is sheer

fantasy unless some totally new means of interplanetary transportation is developed.[16] Even if we succeeded, at the present
rate of population growth within a few thousand years "everything in the visible universe would be converted into people,
and the ball of people would be expanding with the speed of
light!"[17]

The only sensible approach to the population explosion is
birth control. Ultimately birth rates must be brought down or
death rates will soar. Famine, pestilence, war, or something will
reduce the number of people on the earth. Wouldn't it be better
to control the population through limiting births rather than
through widespread suffering?

The answer seems obvious.[18] Yet many still protest birth
control. Some argue that the nation which limits births reduces
its capacity to wage war and defend itself. But in a day of technological warfare a massive population can be a liability rather
than an asset.[19] Others insist that a growing population insures
an expanding economy and increased prosperity. But the most
prosperous nations are among those with low population growth
rates.[20] Some religious groups oppose the most efficient methods
of birth control, labeling them immoral and crimes against nature.[21] But could endorsing birth control be more immoral than
allowing millions to exist in daily torment because of overpopulation? Could the use of contraceptives be more a crime against
nature than encouraging the expanded pollution of the earth's
soil, air, and water under the pressure of overpopulation?

Sometime, somehow the population will be limited. It is
better to do it now than later. It is better to do it by reducing
the birth rate than by increasing the death rate. It is better to do
it voluntarily while we can rather than wait until it is done in-
voluntarily by a totalitarian regime or by starvation, war and disease.

TOWARD LIMITING BIRTHS

Suppose the leaders of the world, or even of the United States,
were to agree that population control through limiting births
is necessary. What would be the best, most efficient, and yet

morally acceptable means of limiting births? A number of proposals have been offered, and some tried.

If the population is to be stabilized, all families must cooperate. Contrary to common opinion, the population boom in the United States is *not* primarily caused by the poor with large families. It is the result of the families in the middle and upper income groups which have more than two children. One of the major problems in population control is that most families want more than two children. Yet population experts insist that two is the ideal number of children in light of the world's crowded condition.

A massive education program is called for to impress people with the need for small families. In fact, those groups and programs which promote large families should be challenged. Large families can provide wonderful benefits for the members. But under the circumstances it is irresponsible to indulge in such selfish practices. Those wanting more than two children should adopt them.

Some writers on the population problem call for a restructuring of attitudes about family life and the role of women. They reason that as long as our culture is family centered and women see their value primarily as mothers it will be difficult to bring birth rates down. On the other hand, if a person is not penalized by tax rates for remaining single, if tax laws are rewritten to favor small families, and if women are encouraged to find fulfillment in a career, the chance of limiting births is increased. The ill effects of such a strategy might, of course, outweigh the good.

An approach more in keeping with the patterns of our society, more readily accepted, and less likely to cause social damage, is to launch an all-out campaign for small families. Such a campaign could stress personal advantages and the larger responsibility to society. This education program should be carried out through the mass media, public schools, religious groups, and other organizations.

The knowledge of birth control techniques and availability of contraceptives is equally important. Most Americans both approve of and practice birth control. There is little public sentiment against distributing birth control information. This is a drastic change from fifty years ago when laws forbade distribution of birth control information and persons were sometimes jailed for violating these laws.

There is a general agreement that so-called family planning clinics are needed in areas where the poor live.[22] Such clinics distribute birth control information and free or low-cost contraceptives. The programs of the clinics are designed to not only lower birth rates but also reduce poverty. Some resistance to such programs exists among the poor, particularly among those who are part of minority groups. The resistance is based on a fear that the birth control programs are an effort by the majority to reduce the number of persons in minority groups.

Even if family planning clinics in low-income neighborhoods succeeded in drastically lowering birth rates among the poor, the population problem in America would not be solved. White middle-class couples planning for three-to-four-child families "will add 100 million people to our population over the next 30 years."[23] There are several reasons why these families have larger families than that needed to provide a stable population. Some, notably Roman Catholics, have religious convictions against birth control. Others choose large families out of personal preference. Millions have unwanted children due either to negligence or failure in the use of a contraceptive technique. Massive education is needed on the importance of population limitations and on the use of the best contraceptives.

Medical science has produced a wide variety of birth control techniques. They fall into two broad categories: those which prevent conception and those which terminate pregnancy before birth. The means used to prevent conception or birth include mechanical devices, chemicals, drugs, and surgery. A couple in selecting a form of birth control should choose one which is effective, safe, simple to use, inexpensive, and inoffensive to both of them.

The two most controversial means of birth control are abortion and sterilization.

Some countries, notably Japan and Hungary, have reduced their birth rate by the use of abortion. Currently, abortion is not considered an acceptable birth control technique by the majority of Americans. However, the general trend in the states is to make abortion more available through normal medical channels than has been true in the past. Abortion no doubt would help check the population boom by reducing the birth rate of unwanted children. Many argue, however, that making abortion available would be morally wrong, that the cure would be worse than the disease.

Voluntary sterilization is also recommended by some population control groups. Couples with two children, for example, would agree for the husband or wife to be sterilized. The operation on the male is safe, simple, inexpensive, and effective. Because the procedure to restore fertility is successful in only half of the cases, this method of birth control has not gained wide favor. Furthermore, the technique has some moral and psychological drawbacks.

What if voluntary measures don't work? Then some type of compulsory birth control program will probably become necessary. A number of measures have been suggested: Require a license in order to conceive a child and limit birth licenses to two per family; add temporary sterilants to water supplies or staple foods with the antidote available only from the government; make abortion mandatory for the unmarried or for married couples with two or more children.

Obviously such programs are undesirable. We should strive to limit births voluntarily so that such measures will never be instituted.

CHRISTIAN RESPONSES

What should be the Christian's response to population problems? The Bible seems to favor large families. On the surface this appears to be an obstacle in the way of Christians working for a reduction of the birth rate. But a careful look at the passages related to population shows that no conflict exists between the Bible and population control today.

Genesis records the instruction of God to mankind to multiply and replenish the earth; we seem to be carrying out this instruction quite well—too well in fact. Genesis 38:4-10 records the condemnation of Onan for spilling his sperm on the ground;

Onan's sin was not birth control, however, but hypocrisy and failure to obey the laws of his people which were given by God.

Old Testament statements about the blessings of many children are in keeping with the culture of the Old Testament period in history. At that time the world was not overcrowded. The death rate was very high for children and many were needed to insure the survival of the family. Children were an economic asset, not a liability. The situation today regarding birth rate and family size is almost the opposite of that in biblical times.

Some argue that the main purpose of sex is procreation and that birth control is therefore wrong. But the Bible clearly indicates that sex in marriage apart from procreation is not sinful; see, for example, Hebrews 13:4 and I Corinthians 7:4-5.

A Christian has a vital role to play in defusing the population bomb. The Christian faith stresses the responsibility of believers to help reduce suffering and pain. Christians are to love and minister to all people. They should help reduce the world's birth rate since overpopulation causes widespread suffering.

Because overpopulation and pollution are interrelated, Christians have an added incentive to work for population control. Christians believe that the earth is the Lord's and that we are but stewards. We have a responsibility to see that the earth is not converted from an oasis in space to a monstrous cesspool.

NOTES AND REFERENCES

1. Ehrlich, Paul R.: *The Population Bomb*. New York, Ballantine Books, 1968, pp. 166-67.
2. O'Brien, John: Population explosion demands worldwide action. *Christian Century*, Jan. 8, 1964, p. 43.
3. Hauser, Phillip (Ed.): *The Population Dilema*. Englewood Cliffs, Prentice Hall, 1963, p. 13.
4. Life expectancy has varied greatly throughout history between different people and living conditions. Two thousand years ago in Rome the average baby had a life expectancy of little more than twenty years. In the province of Hispania it was between thirty-five years for girls and forty years for boys. In Roman Africa it was between forty-five and fifty years. By 1850 the life expectancy of a baby girl in Massachusetts was less than that of one in ancient Roman Africa. After 1850 life expectancy began to increase with a rapid rise after 1900. Har-

rison Brown, Increase in life expectancy due to modern medicine. Louise B. Young, Ed.): In *Population in Perspective*. New York, Oxford University Press, 1968, pp. 49-50.

5. The drop in infant mortality rates has been greatest in the countries with advanced medical technology, education, and sanitation. In the United States, for example, female infant mortality decreased from 110 deaths per thousand births in 1900 to twenty-six in 1946. In Chile the rate went from almost 240 to about 170 during the same period. Within a developed country the rates are lower among the wealthy and higher among the poor. *Ibid.*, pp. 50-52. The control of childhood diseases has allowed more children to reach maturity today than ever before.

6. Control of diseases which once killed millions of young adults—malaria, typhoid, tuberculosis, pneumonia—has progressed rapidly in this century. While mortality rates among infants, children, and young adults have dropped spectacularly in this century, rates for older persons have not decreased much. "Medical science is making it possible for ever-increasing numbers of people to live out their natural life span, the ultimate 'limit' of the human life span is not being increased appreciably." *Ibid.*, p. 55. "The increased life expectancy that has been made possible by the technological developments of the past century has strangely affected two aspects of population growth. First, an increasingly large fraction of newborn girls survive to reach the breeding age. Second, and quite independent of birth pattern, the long life span has resulted in increased population solely because more people are living longer." *Ibid.*, p. 58.

7. Udall, Morris K.: Our spaceship earth—standing room only. *Arizona Days and Ways*, July 27, 1969.

8. See John Calhoun, Population density and social pathology. *Scientific America*, February 1962, for one of many discussions.

9. Ehrlich, *Population Bomb*, p. 87.

10. In 1966 it was, next to Hungary, the world's lowest. This year was abnormal, however, in that it was the "Year of Fiery Horse," a year considered to bring bad luck in marriage and birth. Japan is now easing its birth control effort and the birth rate and growth rate are increasing. World population data sheet—1968, Population Reference Bureau, Washington.

11. See The United Nations and the population crisis. The Victor Fund for the International Planned Parenthood Federation, Spring 1968, No. 8.

12. In 1968 the rates of growth were: Cuba, 2.6 percent per year (one of the lowest in Latin America); China, 1.5 (one of the lowest in Asia); Soviet Union and Yugoslavia, 1.1; Poland, .8; Bulgaria, .7; Romania, .6; Czechoslovakia, .5; Hungary, .3; East Germany, .2. See Jean Mayer and H. Andre Van H. Mayer, Birth control and population policy in the socialist world. *Harvard Medical Alumni Bulletin,* Spring 1967, pp. 2-7.

13. For a brief discussion of efforts in various countries see *A New Look at Our Crowded World,* Public Affairs Pamphlet No. 393; How family planning programs work—will they succeed? The Victor-Bostrom Fund for the International Planned Parenthood Federation, Report No. 10, Fall 1968; Population program assistance, Agency for International Development, Office of the War on Hunger, Population Service, Washington.

14. Presidential message on population. Population Crisis Committee, Washington.

15. Recently, for example, a process has been discovered that turns natural gas into powder that is almost pure protein at a cost much lower than the lowest cost protein available and rich in vitamins. *Look,* February 24, 1970, p. 17.

16. A number of apparently insurmountable obstacles stand in the way of using colonization of the planets as a means of coping with earth's population problems: (1) It is virtually certain that the other planets in our solar system are uninhabitable. (2) The cost and logistics of moving billions of people off the Earth are insurmountable under present conditions. (3) Even if we colonized the nearby planets, at the present population growth rate it would take only about 50 years to populate these planets to the present density of the Earth. We could gain perhaps another 200 years by reaching Jupiter and Uranus. (4) To colonize outside our solar system is even more hopeless. It has been calculated that the United States by cutting down its standard of living to 18 percent of its present level could in one *year* set aside enough capital to finance the exportation to the stars of one *day's* population increase. Ehrlich, pp. 20-21.

17. Ehrlich, pp. 20-21.

18. The editors of *Look* in a special issue on population and pollution wrote, "We have to check the population growth. Without an immediate commitment to an effective program of birth control, the under-developed world is doomed to death by famine, and the affluent world to social chaos." *Look,* November 4, 1969, p. 71.

19. A small population, of course, makes it impossible for a nation to become a superpower. Yet there is a point of diminishing

return in population increase. For an extensive discussion see Philip Hauser, *Population and World Politics,* New York, Free Press of Glencoe, 1958, and A. F. K. and Katherine Organiski, *Population and World Power,* New York, Alfred A. Knopf, 1961.

20. See Young (Ed.), pp. 109-189.
21. Most religions of the world have a heritage of promoting large families. Under the pressures of overpopulation many have begun either to advocate or permit birth control. See Young, pp. 193-243; Religious factors in the population problem, by Arthur J. Dyck, Harvard University Center for Population Studies, Contribution No. 37; Religion, politics, and population—time for a change, by Ralph Potter, Jr., Harvard University Center for Population Studies, Contribution No. 22.
22. How much such clinics are needed, how much they will reduce population pressure, and how much government money should be put into them is a matter of debate. See, for example, *Science,* May 2, 1969, pp. 522-29; July 25, 1969, pp. 367-73.
23. James E. Allen, Overpopulation: challenge to Americans. *Christian Advocate,* October 16, 1969, p. 13.

BIBLIOGRAPHY

Organizations

General Board of Christian Social Concerns of the United Methodist Church, 100 Maryland Ave., N.E., Washington, D. C. 20002.
Planned Parenthood-World Population, 810 Seventh Ave., New York, N. Y. 10019.
Population Council, 245 Park Ave., New York, N. Y. 10017.
Population Crisis Committee, 1730 K St., N.W., Washington, D. C. 20006
Population Policy Panel, Hugh Moore Fund, 60 E. 42nd St., New York, N. Y. 10017.
Population Reference Bureau, 1755 Massachusetts Ave., N.W., Washington, D. C. 20036.
Zero Population Growth, Inc., 330 Second St., Los Altos, Cal. 94022.

Books

Borgstrom, George: *The Hungry Planet.* New York, Collier Books, 1967.
Ehrlich, Paul R.: *The Population Bomb.* New York, Ballentine Books, 1968.
Ehrlich, Paul R.: *Population Resources Environment.* San Francisco, W. H. Freeman, 1970.

Fagley, Richard M.: *The Population Explosion and Christian Responsibility.* New York, Oxford University Press, 1960.

Hauser, Philip (Ed.): *The Population Dilemma.* Englewood Cliffs, Prencise-Hall, 1963.

Paddock, William and Paddock, Paul: *Famine—1975!* Boston, Little, Brown, 1967.

Thompson, Warren S. and Lewis, David T.: *Population Problems.* New York, McGraw-Hill, 1965.

Young, Louise B. (Ed.): *Population in Perspective.* New York, Oxford University Press, 1968.

Chapter 4

BIRTH CONTROL BY STERILIZATION

JOSEPH E. DAVIS, F.A.C.S.

INTRODUCTION

Sterilization as a means of birth control is rapidly becoming one of the most popular means of preventing conception in this country. Whereas in former years, approximately 100,000 men and women chose sterilization as a permanent method of birth control, it is estimated that some 700,000 men underwent the male sterilization operation last year. In this year, there seems to be even a higher rate of increase than last year. Women, too, who desired no more children, are increasingly demanding some form of sterilization operation from their physicians. There may be several reasons for this tremendous growth in the interest in sterilization. Many couples are disenchanted with various types of contraception, including the pill, diaphragm, condoms and others, for various reasons. Many women have difficulty tolerating the pill. Other women find that the intrauterine device is a source of pain. Others are turned off by use of foams, jellies and diaphragms. Many men refuse to use condoms.

For many of the couples the choice of sterilization comes because they have decided they do not want any more children and never will. Increasingly there are young couples who have no children, and who because of their life style, habits, or concern for the population problems in this country and in the world choose to undergo sterilization rather than use other forms of contraception which are temporary.

It is important for us to remember that sterilization is legal in all states except in the state of Utah, where it can only be performed for reasons of medical necessity as determined by the physician. The Utah legislature at present has bills pending to remove the restriction of medical necessity alone.

In olden times, sterilization was a form of punishment. During World War II, the Germans apparently practiced compulsory sterilization on the inmates of concentration camps. But the sterilization techniques that we think of today are purely voluntary. When a couple comes to a physician for consideration of such an operation they do it voluntarily, and the physician usually will discuss and describe exactly what the procedure is and exactly what the effects are in terms of the functions of the body. We will deal a little later with the physical and psychological effects, if any, of the operation, but suffice it to say now that there are usually no other effects of the operation in the male other than to prevent sperm from coming up the male tubes and in the female preventing the egg from coming down the female tube. Sexual desire, sexual behavior, hormonal function and the rest of the sexual parts of the male and the female function without any alteration.

STERILIZATION: WHAT IT IS AND WHAT IT IS NOT

Sterilization is a birth control method achieved surgically by closing a pair of small tubes in either the man or woman so that the egg and sperm cannot meet. It does not involve removal of any gland or organ, has no harmful physical side effects and does not unfavorably effect individual sex life.

While other methods of birth control are effective for child spacing in certain segments of the population both in the United States and abroad, professional studies show that many parents do not want any more children and are seeking a more permanent and reliable birth control method. Voluntary sterilization thus fills the need for a safe, medically accepted, completely reliable method of terminating family fertility.

For a woman, the procedure called salpingectomy is usually performed by making a small abdominal incision so that the ovarian ducts (Fallopian tubes) may be cut and tied, thus preventing the egg from descending from the ovary down into the uterus. In this way the egg cannot meet the sperm. Conception cannot occur. This operation, similar to an appendix operation, is always performed in the hospital. Newer techniques for performing the closing of the female tubes include passing a tube through the abdominal wall and visualizing with a telescope through the lens, the tubes, and then with another instrument put in laterally on the side of the body, cutting and burning the tubes. This operation does not require an abdominal incision but is still being performed in hospitals. Some physicians feel that it may become an outpatient procedure soon.

A second new method of performing the cutting of the tubes involves inserting an instrument similar to the one described through the vagina. This is called the culdoscope. This instrument similarly will allow the doctor to see the tubes and cut them through a cutting device within the instrument.

The male operation called vasectomy involves only the closing of a small tube on each side of the male sac (the scrotum). This tube is called the vas deferens. Usually, a one-half to three-quarters of an inch incision is made on each side of the scrotum so that the tube can be lifted out, cut and tied, thus blocking the passage of sperm. The testicle continues to form sperm which is then absorbed in the body and as far as we know causes no harm. Usually, this minor operation can be performed in a doctor's office under local anesthesia and takes about twenty minutes. There is usually some swelling and discomfort following the operation, but the patient in most cases can go back to work the following day.

Sterilization of the male does not make him impotent or prevent him from enjoying sex. It causes no change in his general health. It is not castration. It does not change a man's ability to have an erection or to ejaculate. Following the operation, the same amount of semen may be ejaculated as before but it simply doesn't contain sperm. There is no change in the production of the male sex hormone. If a man or a woman completely understands the nature of the operation and freely makes the decision to have it, psychological effects are nearly always beneficial. In some rare cases, in patients who have had previous psychiatric history, there may be some deterioration of their condition after the surgery. These instances usually represent situations where the patient was inadequately screened for the surgery.

In females, sterilization does not produce symptoms of menopause. It does not interfere with menstruation. The characteristics which make a woman feminine are controlled by the hormones of the ovaries, and sterilization has no effect on the action of these hormones. It merely prevents the egg from reaching the uterus. A woman's sexual responsiveness also depends largely on the action of hormones and on psychological factors. Often, therefore, when a woman obtains sterilization and the fear of pregnancy is removed, sexual response is increased.

PERMANENCE AND REVERSIBILITY OF STERILIZATION

The operations in the male and the female are ordinarily performed as permanent measures and should not be considered unless the individuals feel sure that they want no more children. Physicians in general present sterilization to patients as a permanent procedure, as well they should. There have been attempts to reverse the tying of the tubes in either the male or the female. Success rates of getting sperm through the newly hooked up male tubes have been reported as high as 85 percent. No reliable figures are available for success in terms of pregnancy. In the female, also, the tubes technically can be reconstituted, but the results with fertility following the fixing of the tubes is less than 50 percent. Therefore, one cannot honestly tell the patient that reversibility can be guaranteed when they come to the physician seeking such an operation.

Several new techniques for making reversibility simpler are being developed. These include the use of valves and other devices which go into the vas deferens so that actual occlusion can be performed without cutting the tubes. Also, sperm banks are just about available in some parts of the country. Under these circumstances a man who will desire vasectomy may give several specimens of his sperm to the sperm bank where the sperm can be frozen for an indefinite period of time, probably as long as ten years. If family situations arise so that the patient may want to have more children in the future, he could then go to the sperm bank, claim his sperm, which would then be sent to his physician where the sperm could then be inseminated into his mate. The results of unfreezing sperm after four to eight years are remarkably good in that the sperm usually regains the motility that it had prior to freezing. Sperm banks then are the first step toward reversibility in the male.

As yet though, the sterilization operations must be considered irreversible. It is hoped that within three to five years several techniques for successful reversibility will be available. Nevertheless, this is still a drawback to the operation in couples who may be dissatisfied with other forms of birth control but yet may want to keep the option of having children in the future. On the other hand, sterilization is probably the most effective means of birth control available.

LEGAL ASPECTS OF STERILIZATION

As stated earlier, voluntary contraceptive sterilization is legal in all fifty states. In Utah it is limited to reasons of medical necessity. The American Medical Association in 1961 brought out the point that nontherapeutic voluntary sterilization, that is for contraceptive reasons alone, until declared illegal by the legislature or the courts in the physician's state is largely a matter of individual conscience and principal. I will go a step further and say that as far as sterilization is concerned, it is strictly a matter of a decision between a patient, married or single, and the patient's physician.

The American Medical Association also states that with regard to civil damages, sterilization does not prevent any greater exposure to liability than other medical and surgical procedures alleged to have been negligently performed. One knows of no case on record of a physician losing a suit brought against him for sterilization when proper consent from the party or parties involved had first been obtained. Refer to Figure 4-1 for the form which the author uses for his patients who will undergo bilateral vasectomy.

The Joint Commission on Accreditation of Hospitals has taken an explicitly permissive position on voluntary sterilizations. Hospitals are free to make their own rules in this matter.

I hereby authorize Dr. Joseph E. Davis and whomever he may designate as his assistants to perform upon _____ the operation known as bilateral vasectomy.

I fully understand that bilateral vasectomy means the removal of a segment of each vas deferens, each of which conduct sperm. I fully understand that this operation(s) will cause sterility in the person operated upon. The word sterility means inability to produce children or cause pregnancy in a female partner. I am fully aware of the implications of the operation called bilateral vasectomy.

I understand that this operation in no way affects sexual potency or the sexual act. I understand that I must present a specimen(s) of my semen following the operation(s) so that the absence of sperm in the semen can be determined.

Signature of patient _____

Signature of person
authorized to give consent _____

Relation to patient _____

Witness _____

State of New York) SS:
County of New York)

On the _____ day of _____ 19 ___, before me came _____, to me known, who being by me sworn, did depose and say that ___he resides at _____: that ___he is the _____ of_____, who executed the foregoing authorization.

Figure 4-1

Three states, Virginia, Georgia and North Carolina, have passed laws affirming the legality of voluntary contraceptive sterilization in those states and clarifying procedures under which the operation can be performed. Recently, three federal government agencies—the Department of Health, Education and Welfare, the Department of Defense, and the Federal and State Medicaid Program—have endorsed voluntary sterilization. At the last count, thirty-two states out of thirty-seven operating a capitalized Medicaid Program reported paying for voluntary sterilization under the program. The great majority of these do not report making any distinction between elective sterilization and that performed for medical reasons.

The Department of Defense has approved voluntary sterilization in military hospitals for servicemen's wives. In a letter to the Association for Voluntary Sterilization from the Assistant Secretary for Health and Scientific Affairs of the Department of Health, Education and Welfare, it was stated that this department does not seek to control the particular medical and surgical procedures to be utilized by any of its grantees in the field of health. The procedures to be followed under any given set of circumstances are for the grantee or its professional personnel to determine. Voluntary sterilization does not differ in this respect from other procedures. In our view, this is a matter of professional judgment in an individual case. Taken together, these evidences of forthright support from important professional organizations and government agencies remove any doubt of the legality of voluntary sterilization in the United States.

STERILIZATION VERSUS OTHER METHODS OF BIRTH CONTROL

The question is often asked, "Why sterilization when other methods of birth control are available?" The answer is that studies in the United States and other countries have shown that a significant proportion of many women do not want any more children. Theirs may not be a child-spacing problem but rather a problem of terminating fertility once and for all in the easiest, safest, and most effective manner. This means sterilization.

To promote the use of a temporary birth control method where a permanent method is needed and desired but can't be utilized is costly. Yet this is often what is done. It may be that this is one of the most unfortunate mistakes that some social workers and population experts make today in their attempts to implement effective birth control programs.

The usual criteria to measure the value of a birth control method are safety, low cost, effectiveness and acceptability. Some rough comparisons of various birth control methods using these criteria are in order. When properly performed by modern medical technique, sterilization of both the male and female is virtually 100 percent reliable. Authorities estimate that the female operation has a failure rate of only .003 with the most used method. One practitioner in Japan cites 5,000 cases by his own technique without a single failure. As to the vasectomy operation in the male, the failure rate is also almost zero.

Other than sterilization most experts list the IUD, the pill, the diaphragm and the condom as the methods considered to have high enough reliability to be acceptable in either an individual or population control basis. The pill, however, is too expensive for many U. S. parents and far too expensive for huge population groups abroad. Both the pill and the IUD sometimes have undesirable side effects despite their general reliability, and the condom and the diaphragm are often not popular for aesthetic reasons or from lack of motivation. Surveys have proved that a large percentage of uneducated or poorly motivated couples cannot use conventional birth control methods effectively for any length of time. Also, there are highly intelligent and well-motivated couples who cannot obtain successful results from temporary contraceptives no matter how conscientiously they try. Such couples of high fertility often find their way to the sterilization method after trying everything else and having failure.

One obstetrician—gynecologist has found in over thirty years of practice that patients in maternity prenatal clinics who already have several children are nearly always interested in the idea of sterilization if it is presented to them. It is very important to spend a few minutes and explain the details of the possibility of tying the tubes right after the woman delivers a child. Postpartum tubal section is very popular and often can be done while the woman is in the hospital having delivered the baby.

RISKS AND COMPLICATIONS OF STERILIZATION

While any surgical operation involves a degree of danger, sterilization in both the male and the female carries an extremely slight risk. One obstetrician—gynecologist said that the risk of the female operation is comparable to that for an uncomplicated appendectomy. A man can have the operation done in the doctor's office in a few minutes and be back to work within a day or two. In the male, complications may be swelling of the scrotum with pain and discoloration for several days. If infection develops there may be even greater swelling of the scrotum, but this usually responds to antibiotic treatment. There are no known long-time complications. There have been several studies on the psychological effects of the operation, but suffice it to say that there has been no proven psychological or behavioral effects in any individual who did not have psychiatric problems prior to the surgery.

Following the operation in the male, he is advised to put ice packs against the area for several days (please see the page of instructions at the end of this chapter). He is allowed to have sex as soon as he desires. It takes at least ten ejaculations of semen to evacuate all the sperm from the duct system above the point where the tubes were tied. Formerly, the patient was told to come back six to eight weeks after the operation so that he could be declared sterile. But newer techniques have demonstrated that most men will be sterile after ejaculating eight to ten times. Thus, the end point of sterility is really a factor of the number of times he ejaculates.

STERILIZATION AS A PREVENTIVE OF ABORTION

Abortion, legal or illegal, is probably the chief method of birth control in the world today, according to experts who participated in the United Nations Conference on World Population that took place in Belgrade in 1965. They estimate that about 30 million pregnancies are purposely terminated each year. Clearly, if the uncounted millions who need and want permanent reliable birth control could obtain it, there would be a significant drop in the annual numbers of abortions with their associated misery and danger. It is indeed strange that with all the clamor of reform of abortion laws in the United States the simple connection between reliable permanent birth control by sterilization and the abortion problem has been lost in the shuffle.

A survey made about twenty-five years ago revealed that in the United States, four out of every five abortions performed were done on married women with children. A more recent estimate for the period 1960 to 1964 puts the proportion of married women obtaining abortions at 59 percent of the total. Obviously, this is still a very significant figure.

A study of maternal deaths between August 1957 and December 1965 reveals illegal abortions as the leading cause of maternal death in California as in many other states. This study defines a composite profile of the usual victim of illegal abortion as a white, married housewife, age twenty-seven, who has had five previous pregnancies, probably none of which were aborted. We often think of the woman in her thirties or even early forties as a typical candidate for sterilization, but it is equally valid to consider a woman in her twenties who wants no more children and has at least twenty years of fertility stretching ahead of her as one who can greatly benefit from sterilization. And she may be very interested in it. Women such as this, if they continue to use temporary methods, may well continue to have contraceptive failures and risk abortion. Would they be better off with a sterilization operation? The question answers itself.

RELIGIOUS AND ETHICAL ASPECTS OF
VOLUNTARY STERILIZATION

Voluntary strilization is a method of birth control like the pill, the IUD, or the diaphragm; the big difference is that it is permanent. Basically, the same ethical criteria apply to sterilization as to other methods of birth control. There is no reason for singling out surgical birth control as being less ethical than any other. Only the Roman Catholic Church is officially opposed to sterilization as it is to all of the methods of birth control except rhythm. In other major religions there is no such official opposition. Leading nonCatholic churchmen have hailed the work of the Association for Voluntary Sterilization in the area of voluntary sterilization as a "beacon of hope and enlightenment."

One prominent Episcopal minister has stated,

> Those who believe that sterilization is wrong or sinful will presumeably not request it but they should not interfere with those who believe our moral stature is raised to the degree that we choose freely to control our natural processes rather than to be controlled animal-like by them. If one method of birth control was morally better than the others, it will be so be-

cause it is more loving, creative and constructive. "Artificial" and "against nature" are meaningless terms here because all medicine and science is an "interference" with nature using it or outwitting it for the sake of humanly chosen ends; everything including sterilization or contraception is good or bad according to circumstances.

Bishop John Wesley Lord of the Methodist Church in Washington, D. C., says that the church has adopted what "I believe is a self-righteous standard about sterilization." "I personally believe that voluntary sterilization if practiced in Christian conscience, fulfills rather than violates the will of God. Indications for or against sterilization should, I believe, include socioeconomic as well as moral factors."

MENTAL RETARDATION AND STERILIZATION

One of the greatest tragedies that can happen to normal parents is having a mentally retarded child. Mental deficiency is probably worse for those who care for the patient, especially if they are the parents, than for the victim himself. As the mentally retarded child approaches maturity, parents become very concerned about the possibility of the child's becoming involved with a pregnancy, especially in the case of girls. No good can come from a mentally deficient person being a parent, only suffering and heartbreak.

It is estimated that approximately 3 percent of the population in the United States are mentally retarded. Many of these are of an I.Q. below 70. Studies have shown that the retarded can often support themselves and a family as well. Their marriages have a quite high rate of success. But their chances for a stable marriage are better if they do not have a large family. Whereas these individuals have the right to the relationships which go with marriage, it is equally evident that the few existing studies of child-rearing practices of mentally retarded parents indicate a large proportion of the children are neglected, mistreated or delinquent. Many are physically and mentally defective. When both parents were retarded, one-third to two-thirds of the children were mentally deficient. Parents with I.Q.s of less than 55 or 60 (equivalent to a 6- or 7-year-old child) are seldom able to provide proper care or discipline for the children. In view of the consensus of experts that marriage can be beneficial to many retarded individuals when not overburdened by children, they become ideal candidates for voluntary sterilization early in their married life or before marriage. It has been our policy to accept these individuals for sterilization in their late youth, after they have been examined by competent pediatricians and psychiatrists and it has been declared that they have reached their greatest level of mental achievement. Of course, it is equally important to have the informed consent of the guardians and parents who usually come forth bringing these children to the physician for such aid. Again, let us emphasize that this is purely voluntary sterilization.

Sterilization may also be of value for those individuals who have inherited diseases which might be transmitted to offspring.

STERILIZATION AND THE WORLD'S POPULATION PROBLEM

In Latin America, where the population problem is approaching the critical stage of India's, voluntary sterilization is almost unheard of among the masses, due to the influence of the Roman Catholic Church. Puerto Rico is a significant exception, with high acceptance of the female sterilization operation. While the American cultural influence might be a major factor in Puerto Rican attitudes toward sterilization, the success of the method there is nevertheless worth close study to determine whether and how similar progress can be made in other Latin American countries. Despite obstacles, voluntary sterilization is making substantial gains with increased utilization in the United States, India, Pakistan, Britain, Japan and other countries.

On the premise that we must all use effective means available to win the war on poverty that has now become a desperate worldwide struggle, it is clear that voluntary sterilization should be included in all birth control programs. To make known the benefits of sterilization will require greatly expanded programs of education in the public and professional agencies and of governmental officials, particularly in underdeveloped countries.

Finally, qualified medical personnel must be organized and assigned to implement voluntary sterilization programs on a crash basis in the most critical areas of the world.

CONCLUSIONS AND SUMMARY

We have discussed voluntary sterilization as a method of birth control. This method requires simple surgery. The operation for the male can be performed in the office. The operation for the female requires hospitalization. In both cases, the tubes which conduct either the egg or sperm are cut. There are no effects on the psychology, sexuality or the physiological functions in men or women. The operations are legal in practically every state of the United States. Increasing numbers of individuals, regardless of their age or marital status, who are disenchanted with temporary means of birth control, who do not want any more children, or any children, are becoming increasingly interested in this form of birth control. It is being widely accepted throughout the United States. Besides the many practicing urologist, gynecologists, general surgeons, and general practitioners who perform sterilization on males and females, there are now more than fifty-two vasectomy clinics, many associated with Planned Parenthood Centers throughout the United States. Whereas one said that as of last year approximately 2 million living Americans had been sterilized and approximately 100,000 men and women were sterilized each year, in the past year "the sterilization revolution" has occurred in effect so that it is estimated that over 700,000 men underwent vasectomy last year.

The instructions for the operation and a typical consent form are included in this chapter. We have also covered the relationship of sterilization to abortion, religious considerations and other factors relative to sterilization.

The cost of sterilization is low in comparison with continued use of the pill over a number of years. It is less expensive than all other methods of bitrh control if the higher failure rates of other methods with their attendant costs in both money and misery are brought into consideration. Sterilization is a one-shot permanent procedure with a limited and simple medical checkup period required only in the case of the male. Voluntary steriliza- tion is by and large not sufficiently understood either in the United States or abroad. This is the result of social and educa- tional obstacles rather than any fault of the method itself.

INSTRUCTIONS TO PATIENTS WHO WILL UNDERGO VASECTOMY

Your operation is scheduled for _____.

In order to prepare your skin for better antisepsis during the vasectomy procedure, it is advised that you take a *daily shower for three days* preceding the day of your appointment. *Use Dial soap, or phisoHex.*

Lather the genital area (the scrotum, penis, and pubic hair) for about three minutes with the soap at each showering. If you are not circumcised, retract the foreskin fully during the wash- ing period.

On the day of the operation, shave the scrotum (the skin bag behind the male organ) carefully and then shower as di- rected above. Be sure to bring with you an athletic supporter (jock strap) or scrotal support to wear after the operation. BE ON TIME FOR YOUR APPOINTMENT (If you arrive late, another patient may have to be scheduled in your place.) On the day of the operation it is advisable for an adult to accom- pany you during your journey home, preferably by car or taxi. *Do not plan to drive yourself.*

Bilateral vasectomy requires two small incisions in the scrotum under local anesthesia. Only a needly prick on the skin is usually felt, similar to the injection given before dental work.

After the operation, which usually takes 30 minutes, there may be some minor local discomfort. This can usually be re- lieved by aspirin or any common analgesic.

The tissue in the scrotum is much like the tissue around the eye in that it is easily bruised, bleeds easily, and swells. There is a definite risk of swelling after the operation. It is advisable that you rest one to two days at home and use cold compresses or ice packs intermittently for several days thereby tending to minimize swelling. The suture in the scortal skin will absorb and in seven to ten days will drop off often before the edges of the wound have closed. Therefore, you may notice some gaping and some discharge. The area should be protected and baths and showers should not be used for about a week to ten days.

You should be able to return to your normal occupation within several days. However, as in all cases of surgery, the recovery period greatly depends on the recuperative powers of the individual, and therefore varies substantially from person to person.

In case of any doubt or problem, do not hesitate to call or speak with the doctor before the operation.

Please remember that *you will not be sterile immediately following the operation.* As soon as there is no discomfort from the operation, you may resume normal sexual activity *with contraceptive technique* until you have had ten ejaculations. You will then collect a semen specimen by masturbation into a clean dry jar for examination at this office to determine that you are sterile. The specimen should be *no more than six hours old.*

Chapter 5

PROBLEMS IN MEASURING CHILDREN'S DISTURBED BEHAVIOR

Benjamin C. Hammett, Ph.D, and Harold C. Batchelder, ACSW

The average American parent is accustomed to obtaining almost immediate service for his everyday living. If immediate service is not forthcoming, he can often expedite matters by complaining, pulling strings or actually taking his business elsewhere. This same citizen when faced with the need for treatment for his emotionally disturbed child can be stymied. If alternate services are not available all his efforts will be in vain.

It is difficult for the parent to understand the shades of difference between the type of child an agency can serve and a child who can be better helped elsewhere. Every agency treating emotionally disturbed children has more or less objectively defined and agreed upon criteria as to the type of emotional problems they feel they can help. By way of example one agency may be a crisis clinic. A second might be equipped to treat children in need of long-term residential care. Still another agency might offer day-care programs for children needing a therapeutic milieu but who are able to live with their families. Parents may approach a crisis clinic with a crisis, "Johnny won't go to school." The clinic says, "this is not a crisis." It is not until a parent starts hunting for a treatment facility that he becomes aware that institutions' programs are often explicitly spelled out in charters, the law and, all too often, limited by finances, staff and structure. The parent does not understand and probably is not interested in fine points, definitions and studying what problems are handled by different types of agencies. All he knows is that he has a problem on his hands.

No clinician likes to be in the position of having to say "no" to a request for service. He is acutely aware of the need for immediate intervention, as well as being even more cognizant than the parent of the implications of delayed treatment. The challenge to the clinician or agency is to provide treatment as soon as possible. However, before this can be done there is a twofold responsibility: to assess the needs of the child and to determine whether that child's problems can be best served by their institution. The task for the agency is to provide the parent with a firm decision which is both immediate and equitable. If the intsitution feels it cannot meet the child's needs, then it should interpret the decision to the parents and if possible make a referral to a more appropriate service.

In spite of carefully stated criteria regarding the service an agency can best offer, each applicant presents a multitudinous number of variables, in varying degrees, making a simple yes or no answer to the request for service difficult. The clinician often feels he has been too arbitrary unless he has had the advantage of being able to base his decision on a sufficient number of pertinent facts and direct observations. However, it is often impossible for the clinician to have either the time or resources available to personally make a large number of objective observations. People who have been able to observe the child in various areas of his living, such as parents and teachers, are in an excellent position to do this. However, their efforts need channeling so they report only those observations which they can make objectively and reliably. This can be accomplished by the development of a parent or teacher-rated child behavioral questionnaire.

If designed correctly, such a questionnaire can also be utilized to great advantage in following a child's progress in therapy, in assessing postdischarge adjustment, and in research. An instrument which can be used by persons who are in close contact with the child can serve to supplement the therapist's feelings and impressions. It has the added advantage of pooling information from other areas of living experience. This makes it possible for the therapist to verify his own observations in therapy and to assess the extent to which the child's improved behavior in therapy is maintained outside.

Over a given time period in therapy there should be certain

key behavior changes indicating the degree of progress, emergent strengths, regression or the appearance of new problem areas.

The assessment of a child's readiness for discharge and its timing are as difficult as the decision whether to admit the child into residence. Premature discharge can expose the child to situations he is not quite ready to handle. Equally traumatizing is any insistence in continuing the therapy program beyond its optimal length. Holding a child back when he is ready to progress on his own can result in resistance, regression or apathy. The child can lose his initiative to get well, become demoralized, institutionalized and may regress, since improvement is perceived by him as keeping him hospitalized. Just as in the screening procedure, there is no easy yes or no in the decision to discharge. A wide variety of objective measures in a questionnaire can be most helpful in reaching a decision.

Another reason for measuring behavior is the facilitation of postdischarge follow-ups. Often the child is geographically inaccessible to the direct observations of the therapists. Since parents and teachers may not always recognize or remember to share the beginning signs of regression or new problems by their occasional phone or personal contacts, the routinely mailed questionnaire can be of inestimable value. The therapist, using this method, has the advantage of being able to compare the most recent questionnaire responses with previous ones. This, coupled with his recollection of the child's behavior in therapy, places the therapist in a better position to assess the degree of continuing progress and to spot problem areas. He will be able to focus on all areas necessary in recommending future treatment plans, if indicated. For example, recently a follow-up team discovered a former patient who had not been in school for two years. This situation would have been uncovered much earlier if a periodically mailed questionnaire had been used. There are inherent disadvantages in using a mailed questionnaire, such as a low rate of return. It has been countered by making a verbal contract with the family when the child enters the therapy program. The parents see the questionnaire as both their contribution in helping meet the needs of emotionally disturbed children and as part of the therapeutic process for their own child.

A final advantage in the development of a questionnaire lies in its usefullness as a tool for the much needed research into the causes and methods of treatment of emotional disturbance in children. It is equally useful both in sophisticated research requiring computers and in aiding small agencies concerned with emotionally disturbed children. Every program should have some measure of its effectiveness to guide it in approving its services to children, their families and communities. Every agency, regardless of size, must assess its program in terms of its stated goals in order to meet ever-changing community needs and thereby to determine redirection of goals. This assessment is essential in providing justification to the staff and governing body for the continuation or redirection of programs, and to do this there has to be available comprehensive objective data.

When an agency or institution decides to undertake any research project, it is recommended that the initial step should be the formation of a research committee. This committee should be composed of representatives of each of the agency's departments. This is reassuring to staff and underscores the importance of research as part of the agency's function. It is vitally important that if effective research is to occur, the researchers must not only have the backing of the administration but the interest and support of their colleagues. All too often research becomes the stepchild of an institution, when in reality it is as vital to its growth as any other service offered. The research committee should be charged with the responsibilities of aiding in research design, obtaining computer services, funding, grants and publication services. It should stimulate movement of the project as well as coordinate project efforts, both within the institution and in cooperation with other institutions engaging in similar research. Finally, this committee should be responsible for assuring that the confidentiality and rights of patients and their families are respected.

If an agency or institution decides to develop its own questionnaire to measure emotional disturbance in children, it must be prepared to commit fairly large blocks of staff time for an extended period. This will include an adjustment of schedules so that those involved in the project do not become overly burdened and frustrated. The entire staff should be involved in varying degrees. The project then becomes theirs and takes on a personal interest. One possible way of involving personnel is to have all those who work directly with the children complete the questionnaire and invite their comments. This should be interspersed with both formal and informal meetings by the principal researchers with the staff to discuss progress, problems and invite suggestions.

The nature of the research is going to be determined by the size of the sample of children available. The researchers should be assured that they will have a sufficient number of cases to justify the expenditure of time and money. Although a researcher might be interested in studying the child-rearing antecedents of school phobia, for example, he might be able to collect only six cases a year and therefore be unable to derive statistically stable results. This individual might, however, contribute a very meaningful, descriptive clinical paper on school phobia rather than a statistical study.

A pilot study is one of the researcher's most valuable tools and should never be underestimated. The relatively lower time and energy expended in it can save the researcher much time and wasted effort later. It affords the opportunity to testing one's theories and pinpoints the strengths and weaknesses in the research design. It therefore affords the researcher the opportunity to make valuable corrections early and avoid costly mistakes. The researcher is more likely to abandon or alter an unfruitful idea if great time and effort have not been expended. (It is less embarrassing, too.)

The breadth and sophistication of any research project is determined in part by the availability of certain resources to the team. Researchers certainly have an advantage when they have easy access to large libraries with research journals and centers for computer consultation, programming and calculation. Probably the most fortunate of all is the agency which has connections and accessibility to a university with research-orientated graduate departments such as psychology, sociology and statistics. There are additional resources such as state and federal libraries which will aid in literature search. For example, the National Library of Medicine in Bethesda, Maryland (MEDLARS) will furnish printouts of all their computer-stored research studies. All one needs to do is list on the MEDLARS form a few references to relevant research projects.

A review of the literature is essential in order to avoid duplicating the construction of a questionnaire which has already been developed and extensively proven. Also, the review serves to guide the researcher in establishing a perspective of his efforts in relation to work that has been done and work still needed. It was our experience in developing a questionnaire for untrained raters, such as parents, that a review of the literature was an invaluable guide in determining for our questionnaire the item content, language, format (appearance) and length.

Bearing in mind that we wanted to construct a questionnaire that could be managed by the untrained observer without professional help, we decided to limit ourselves to behavior that was observable not inferential and present not past. The professional rater can answer inferential questions. The untrained person will have difficulty in doing this, and so all our items have to do with present, observable behavior, for instance, "wets bed," "physically attacks adults," "sets fires," "will not leave own room." A wet bed, black eyes, a grass fire and a pubescent "Peter The Hermit" are observable.

High agreement among raters is better obtained by the use of presently observable behavior items. Historical data, which is subject to the vagaries of memory, can better be discussed during the social history. It is possible that some of the past behavior has changed in intensity so is no longer present or relevant. Frequently, parents who have a number of children will become confused in trying to recall which child did what, how much and when.

Through an intensive review of a wide variety of child behavior questionnaires we arrived at what we felt would be the essential characteristics of an instrument that would be suitable for an untrained rater, yet still include the variety of desired measures. The problem was complicated by the fact that the parents were under stress, were applying for treatment on behalf of their child and not for participation in a research project. Therefore we wanted to avoid, at all costs, making the application procedure any more complex and arduous than necessary. Even the most innocuous of questionnaires can be very threatening to some people. We reviewed a wide variety of questionnaires, some of which we had considered either using or adapting to our particular needs. A number of our colleagues tried them with their families. Through their comments we obtained further insight into what would be needed for the untrained respondent. Many of the questionnaires review needed a professional rater. The language was too technical and the behavior was inferential rather than observable. For example, feeling states in children rather than measurable frequency of behavior were concentrated on. Many of the questions required remote memory for past events rather than recent recall of present observable behavior. Some were found to have a combination of styles and were inconsistant from section to section, thereby making it necessary for the rater to constantly readjust to new directions. For example, some questionnaires would move from a five point rating scale to muptile choice questions, to a true-false format, and finally to a sentence completion type test. It seemed to us that a complex format would increase the rater's resistance and his margin of error due to distraction and confusion. In other instances, there were so many questions and the pages were so crowded that the task looked formidable and the rater would become discouraged before he even began. Furthermore, some questionnaires used a contingent item format and rating became a real test of direction following intelligence. For example, there is nothing more aggravating when completing a form than to be confronted with something like the following: "If you answered question 18 on page 2 yes do not answer questions 27-39, but move on to questions 40-69, omitting questions 48-53." Although these directions were not taken from any specific questionnaire, they are about as lucid as some of the directions seen in our review of the literature.

We were faced with the problem of screening children for the services that our particular program had to offer. Therefore, we selected a variety of commonly accepted dimensions which connote emotional disturbance in children, such as aggression, depression, withdrawal and learning disturbances. We then translated these into simple, unambiguous language which was readily understandable by the untrained rater. In addition, we had to find a method for determining the intensity of the child's behavior —whether this behavior occurred constantly or only in isolated incidences. The parent, for instance, might become very upset over a child's occasional rebellion or untidiness, yet discount his accident-proneness or peer withdrawal. We had to provide the items which would represent real emotional disturbance and structure them in such fashion as to obtain an actual picture of the intensity of the problems. The intensity of the problems could be more objectively assessed by asking the parents how frequently the pertinent behaviors appeared. Asking general questions requiring yes or no answers provides no graded measure, other than to say that the child has or has not done something. To force parents into making a yes or no subjective and arbitrary statement can either cause them to exaggerate or deny the problems. On the other hand, when we provide them with the opportunity to report the frequency of observable behavior on a five point scale, they can more nearly approach an accurate statement.

Our behavioral items are rated on a five point scale, "never," "almost never," "occasionally," "often," "constantly," and always deal with the child's present behavior. In addition to reducing the vagaries of memory, an advantage in using only present behavior makes it possible for the questionnaire to be repeatedly administered at specific points in time. Therapy progress, lack of it, regression, problems or new strengths can all be measured by comparison of consecutive questionnaire ratings.

Only one parent is requested to fill out the questionnaire as part of the application procedure. We have followed the procedure of sending only one questionnaire, feeling that parents will tend to consult with each other. More recently, we have wanted to examine how the individual parent separately sees the youngster. Therefore, we have started asking both parents to complete a questionnaire. This is done in a controlled situation where they are unable to consult with one another. On the day of the child's diagnostic evaluation at the clinic the parents are assigned separate rooms in which to rate the questionnaire. The foregoing illustrates a research problem—a need to obtain independent measures of the same child's behavior. If parents can consult with each other, then one or more contaminating circumstances can occur:

one parent can refuse to participate, the more forceful parent may insist that the questions shall be answered as he sees the child, and parents may consult with and rely on the observations of some other unspecified person. When we have obtained independent ratings of the same child's behavior, and these measures are in near agreement with each other, only then can we be confident that the ratings are both objective and accurate measures of the child's actual behavior. If the parents are not in agreement on certain items, then we are in a position to examine whether one parent is too threatened to expose his feelings, tends to exaggerate, or shows undue anxiety concerning particular areas of behavior. Many parents of emotionally disturbed children feel most vulnerable. They may have great feelings of inadequacy and guilt, because they feel they have failed as parents, a supposedly natural or instinctual occupation. They are often quite startled when it is pointed out to them that they are formally schooled or trained for almost every facet of their lives except for one of the most important, that of being a parent. This is left to intuition, instinct and experience. In addition, many of the parents have had difficult childhoods and their experiences have therefore been more of a hindrance than a help.

The questionnaire is completed a third time just prior to the interpretive interview. (This is the interview in which the professional staff summarize for the parents the results of the diagnostic evaluation and make recommendations for a treatment plan.) Our staff can examine changes in the ratings and measure the extent of spontaneous behavior changes before a formal therapy program is instituted.

Once a therapy program is initiated, questionnaires are simultaneously and individually completed every three months by parents, therapists, teachers and child care staff. Upon discharge from the program, the questionnaire is completed at six-month intervals for a period of two years by parents or parent substitutes and teachers.

The frequency of the data collection and the number of different persons filling out a questionnaire at a given period of time can be dependent on the purposes of the program. For our purposes, the number of questionnaires collected for each child is large. We are attempting not only to obtain measures of change in a child over a period of time but also to develop and standardize a questionnaire. The standardization of a questionnaire requires obtaining measures of agreement between different raters from all representative areas of the child's life. In addition, we are also interested in fully assessing the behavior of each child in a variety of life situations and the behavioral changes in each.

The large amount of information on a questionnaire must be reduced into a usable and efficient summary. There are various methods of combining the ratings from the many items. In our case, the total items on each questionnaire number 105; although all items are scored, these scores can be then combined into eighteen summary measures. Three methods that can be employed to combine large amounts of ratings into manageable scales involve grouping the items (1) by an examination of their content (wording), (2) by their power to distinguish between personality types, or (3) by computer.

The content method merely requires several clinicians to agree on groups of items that in their judgment measure the same thing. For example, they might group together all items they felt measure physical aggression. Other groupings (scales) might be verbal aggression, depression, withdrawal and learning disturbance. A child's score on any one of these scales is merely the sum of the ratings of the individual items making up the scale. Then each scale is validated using independent measures of the same personality trait. For instance, scores on the physical aggression scale can be checked against observations of the frequency of attacking behavior during school.

The second method of developing behavior scales essentially involves selecting a group of items which are best able to identify children who are characterized by some common trait. To illustrate, all items in the questionnaire that are usually given high ratings for physically aggressive children are combined into a scale. This scale is then checked for its power to distinguish a new group of aggressive children for a group of normal children. Items are retained which are still able to distinguish in this new group the presence or absence of the personality trait.

Factor analysis is a third method of developing behavior scales and requires the service of a computer. The computer makes it possible to discover the clusters into which related the behavioral items on a questionnaire can be classified or grouped. In our case, the computer grouped the items on our questionnaire into eighteen clusters (factors) of items. From an examination of the wording of the items in each factor we were able to assign such names to them as psychopathy, verbal self attack, school phobia, and regressive withdrawal. A child's score on a particular factor is roughly the sum of its component item ratings with some items given more weight or importance than others. In our study each child received eighteen scores, one for each factor.

The content method of scale construction is both easy and inexpensive. However, since items are selected on the basis of their content, what they measure tends to be obvious to the rater. For example, an anxiety scale might be composed of items such as "I am a worrier." If the rater has reason to be defensive in his answers, the scores may not objectively reflect the person's actual behavior. Therefore, the content method of scale construction is probably best confined to questionnaires rated by professional staff who, through their training and experience with a variety of children, can be more objective than parents.

The second and third methods of scale construction rely on mathematical procedures for selecting items without regard to content. Therefore, the untrained rater may be wholly unaware of what an item measures. The questionnaire can then become less threatening. The second method is less expensive than the third (factor analytic technique) and seems to us preferable when the questionnaire has been constructed to measure specific types of problem behavior. Factor analysis, on the other hand, seems the preferred method if the researcher is interested in discovering the less obvious or otherwise hidden dimensions inherent in his particular questionnaire.

Research is greatly needed to help improve both our methods of recognizing emotional disturbance in children and our methods of treatment. Although there are many excellent research questionnaires, there is still the need for improvement and new methods. For example, questionnaires measuring family interaction have yet to be developed. Some agencies will need questionnaires suited to their unique purposes.

The foregoing has been a brief digest of some of the problems we encountered in attempting to measure emotionally disturbed behavior in children.

Chapter 6

DRUG ABUSE AND MODERN YOUTH: A PSYCHO-SOCIAL VIEWPOINT

JAMES L. MATHIS, M.D.

Revised version of "Psycho-Social Aspects of Drug Abuse by Modern Youth," published in *Medical College of Virginia Quarterly*, 6:187, 1970.

All human behavior is so complexly determined that the type of scientific research which leads to simplified cause-and-effect answers is virtually impossible. Certainly that is true of behavior which involves an interacting combination of social and psychological factors such as is seen in drug abuse by modern youth. Most observers agree that drug abuse by youth has become a major problem, but differences immediately arise when the varied sociological, psychological, and even ecological factors of etiology are discussed. The many concepts of causation become more or less the products of the individual observer's past experience, present orientation, and future expectations and, therefore, they rarely are subject to cross-validation.

The more one learns about the problems, the more obvious it becomes that an open and skeptical approach is necessary. A single-minded, dogmatic view may lead to oversimplification and to corrective moves which are doomed to failure and which may even further compound the situation. We have already seen that the over-hasty response of more stringent legal and punitive measures made by many of our communities not only has failed but has led to further alienation of those whom we wish to protect.

The problem itself is far from being well defined. One can debate whether or not drug abuse is a distinct illness, a symptom of an illness, or even a relatively normal response to a complex and changing social situation. The adolescent drug abuser might disagree with all of these possibilities and see it as normal and logical behavior.

When does drug use become drug abuse? The average adult answer, by and large, differs markedly from that of the average adolescent. A high school student who smokes marijuana only on Saturday night or at special parties does not classify himself as a drug abuser, but even he might so term an acquaintance who used the drug three or more times a week or who used narcotics at any time.

Despite this apparent confusion, there appear to be some areas of general agreement. It is obvious that the per capita number of youthful drug users has risen markedly in the past decade. Drug use is seen at earlier and earlier ages, and there has been a change in the socioeconomic status of narcotic users. For example, heroin use among middle-class teenagers was quite uncommon four years ago and it was an extreme rarity five years ago. It is now estimated that from 1 to 2 percent of college students on the Northeastern seaboard have used heroin to some extent, and that the number of high school users from middle-class families is continuing to rise. The major concern of those of us working in the drug field was at the college level in 1964; by 1967 it had become a problem in high schools, and today it is increasingly noted at junior high and grammar school ages. Parenthetically, the increase in the abuse of mood-altering drugs by the young people has been paralleled by a rise in the suicide rate of adolescents in the last decade.[1] Drugs were the major cause of adolescent death in New York City in 1969.

Let us examine some of the phenomena that may be operative in the behavior and attitudes of today's youth and relate them to drug use and abuse. Specificity and completeness are patently impossible and not only may each factor be debated but also may bring to mind others of equal importance. Let us begin this examination with a look at some of the variables which may have influenced the basic concepts and attitudes of the modern young person.

Television is an ubiquitous form of sensory input which must have far-reaching effects upon development which are still largely hypothetical. It has been estimated that the average sixteen-year-old has spent about 20 percent of his waking life watching television, and that the figure is over 50 percent for the child over age six. This readily makes it quantitatively the greatest single influence impinging upon the developing central nervous system throughout those most crucial years. It is doubtful that parents, school, or any other person, thing or agency can claim to have been in direct contact with the youth for this amount of time. This influence begins virtually at birth, and it may be capable of programing the individual nervous system with attitudes, values and expectations which form the base of all future learning and behavior. (In the early years a child can learn a complex language perfectly with little conscious effort. This is no longer true after six years of age.)

Lorenz and others have shown that imprinting occurs in lower animals at a very early age, and that these early experiences influence future self-concept and behavior in an irreversible manner.[2] This concept cannot be translated directly over to human behavior, but there is some evidence that a similar phenomenon occus in man spread over a longer period of time and perhaps somewhat less definite. For example, it has been shown that the basic concept of gender identity, the knowledge of being male or female, is fixed before three years of age, and that a change rarely can be produced after this time even when the genitalia contradict the assigned gender.[3] This unfortunate circumstance occurs more frequently than is generally known. Also, there are basic personality disorders which appear to be products of the early years and which resist our efforts to change them. It seems probable that many other attitudes toward and ways of approaching life may be equally indelible and even more fundamental to the total behavioral pattern.

Television may imprint the developing child with the concept that pleasure and gratification of his senses can occur instantaneously without his active involvement or expenditure of energy. The development of the basic sense of reality testing may be delayed because the possible and the impossible are not sharply defined in the world of television. There are no reality limits to this world of fantasy, and magic beginnings and endings become an accepted part of living. The machine is turned on, and ergo, one lives with an ever-available and inexhaustible Aladdin's lamp. It may be more than accidental that the drug culture has adopted the phrase "turn on" as indictive of an approach to life which includes gratification without effort or responsibility. "Tuning out" is another phrase adopted from this modality by the drug culture to indicate a voluntarily controlled escape from reality living. We cannot dismiss lightly the possibility that one of the earliest, the deepest, and the most indelible concepts imprinted upon the mind of today's youth is that of the ease and the desirability of escape from reality through instantaneous and passive sensory gratification.

Television also furnishes the child with an unlimited and ever-changing supply of identification figures and role models which are far more tangible and believable than those found in a book or developed from fantasy. These identification figures may become parent substitutes, and the incorporation of them and their unreal or deviate characteristics undoubtedly produces a major effect upon the development of basic ideals, self-identity, and value systems.

Present-day youth, reared as they were in a television-dominated civilization, also have grown up in a nuclear family in which there was a decreasing ability to escape the intensity of the family triangle. Industrialization, urbanization, and geographic mobility have all but destroyed the extended family of the past. There was a time when the geographic proximity of grandparents, uncles, aunts, and cousins furnished an ever-present safety valve for the condensed tensions of a nuclear family consisting only of parents and children. This extended family furnished innumerable role models for the growing individual, and it was a microcosmic world in which to experiment with growing up, and from which one obtained the basic patterns of culture. The television world in the first few years, then later the peer group and the school system with its teachers, counsellors and social workers have become inadequate and perhaps sometimes even detrimental replacements for this old extended family. The peer group, always of major significance, has become of more and more importance to the developing child as a source of learning, support, guidance, and as a repository of values and standards.

A generation of unlimited affluence and complex technology

has gone hand in hand with the above forces and social changes. An abundance of material goods and increased bodily comfort are obvious products of affluence, but one of its side effects may be of even more importance in molding the growing child. This side effect is the loss of opportunities for the growing child to achieve mastery. Mastery here refers to the growing child's experience of meeting and overcoming graded frustrations and of achieving desired goals by its own energy and activity. Self-esteem is derived from many sources from birth onward, but this source may be relatively essential to normal maturity. The more affluent the society, the less the opportunity exists for constructive mastery on the part of the young. Not only are the opportunities simply not so available, but society will, in fact, actively discourage attempts at mastery when they conflict with that which passes for progress, advancement and social status. There is virtually no constructive role for the young person to play in an affluent and crowded society which literally does not need people. There always appears to be an easier and more efficient way of doing things. For example, one junior league baseball team met one Saturday morning in early spring to clear a field of weeds with hand blade and sickle. This was vetoed by the adult leaders who quickly and efficiently cleared the field with power mowers. This well-intended and apparently thoughtful gesture denied the children an opportunity to master a task of great relevance to them and to achieve a step upward toward self-growth.

"Relevancy," a much overused word for the past few years, must not be dismissed lightly. Whether or not an action is relevant to the individual may determine its value as a growth-promoting factor. An event or action which contributes fundamentally to the welfare of the family, the social group, or the individual is worth far more than one contrived by well-meaning adults to furnish the youngsters with an activity simply designed to keep them out of trouble. Many of the activities of youth in an affluent and urbanized society are either contrived, pointless, or totally hedonistic. Not only do they rarely contribute to the welfare of the social unit, but they usually are obviously an added expense and burden and/or they furnish vicarious pleasure for the adults involved and are therefore self-defeating at the best and harmful at the worst.

Now let us combine these observations and theories with some aspects of "normal" youth. Peter Blos, in his book *On Adolescence* states that the period from puberty to adulthood primarily is the time for experimentation and trial which leads either to a mature resolution of childhood conflicts or to some form of compromise which ranges from a mild behavioral disorder to a complete disaster.[4] He elaborates upon the heights of creativity and imagination which the adolescent may reach during these vital years. He foresees a permissive and totally unstructured adolescence as producing adults of almost unlimited potential for creative thought and imaginative living. He contrasts this with harshly limited and controlled adolescence which produces an adult characterized by rigidity, inflexibility, a lack of imagination and creativity, in other words, one whose need to conform to authority makes us uncomfortable to contemplate. It sounds, therefore, as if a totally permissive adolescent period is very desirable unless one wishes to crush and wrap those traits which symbolize progress and advancement of human interactions. There is, as one might well expect, a catch to this otherwise obvious choice. It appears that there is a price to pay for the totally permissive and unstructured situation, and that price is a certain casualty rate among the young experimenters. A total lack of reasonable structure and flexible protective limits produces a high-risk high-gain situation in which many of the young people simply will not survive into adulthood unscathed. Their wounds will be largely psychological in nature and frequently manifested by antisocial behavior. Our generation may be witnessing a massive sociological testing of this hypothesis by Blos.

Eugene Pumpian-Mindlin adds to this the concept of omnipotentiality which he describes as a normal characteristic of adolescence.[5] This refers to a boundless feeling of invulnerability, invincibility and power not dulled or contradicted by conflicting reality. Combine this idea with the concept of Blos and you have a situation in which boundless energy, creativity and imagination are urged onward by a sense of power and invulnerability which does not recognize reality limits or time boundaries. All things are possible and future consequences or present behavior simply do not exist, or they must by definition exist only for others. This should tell us something about the value of danger, threat, and punishment as deterrants to adolescent behavior!

The concepts of these great students of human behavior imply that the adolescent tends to ignore and deny reality factors when they conflict with his fantasies and/or his desire for the pleasure principle, and that he tends to depend more upon his own private interpretation of a situation. The process of maturing necessitates some degree of structure and guidance, thoroughly flexible, to prevent damage and/or deviance in development. Unfortunately, the post World War II years have seen a rapid decline in parental guidance and acceptance of responsibility. By and large, the youth of today have been left free to explore, to experiment, to act without constructive discipline and regulation. The old standards and values were dethroned long before heirs were chosen to take their places. Society approached, or perhaps has reached, a state of anomie; a state in which normative standards of conduct and belief are either weak or lacking. Durkheim spoke of anomie in the individual as being a lack of society's influence on the basic passions, therefore leaving the individual without a checkrein on his behavior.[6] He felt that this was a major factor in much self-destructive behavior. The phrase so commonly heard, "doing one's thing," may be a concept which stems from a positive value upon and a desire for individual freedom, but more frequently it may be an anomic concept derived from the lack of social and cultural guidelines which give one a sense of belonging. Certainly this latter concept appears to be more accurate when "doing one's thing" refers to behavior which is destructive either to the individual or to his society.

We have examined some of the factors influencing the developing child, and we have attempted to combine them with some basic concepts of adolescence. Now let us examine how these psychological influences and social contingencies may interact with some reality factors of today.

We live in a culture which places great value upon the alleviation of discomfort and anxiety by external means. Madison Avenue has capitalized upon this trend and has flooded the media with encouragements to take compose® for tension, Sominex® for insomnia, No-Dose® to awaken the next morning, and Alka-Seltzer® for discomfort caused by the other medications. Millions of dollars worth of tranquilizers are sold annually, and our most financially rewarded citizens are those who amuse us in the entertainment world.

The youngster, with a nervous system which was attuned from birth to the reception of television messages, has incorporated both the desirability of and the means of escape from discomfort into his basic concept of living. He learned so well to alleviate anxiety by oral means that he discovered new and more effective ways, and he improved upon the adult example by developing his own brand of tranquilizers and stimulants. One of his major methods of tranquilization, marijuana, has been known almost throughout recorded history as a drug highly effective pharmacologically. Our young people quickly became aware of this, but they also discovered an extremely important side effect was that the use of this drug increased the anxiety and tensions of the adult world while it decreased that of the user. The user simultaneously thoroughly agitates his parents and other representatives of authority while becoming the central focus of society and its communication media. Herein are all the needed ingredients for positive reinforcement of behavior and therefore assurance of its continuation.

The adolescent not only is able to defend his position on drug use with strength derived from adult examples, he simultaneously cannot develop the type of world perspective common to his elders. There are many factors operative here, but one is that today's youth are part of the first generation to see history unfold before them as it occurs. Past generations learned of the major events of civilization after they had been embellished and distorted so as to obscure motives and to rationalize behavior. Good and bad were divided into definite camps in which the hero always won and the stranger was the villain. This can no longer be done to those who have a ringside seat to history on the television screen. All the frailties of adulthood and its world are laid bare so as to destroy the idealized images and fantasies of childhood and to leave no God in their place.

There have been other perfectly realistic factors new to this generation which have crashed in upon the young person so as to disenchant him with adult values and goals. The word "ecology," new to most of us, has erupted into importance. Concepts barely thought of a few years ago, environmental pollution, population explosion, a raped planet, all have become common knowledge to this generation. These concepts, rapidly becoming axiomatic, were not invented by the youth, but they were quick to realize their validity and to look with a degree of just accusation and mistrust at an adult world which had left them this heritage.

It would appear that the markedly increased use of chemical measures, either as a negative escape from reality or as a positive flight to the pleasure principle, is understandable if these hypotheses are accepted. This by no means indicates that it is desirable unless one wishes to assume a completely hopeless stance. On the coutrary, survival in the future and the correction of these ecological "sins" undoubtedly will require a degree of maturity and stability greater than ever before. This maturity requires the process of adolescence with its mastery of anxiety-provoking situations, its search for a role in life, the amalgamation of sexual identity, and all of the attendant pain and discomforts. This period of life is one of emotional lability and transition during which the teenager must come to grips with conflicts and confusions which, by their solution, will solidify his self-identity and his future social role. This means that at no other period of life is a brain-disorganizing drug more contraindicated. It is doubly dangerous if that drug presents an artificial solution to problems and allows an indefinite postponement of this essential process so that mature adjustment keeps receding into the future. It appears neither logical nor profitable to encourage an escape from this process or maturation.

Neither does it appear logical to fight an enemy whom one does not understand and cannot readily identify—an enemy with all the cards in his favor. This is as illogical as it is for a physician to treat only the symptoms of illness. If we are raising a group of sick youngsters, which is doubtful, then we must assume that the contagious carrier is society and that drug abuse is only a symptom. If it is not true that we have a generation of sick youth on our hands, then it is possible that their behavior may represent a relatively rational response of preprogrammed minds to social and environmental changes of cataclysmic proportions. If that is so, again our attention must focus upon our social structure and patterns of living. There is a need for those who treat the individual youngster in trouble with drugs, just as many of us treated the polio victims of the early 1950s, but just as with polio, we must keep in mind that the ultimate goal is the understanding of and therefore the control of the pathogenic process.

REFERENCES

1. Ross, M.: Suicide among college students. *Am. J. Phychiatry, 126*: 106, 1969.
2. Lorenz, K.: *King Solomon's Ring: New Light on Animal Ways.* New York, Thomas Crowell, 1952.
3. Money, J., Hampson, J., and Hampson, J.: Imprinting and the establishment of gender role. *Arch. Neurol.* 77:333, 1957.
4. Blos, P.: *On Adolescence.* New York, Free Press, 1962.
5. Pumpian-Mindlin, E.: Omnipotentiality, youth and commitment. *J. Am. Acad. Child Psychiatry, 4*:18, 1965.
6. Durkheim, E.: *Suicide.* (Translated by Spalding, J. and Simpson, G.) Glencoe, Free Press, 1951.

Chapter 7

PEOPLE WHO CHOOSE TO DIE

Herbert Waltzer, M.D.

Suicide, the act of conscious and willful self-destruction, has been an enigma that has befuddled and perplexed philosophers, sociologists, and physicians, particularly psychiatrists. In recent years there has been an attempt made to distinguish the attempters from the successful doers. Individuals who were successful in destroying themselves were felt to be a different breed, have a different personality structure, and different conscious and unconscious psychodynamic motivations as compared to those who make gestures, overtures, or aborted attempts. A distinction was thus being made on the basis of the end result. This loses sight of the fact that there are accidental suicides, e.g. where the individual really never intended his death, and conversely, accidental survivals, e.g. where death was seriously intended but was averted by chance, luck, or unforseen circumstances. The girl who takes six aspirins to scare and manipulate her mother or boyfriend and has a paradoxical reaction and dies, or the man who jumps from the fifth story of a building and survives the fall are examples of accidental death and survival.

At best, after a successful suicide one can only speculate, in the form of a "psychological autopsy," a retrospective analysis, using all the available history and data about the person to explain the precipitating stresses and other psychological factors. Such material as suicide notes and interviews with relatives and friends help reconstruct events and give rationality to, at times, seemingly irrational acts. Often, in spite of all efforts, no explanations are forthcoming.

Every human being, at one time or another, has felt the urge to end his life or has wished that it was over. This represents a normal reaction or response to stress; be it the loss of someone dear and close, the loss of one's self-esteem after losing face or failing at something. Some individuals cannot tolerate even minimum failure, an important and necessary maturation ingredient of every human being's life. Most of us, through rational and logical thought processes, are able to place the event in the proper perspective and go on.

About 50,000 of our fellow citizens do not wish to go on and destroy themselves annually in response to either an external stressful event or in response to a severe internal conflict.

About another 100,000 make some attempts or gestures at ending their lives. In 1962 the United States Office of Vital Statistics reported 20,890 deaths resulting from suicide. Suicidologists, those who study the subject of suicide, readily concede that the statistics are wholly unreliable and grossly underreported. In some areas of the country there is a marked reluctance to label the cause of death as suicide. Some communities require the presence of a suicide note before the death is so labeled. The social, moral, and religious stigma associated with suicide frequently serves as a deterrent to the family, the coroner, or doctor from reporting it as such. Furthermore, many suicides are disguised as accidents. Not infrequently, the death is classified under a different heading if it results only indirectly from the suicidal attempt, such as in the case of bronchopneumonia secondary to barbiturate poisoning. Another reason for trying to cover up a suicide is the reality that life insurance claims are not paid when it is declared as the cause of death.

It has been estimated that about every three minutes a completed, successful suicidal act occurs in this country, and for every suicide at least eight unsuccessful attempts have taken place during this period.

PERSONS WHO SUCCEED

As stated previously, the potential for self-destruction resides in all of us. However, studies have shown that certain individuals have a greater propensity for suicide or are considered higher risks. Whereas younger people, particularly female, make abortive suicide attempts, older people are most likely to succeed. This is particularly true of the older male, who may be isolated and alone, in poor health, and with few emotional or economic resources to handle these stresses. The impetus towards self-destruction is particularly great in the surviving partner of an old married couple. This is especially true when there has been an extreme degree of dependency of the survivor on the one who died. The absence of other meaningful relationships, goals, family ties, or interests frequently causes profound depression, apathy, and suicidal preoccupations. This occurs often after mandatory retirement from gainful employment. We are a youth-oriented society and encourage the elderly to collect themselves in retirement villages, nursing homes, and so on. They make us anxious and aware of the aging process, which we fear. We don't like it, and so we put them out of sight. It is our way of saying "Disappear." Our society is unconsciously encouraging the dependent elderly to commit suicide and thus relieve us of the responsibility for their care.

The risks of suicide are greatest in individuals who have a repeated history of having made suicide attempts. They are particularly strong in individuals who suffer from severe alcoholism, and the act is frequently carried out under the uninhibited state of either partial or total intoxication. Narcotic addicts and persons who use drugs in a very dependent and abusive fashion have a strong potential towards self-destruction. The incidence of suicide is high where there is a history of suicide in the family. The individual who has obsessive thoughts about dying carries a greater hazard than the person with occasional transitory thoughts. The incidence of suicide is somewhat higher in people with a history of having psychiatric treatment or hospitalization previously. This is particularly true where feelings of alienation from oneself and external reality are pronounced.

It has been said that persons with strong religious ties are less likely to carry out suicide. This no longer appears to be true, with the possible exception of Roman Catholics, since ties to religious institutions and teachings have become appreciably weakened in our society.

At one time suicide among the black was considered rare, and homicide occurred about ten times as frequently. The homicide rate continues to be high but, interestingly, a significant rise in the suicide rate has been noted. This is particularly true of the young black male who grew up in a disorganized and deprived home, in which the father was absent and the mother was the major dominating force. There usually have been frequent uprootings and shifts in the care of this person when he was small.

Among American Indian tribes, particularly those confined to the reservation, cultural deterioration has taken place. There is a high rate of alcoholism and an exceptionally high incidence of violent injuries, which include suicide, homicide, and accidents. These findings were observed in a study of the Cheyenne Indians.

Successful suicides have occurred in epidemic proportions, particularly when an important figure died suddenly and unexpectedly. Many suicides were reported after the death of Marilyn Monroe and John F. Kennedy. In psychiatric parlance, an over-identification with that famous person took place. There was a rash of drug overdoses and successful suicides by young women, between the age of 17 and 25, after Marilyn Monroe's death by overdose.

In the past, it was in keeping with the Japanese culture for an individual, and expected of him, to commit hara-kiri in order to "save face." This is no longer acceptable by the Japanese.

Self-immolation, or self-burning, has occurred with increasing frequency. It represented a form of self-sacrifice that was carried out by Buddhist monks in the Far East in an attempt to express their anger at some institutional or social injustices. The practice spread to other countries and we have seen it occur in the United States. How a person chooses to destroy himself is dependent on three factors: what he or she has available as instruments of death, methods suggested by others or read about, and the specific unconscious meaning of the particular act or method.

Some individuals cannot kill themselves directly, but achieve their own self-destruction through provoking others to destroy them. There have been several instances where a husband, during a fight, hands his wife a knife and then prods her, through constant needling and insults, to use it. One husband told his wife, "You don't have the guts to stab me, you whore." She did.

Recovery from an illness may upset an equilibrium that the

individual had established with those close to him. Several cases have been reported where individuals who were blind committed suicide after the blindness was removed. In these instances, the patient had received care, attention and love while relatively blind and now felt abandoned, since with recovered vision he was expected to be independent. Similar reports have been written in relation to individuals who have had their hearing restored. These cases represent the unusual response to recovery from a prolonged impairment or disability.

CONSCIOUS VERSUS UNCONSCIOUS SUICIDE

When we speak of a suicidal patient, we are talking of an individual who directly expresses self-destructive thoughts or wishes or who knowingly and consciously attempts to destroy himself. In contrast, there are vast numbers of people who are grossly unaware of their self-destructive behavior or will deny its existence when it has been clearly demonstrated. Think of the person who drinks excessively, is warned not to drive his car, and then drives it at excessive speeds. Then there is the individual who has suffered a severe coronary and is put on absolute bed rest and walks about and is physically overactive, or the patient who stops his kidney dialysis treatments.

What about the individual who makes it a hobby to flirt with death! There are such sports as parachute jumping, speed car racing, mountain climbing, aerial acrobatics, and so on. We read in the newspapers about Russian roulette. If interviewed, these individuals would categorically deny any self-destructive urges or impulses. They would speak of the feeling of jubilation or exhiliration at succeeding. The measure of success is the ability to avoid death. It gives the individual the feeling of power or control over his own life. Characteristically, they minimize the gamble involved, in which their lives represent the stakes. With it is frequently the feeling of invulnerability to death. It is as though the individual is trying to demonstrate over and over again to himself his indestructability and immortality. If we were to sit and think or dwell on our own demise, it would almost invariably create feelings of uneasiness or dread, if not outright anxiety or panic, which might then have a paralyzing effect on our capacity to function.

Some people kill themselves as an exercise of their own power to control the time, place and method of their demise. The prospect of growing old, with its concomitant diminished physical capacity for activity, excitement and pleasure, is what drove Ernest Hemingway to take his life. Many people fear, dread, and equate the aging process with pain, suffering, and aloneness. Which is it going to be—a stroke, a heart attack, or cancer?

Characteristic of the suicidal person is the presence of what we call ambivalence. It is the simultaneous unconscious wish to live and to die. In studies of many hundreds of attempts at suicide, it has been demonstrated that whenever a reasonably detailed account of the individual's behavior is available, there is evidence of the fantasy of rescue. The "cry for help" is frequently expressed directly and in verbal form. The communication for help or rescue may take the form of a note, a farewell letter, the sudden writing of a will, the working out of a suicidal plan, or the actual suicidal gesture or attempt.

The response to the communication by the family or the physician frequently will determine the outcome of that crisis. A major fallacy that exists in the minds of most people, including physicians, is that people who talk about suicide do not carry it out. Other misconceptions pertaining to suicide are the following:

1. Suicide happens without advance warning, either verbal or behavioral.
2. All suicidal individuals are mentally ill or psychotic.
3. Suicidal individuals are fully intent upon dying.
4. Once a person is suicidal, he is suicidal forever.
5. Motives or causes of suicide are easily established.
6. A person who is very ill, even in a terminal state, is not likely to commit suicide.
7. Improvement following a suicidal crisis means that the crisis is over.

As stated previously, there is a need within us, also within the physician, to deny and to minimize the potential for self-destruction in family members, friends, and patients. It evokes too much anxiety in us. Most of us are identified with religious or philosophical systems or beliefs which assert that there is really no such thing as death, but only a transition from one form of existence to another. There is a tendency to divert the discussion away from death to another topic, when in actuality it is best to let the person discuss the suicidal feelings, the feelings of depression and aloneness, or the feelings of estrangement. By discussing these frightening themes the individual in crisis feels that you have some grasp as to the depth of the struggle going on within as to whether "to live or to die."

SUICIDE PREVENTION SERVICES

It became apparent to many that the response by friends, family members, clergy and physicians to the suicidal communication was frequently inappropriate or inadequate. The result was the establishment, over the past fifteen years, of about sixty Suicide Prevention Centers throughout the country. An important part of these services is the existence of a telephone number which the suicidal person can call when overwhelmed with suicidal thoughts, ideas, or impulses.

One must be fully aware that an individual who has determined to destroy himself will do so, and nothing can be done to prevent it. Individuals have been known to destroy themselves in closed psychiatric wards as well as in maximum security prisons. They will use whatever is available as instruments of death. Fortunately that force, called ambivalence, is usually present and crying out for a rescuer.

The goal of these services is to act as rescuer and to avert the carrying out of the suicidal act. It is felt, and rightfully so, that if the person can be helped over the crisis period, an unnecessary death can be avoided. At times, the most appropriate place to render the care is on a closed psychiatric ward. Often the individual responds with tremendous relief when he is in a setting which hinders his potential to yield to these impulses. Very depressed and almost mute suicidal patients frequently require a course of about ten electroconvulsive treatments. The subsequent changes noted in thoughts and functioning are remarkable.

THE RIGHT TO SUICIDE

There are many people who are of the persuasion that an individual has the right to commit suicide and that intervention is inappropriate. This argument has been set forth by some outstanding lawyers and psychiatrists. There are instances in which suicide can be viewed as reasonable, understandable, and perhaps justifiable. One can readily understand suicide as a choice in prisoners-of-war about to undergo torture and in patients suffering from intractable pain, resulting from terminal cancer. However, the vast majority of attempters are responding to a stress, are in crisis, and are limited in their capacity, because of their distorted perspective, to find alternate methods of coping with life. Should we ignore their ambivalence or their cries for help and assume that this final and irreversible act was the product of a well-thought-out and rational approach to a specific problem? The answer must be no.

Euthanasia, or letting someone in great suffering die, is another issue that has stirred much debate in the medical community. In essence, the physician must then determine whom he wishes to save and whom he wishes to let die. In a sense, it is now being done, however, on an unconscious level. The physician who chooses to devote his precious time and energies to the young man who has severe pneumonia in favor of the very old man who is in coma after a stroke might be practicing euthanasia without ever knowing it. The formalization of the practice of euthanasia is a frightening concept. Can one visualize a medical conference in which the doctors determine whom they will try to help and whom they will let die? What of the possibility of a misdiagnosis or the imminence of a specific cure?

As the population grows, the worth of the individual shrinks. Wars make life seem very cheap. A dead young man becomes a number, a statistic. The preservation of life is a reasonable goal, lest we, as physicians, take on the god-like role of determining who is to live and who is to die.

ADDITIONAL THOUGHTS

The United States is a violent nation. The number (750,000) of Americans in the U.S.A. killed by guns over the past sixty-seven years exceeds the number (550,000) of Americans killed in all wars—from the Revolution to Viet Nam—that this country has ever fought. Yet this tool for destruction is easily accessible to individuals with strong homicidal or suicidal potential. This nation seems powerless or uninterested in introducing stricter gun control measures.

Unfortunately, there are individuals who choose to take the lives of others in addition to their own. This is the combination of homicide and suicide and is quite often seen in lovers and in families. Not infrequently one reads of the mother who kills her child and then herself. Another example is the person who drives his car deliberately head-on into another car. The Japanese pilots in World War II, the kamikaze, directed their planes to crash into American warships. These are the altruistic deaths, where the individual is making a sacrifice for a greater cause.

What about the kidney donor? Is he enhancing the dangers to his own survival in order to give another a chance to live?

Many people associate living with pain, turbulence, anxiety and suffering whereas they view death with calm, peace, and tranquility. The emotional struggle consists of making a choice. Unfortunately, many in our society choose the latter.

Chapter 8

SUICIDE, CULTURE AND RELIGION

ROBERT L. GARRARD, M.D., AND GERTRUDE P. GARRARD, M.D.

INTRODUCTION

Suicide has been a controversial topic since ancient times. Religious and philosophical debates have occupied the minds of thoughtful men, conclusions were made and later discarded. Research has provided some answers to the problem of suicide, but at the same time has posed new questions. For example, does a man have the right to dispose of his life as he wishes? Is a physician ever justified in his decision to withhold vigorous treatment and heroic measures to prolong a life of hopeless suffering? Is there any justification for mercy killing or euthanasia? When is suicide justified? Shakespeare entered the discussion when Hamlet asks, "whether 'tis nobler in the mind to suffer the slings and arrows of outrageous fortune". Is suicide a manifestation of courage or cowardice? Or is it simply madness? Where does religion enter in? Is suicide a sin?

Answers are not readily available. Various explanations can be found, and throughout this chapter efforts will be directed toward giving some of the background in suicide investigations in the hope that greater knowledge and understanding of this vastly complex problem will provide some answers.

In the United States about 25,000 suicides are reported each year. Probably two to three times that number actually occur, although these statistics cannot be confirmed. Many equivocal cases are reported as "accidental deaths" when they were really suicidal deaths. Some times, in order to protect families significant information is withheld, and a suicide may be reported as an accidental death or even a natural death. Also, some suicidal

111

deaths are delayed or result from complications of the original suicidal act, all of which adds to the confusion. In some areas suicidal deaths cannot be recorded as such if the victim failed to leave a suicide note. Regardless of the statistical evidence, suicide is a major public health problem.

The tragedy of suicide is brought into focus when we observe that it is ranked as the tenth leading cause of death in the United States, and the fourth between the ages of fourteen and forty-five. It ranks third among teen-agers and second among college students. There are three or four times as many suicides as homicides each year. The suicide rate appears to be increasing and clearly we are losing too many people who have contributions to make to the world.

Suicide frequently strikes in unexpected places. Probably no one is immune, and given enough stress almost anyone would be vulnerable. The usual reactions to a suicide are shock, dismay and disbelief, not only among close relatives but among friends, associates and the attending physician. Suicide inevitably produces guilt in the survivors. The physician, who is totally committed to the preservation of life, is faced with the shocking reality of a self-induced death, and he must struggle with his own guilt and sense of failure. He joins the layman in asking, "Where did I fail? Would the results have been different if I had done differently?". There is some consolation in the thought, "Maybe it is best this way. He suffered so much. He wouldn't have wanted to live in such misery." Strangely, the survivor, frequently a spouse, may be held responsible for the suicidal death and be subjected to hostility and anger. Occasionally there is a tendency among relatives to deny the certification of a suicide and to take refuge in the more comforting thought that "it might have been an accident". Punitive attitudes may be markedly reduced in the case of an aged invalid, although regret and guilt may be increased. Public reaction can be especially strong to the suicidal death of a highly respected person, a successful business or professional man, a young mother, or a college student. The tragedy is more obvious in such cases. One physician commented that an unexpected suicide in his practice left him with "a permanent streak of humility".

HISTORY AND CULTURE

Suicide has been with us since the dawn of time. It is mentioned in the Old Testament five times, recording the suicides of Samson, Saul, Abimelich, Ahitophel and Zimri. In marked contrast to the attitude toward suicide in our culture, these deaths did not seem to meet with rejection or criticism, but were accepted as appropriate actions in their particular situations. History indicates, however, that attitudes toward suicide have undergone many changes over the past 2000 years. There was approval and acceptance of suicide by the Stoics of ancient Greece and almost total rejection of it by the early Christian Church. Over the centuries, different societies have responded to suicide by various crude and cruel means.[1] In medieval times, the bodies of suicides were dragged through the streets, hung naked upside down for public view, and impaled on a stake in public places. Although the dead man could no longer be punished, his widow and children were made to suffer. It was early English practice to censure the suicide's family, deny the body burial in church or city cemetery, and confiscate the survivor's property. As a violation of one of the Ten Commandments, suicide has been called a crime against God, a heinous offense, punishable not only in hell, but also in the courts of man.

Suicide has had many cultural implications. Hara-kiri, the most acceptable form of suicide in Japan, was used as atonement for wrongdoing, to achieve an honorable death, or to wrench moral victory from defeat. No stigma was attached to such a suicide—on the contrary, it was considered an honorable and worthy way to die. Similarly, prior to World War I German military men and members of the nobility could avert disgrace by commiting suicide—the so-called *Ehrentod*, and this restored their honor and good name. Traditionally, Hindu widows were expected to leap upon the funeral pyre of their husbands and cremate themselves. Until recent years, in their culture such a self-inflicted death was considered appropriate, and to continue living would be disgraceful. In Eskimo and other folk cultures the aged and infirm were expected to kill themselves to avoid being a liability and a threat to the survival of the tribe. In such cultures society prescribes the action and an individual would not dare to defy long-standing customs.

In our present civilization, suicide[2] varies widely in different parts of the world, depending upon the culture, religion and values of the particular nationalities. Suicide is treated more tolerantly and accepted more readily in the Scandinavian countries and in Japan, in contrast to such countries as Italy, Ireland and Portugal, where there are powerful proscriptions against suicide. In Europe generally, the suicide rate among Protestants is higher than among Catholic and Jews. The Catholic Church is thought to have a marked influence in the low rate of suicide in Italy, Spain, and other strongly Catholic countries, yet Austria, also a strongly Catholic country, has one of the highest suicide rates in the world. Suicide in South America is generally rare, and it is almost unknown among the Moslems, who seem to accept suffering and privation as "the will of Allah".

In most north and central European countries suicide ranks sixth or seventh as a cause of death, while in Norway, Britain and Australia it ranks tenth, similar to the United States and Canada. In Denmark, Sweden, Hungary and Japan the suicide rate is approximately twice that of the United States. Some researchers have suggested that "cradle to the grave" social security systems in Denmark and Sweden may eliminate challenges, reduce ambition and cause frustration which could contribute to suicide. However, Norway, also a highly socialized land, has a much lower rate. Moreover, the high rate in Denmark goes back a century or more, predating the welfare state. Some observers believe that basic personality differences account for these variations. Highly industralized nations, with correspondingly high standards of living and adequate health care, tend to have a higher suicide rate, explained in part on the basis of a longer life span which leads to the increased suicide potential associated with old age.

A very low suicide rate is found in certain tribal societies of Africa. In West Nigeria it has been reported as less than one per 100,000. The starving, ill-housed millions in India and other Asiatic nations cling tenaciously to life. Perhaps their precarious survival makes suicide superfluous, since death by disease or starvation is apt to overtake them before they reach an age when suicide becomes more prevalent. Underdeveloped countries with a high peasant population have stronger family or tribal ties and more stringent social controls, which tend to act as a suicide deterrent. A tightly knit family or social group tends to maintain low suicide rates.

In our country there has been a shocking epidemic of self-destruction among the Cheyenne Indians. Psychiatrists have attributed this to a "cultural dead-end" imposed on a once proud, strong people. The rate was roughly ten times the national average, and while the age range was from fifteen to fifty-five, only two of the fifteen deaths studied were in persons more than thirty-five years old, and seven were aged twenty or younger. More than half the deaths occurred in off-reservation jails in towns where, according to one boy, Indians are regarded as "drunks and bums". Dr. Dizmang states, "These terribly beaten people hold on to a code or pride and self-respect. They are industrious and intelligent people, and if their latent internal resources can be tapped, a culture pattern of self-renewal can replace the present pattern of self-destruction."[3]

In the United States generally, three out of four suicide victims are white males. The Negro suicide rate has always been low, especially among Negro women, but as Negroes migrate to northern industrial centers, the rate among Negro men is beginning to climb. In relatively affluent Britain, there has been a shift toward a higher suicide rate among unskilled classes, and in some parts of Britain these workers now account for the highest rate of all. Suicide in general is a problem of affluent rather than underdeveloped countries, but it cannot be considered the disease of the wealthy only.

The relative constancy of the suicide rate in any country was first observed by Madame deStael (1766-1817) who became interested in the subject and wrote her *Reflexions sur les Suicides*. She noted that the constancy of suicide is a mark of other social indices as well, demonstrated by the fact that the number of divorces in the Canton of Berne and the number of murders in Italy remained more or less unchanged from year to year. Nineteenth century sociologists considered these social phenomena to be subject to "natural law".

CLASSIFICATION

Suicide, by its very nature, defies accurate classification. It is a highly personalized and internalized phenomenon, and it is safe to say that there are almost as many variations as there are individual suicides. However, clinical investigation reveals two basic entities: the *actual suicide* and the *suicide attempt*. Although there is considerable overlap, the successful suicide usually intended to die, and if he lived, it was mainly because he bungled the attempt or was unexpectedly rescued. The suicide attempter usually intended to live and died only if some prearranged rescue plan failed or a normally harmless agent proved unexpectedly lethal. Some serious suicide attempters repeat their effort until they finally achieve the intended fatality. Chronic attempters occasionally change their pattern of nonlethal, dramatic methods to lethal ones. This occurs in some immature, hostile persons whose suicide gestures are a way of life, an adjustment to frustration. When a serious emotional crisis overwhelms them, they resort to their customary pattern—suicide attempt—but may change the drug or method to assure a fatal outcome. The seriousness of the suicide attempt may be ascertained by the "point of no return," when rescue is no longer possible. Obviously, a person jumping from a high building or firing a bullet into his head does not expect rescue, while a "pill taker" has assured a wide margin of safety.

In the late nineteenth century, Durkheim[4] described three types of suicide. The first he called *altruistic* suicide, a type literally *required* by society. Hara—kiri in Japan and suttee among Hindu widows as well as the suicides of aged Eskimos are all examples of altruistic suicide. Durkheim's second classification, *egoistic* suicide, includes most of the suicides in the United States. This type of suicide occurs when the individual feels alone and lost and has only slender ties to his peers or to the community. The third classification, *anomic* suicide, occurs when an accustomed relationship between an individual and his society is suddenly destroyed. The shock of losing a job, a close friend, one's life savings—all may be precipitating factors in anomic suicide.

Psychoanalytic theory postulates a built-in death wish as part of the original biological endowment of man. Freud considered suicide to be essentially within the mind, the failure to externalize aggressive feelings. Menninger believes that there are three components to suicide: the wish to kill, the wish to be killed, and the wish to die, all of which are characteristic of suicide. It is generally believed that the pairing of at least two of the three, in any combination, would constitute a serious suicide threat. Others, like Herbert Hendin, look on suicide as a "barometer of social tensions." Psychologists understand suicide in terms of various levels of pressure on people, such as traumatic experiences in childhood and youth, a physical handicap, psychological disturbances, etc. During a war suicide rates seem to be generally down, and during the depression of the 1930's, the rate was up.

The usual legal classification of death, the so-called NASH classification, includes *natural, accident, suicide* and *homicide*. Authorities in suicidology[5] believe there should be an additional classification to allow for *sub-intentioned* death. No one knows how many accidental or natural deaths are caused by the sub-intentioned wish to die. There are people who want to die but have not reached the state where they will consciously act on this suicidal desire. Yet they are slowly destroying themselves. A chronically ill person may forget to take medication he needs to keep living. An alcoholic with cirrhosis may continue drinking. These people are killing themselves by inches—fractional suicide, or they may allow some disease to kill them—passive suicide. They may become careless and thereby unconsciously endanger their lives. Accident-prone persons may have strong, unconscious death wishes. If they do not have the determination to commit suicide overtly, or if they have some deeply ingrained prohibitions against suicide, they can take wild risks with their lives. Many reckless drivers constantly gamble with death, leaving the outcome to fate. This is often characteristic of teen-agers who challenge fate but give death the edge. Russian roulette also falls into the category of gambling with death. Sooner or later they will succeed in terminating their lives, and whether they are certified as accidental or natural deaths, they are the result of death-oriented behavior. In most of the destructive behavior patterns there appears to be a subtle death wish. When death occurs in such cases it is usually classified as accidental, yet this is clearly not an accurate or complete description of such a death.

It has been proposed that the *attitude* of the deceased toward his death be evaluated and described as *intentioned, sub-intentioned,* or *unintentioned,* and that such an entry be made on the death certificate, in addition to the actual cause and mode of death.

THE PROFILE OF SUICIDE

The word "suicide" means killing of the self, or self-destruction. The term has often been misused or loosely applied, which has served to confuse the problem. People are called "suicidal", even when the attempt at self-injury does not result in death, when the action is not even intended to end in death. People may be considered suicidal if they express thoughts or wishes for dying, or if they threaten to kill themselves. Suicide, used legally, is applied where there is a conscious awareness on the part of the person that his actions will result in death by his own hand. There are many forms of human functioning and behavior which are destructive and "suicidal" in that a person is living his life with unconscious forces directing him gradually downward toward inevitable self-induced termination. Such unconscious aspects of the person's "suicidal behavior" are difficult to understand and evaluate and yet may be more important than conscious factors.[6]

As already mentioned, attempted suicide usually represents an entirely different clinical entity from committed suicide. Suicide, attempted suicide, and suicidal gestures and thoughts, may be considered in terms of three basic categories of disorders: (1) depression of varying severity; (2) character disorders, i.e. hysterical, sociopathic, manipulative types; (3) disorders combining elements of both (the "cry for help").

The most common clinical picture preceding a suicide is depression. Research during the last fifteen years has shown that there are certain high-risk groups, with professional and white collar persons constituting the most vulnerable socio-economic group. Physicians, dentists, lawyers, ministers, executives—generally those carrying more than average responsibilities—are more predisposed to suicide.[7] The highest rate of all is found among psychiatrists. The conclusion must be that the personality of individuals choosing any of these professions, with their attendant responsibilities, may explain this high suicide rate. Successful men, often in the prime of life, may be subject to severe depressions and end their lives. Sometimes the thought of approaching age or retirement is devastating to an intelligent, vigorous man; or an ambitious man who has reached the pinnacle of success sees no further goals and cannot face life without the stimulation of new challenges. Tragically, suicidal depressions are generally short-lived, and with prompt treatment, the suicidal person might have been salvaged.

Although suicidal depressions are far more prevalent in men, women in the menopausal or involutional period are often in danger. Psychologically the problem is complicated by their fears of being less sexually desirable or attractive, of having reared their families and being no longer needed, or of losing their husbands and their security. Not infrequently, younger women in the post-partum period also suffer severe, psychotic depressions which may end in suicide.

Since alcohol is a factor in a large percentage of cases, alcoholics are a very high risk. Possibly alcohol is a factor in at least 85 percent of all suicide, if only as a means of seeking forgetfulness for intolerable problems, or bolstering courage for the final act.

The suicide risk is high among divorced, single and widowed people—those who have no real ties or who have suffered loneliness through personal losses. Among single men the suicide rate is about twice as high as among married men of the same age. Divorced or widowed men have nearly four times as many suicides as married men. Suicide increases with aging, when loneliness, feelings of rejection and fear of being a burden are combined with ill health, economic insecurity and helplessness. Among white males suicide climbs steeply with advancing age, until at age seventy-five there are about four times as many suicides as at age twenty-five.

Manipulators use the suicide attempt to gain their way or influence or control the behavior of others. These are the ones physicians see most frequently. Clinically, this person is usually a young woman, in conflict with parents, boy friend or husband.

In order to get sympathy or force them to give in to her, she swallows a handful of tablets or nicks her wrist, making sure that the individuals involved are aware of what she has done so that rescue will be assured. She does not intend to kinn herself, although in some instances plans for rescue failed and death resulted. Sometimes the victims of this emotional blackmail became so accustomed to threats or suicide gestures that they paid little attention, failed to act on cue, and thus a fatality resulted. Often adolescent girls[8] who attempt suicide are victims of a chaotic, disrupted home, with pathological child-parent relationships. Studies have shown that two-thirds of such families were broken by divorce or separation, and the fathers were frequently absent or indifferent to their daughters. These adolescents had long and bitter clashes with one or both parents, felt rejected and subjected to unjust parental demands. If rejection by a boy-friend is added to the prior emotional trauma, a suicide attempt may follow. About 75 percent of such suicide attempts are by drug ingestion, and fortunately many of these drugs are relatively innocuous. Sometimes this immature behavior is continued into later life, and there are many middle-aged women who have threatened suicide hundreds of times and have made many suicide gestures. This is a pathological adjustment to frustration and usually evokes little sympathy.

In more recent years young people have felt greater social pressures, with competition and parental exhortations to excel. Failure is unacceptable to parents and represents humiliation before peer groups. These adolescent maladjustments have been complicated further by the use of hallucinogenic and other dangerous drugs, rebellion against authority, inconsistent parental restraints, more liberal sexual practices, and the excitement of protest movements and demonstrations. While a predisposing background makes these adolescents more vulnerable and more accessible to harmful influences, some suicidal deaths have occurred while in a state of drug-induced ecstacy, during a hallucinatory experience, or as a result of misplaced idealism. The recent cases of self-immolation illustrate the latter problem.

The third category—those combining elements of depression with hysterical, manipulative features—offers the most hope in a treatment program. These people are trying to communicate that something in their lives has gone wrong and they need help. Sometimes a suicide attempt will call attention to a problem which demands ameliorative efforts. This action shows a person with few inner resources, but it often produces results in a family, especially where communication has been difficult. Fortunately, if appropriate treatment and counseling are instituted, and this should involve all persons in the family constellation, such an attempter may attain sufficient emotional maturity to handle problems and may never try suicide again, may not feel the need to "cry for help" in such a dramatic and dangerous way.

Every individual has a so-called "suicide potential[5]" which varies in degree from one person to another. Each individual, to some extent creates his own environment, and thus the suicidal person helps create the very condition from which he seeks escape by suicide. The internal unconscious factors are more complex and more important than the external stresses.

When an individual has suicidal impulses, his perspective is distorted. There is usually considerable ambivalence about dying, and the will to live is pitted against the wish to die. The potential suicide is unconsciously hoping for rescue, for someone or something to come along to solve his problem so that life may become tolerable again. Although bewildered and frightened to the point of panic, a suicidal person is not always insane in the legal sense. A suicidal crisis presents a severe emotional turmoil, but it is generally temporary, and if it is recognized and treated promptly, the suicidal person can usually be brought through safely.

The most significant alerting clue[9] is depression, overt or veiled. In fact, depression and chronic alcoholism, often in combination, are the most frequent suicidal precursors. Studies have shown that nine out of ten people committing suicide suffer from an emotional illness, which is depression half the time and chronic alcoholism one-fourth of the time. In a rigid person the most common causes for suicide are disappointment and frustration with which he cannot cope. Suicide is also relatively frequent in schizophrenic and paranoid patients, especially those whose mental content includes a component of depression. A family history of suicide should not be dismissed lightly, for this does increase the probability of suicide.

Almost all persons who commit suicide give some indication of their intentions in advance. These "cries for help" must be understood and heeded if the patient is to be protected until the suicidal crisis is over. Warnings are to be found in frequent talk of suicide. Contrary to common belief that people who threaten to commit suicide never do, it is quite likely that a suicidal individual has given verbal expression of his intent. Statements to the effect that one is a burden, has nothing to live for, no one cares, is tired of living, should be taken seriously. Other clues might include detailed preparations, as if for a long absence, making a will, giving away personal possessions, along with such physical symptoms as fatigue, loss of interest, apathy, depression, poor appetite and disturbed sleep pattern. If failing health, real or imagined, is added to these symptoms, the danger of suicide is greatly increased.

Suicide notes are often interesting illustrations of the emotional turmoil in a suicide's mind.[6] He is confused, often irrational, and his logic is faulty. He can see no way out, but still hopes for some miraculous change in his status. Even during his last moments he tries to write down his feelings. Some suicide notes show much self-pity, others give detailed instructions, with the implication that the writer will be present to see his orders carried out. Many notes[1] indicate the suicide's morbid desire to punish persons close to him, suggesting that he will observe the pity, tears and consternation he has created. Often tremendous hostility is expressed in suicide notes, trying to punish someone or get even for real or fancied hurts. Sometimes these accusatory notes leave innocent recipients permanently scarred. Young people seem unable to associate suicide with being dead and gone, and in their fancies they play the role of the suffering hero and enjoy the attention, pity and admiration of others.

ATTITUDES TOWARD SUICIDE

Education and mental health advances over the past few years have promoted greater understanding of the suicidal personality, along with more effective detection and prevention, but attitudes are slow to change. The suicide has permanently removed himself from any further medical or psychiatric care. So it is the family—the wives or husbands, siblings, parents, and especially the children of a suicide who suffer most. There is still a stigma associated with suicide, and if possible, discussion of the mode of death will be avoided by the family. Most survivors would rather their loved one died of almost any other cause, regardless of suffering or expense, than face the harsh judgmental attitudes still so prevalent. There is an atmosphere of shame surrounding the family of a suicide which affects close friends and associates as well. All feel compelled to make apologies or explanations, and those who have experienced a loss through suicide find it difficult to be objective. In most cases, suicide remains a taboo topic.

To a physician suicide is inconsistent with his basic philosophy. Although the suicide is beyond his help, he should turn his attention to those who must bear the burden of sudden, shocking death. Often a family may be overwhelmed by feelings of guilt, frequently not justified, and they need understanding and support, especially from physician and minister.

There is a psychic contagion in suicide and sometimes the children or the spouse of a suicide will also commit suicide. Often they will repeat the same method or will use an anniversary date to arrange their own demise. The suicide of a prominent person, or a particularly bizarre method, may precipitate other suicides, frequently using a similar method.

SUICIDE PREVENTION

Most authorities insist that suicide can be prevented. This may be true in the majority of cases, although physicians and hospital authorities regretfully admit that some suicidal persons are so determined to end their lives that they succeed in spite of precautions and constant vigilance. These suicides may resort to bizarre means, since all conventional instruments of self-destruction have been removed. We recall one woman who choked herself on a bolus of breakfast food, and a recent newspaper item reported a teacher in France who allegedly drank water incessantly until she managed to asphyxiate herself, resorting to a method used as torture in the Middle Ages. These extreme cases are fortunately rare. The ambivalence—the will to live opposed to the wish to die[1]—is the most powerful factor in the survival of seriously suicidal persons.

Early recognition of suicidal tendencies is the best preventive. Surely suicide should be easier to prevent than automobile accidents or any of the other major causes of death. Many suicide or crisis intervention centers have been established, and their number is growing, giving recognition to the gravity of the problem. Some of these centers are operated in connection with hospitals, mental health clinics, churches or social agencies. Although a few are staffed by professionals, the majority are operated as a telephone service, using trained volunteers[10] to evaluate the seriousness of the caller's suicide intent, his degree of "lethality," and refer the troubled person to an appropriate counseling or medical facility for therapy. Often clergymen operate such services and give spiritual counseling if this is indicated, but a caller who feels completely alienated from God and man may be unable or unwilling to talk to a clergyman. Some ministers who serve in suicide prevention centers agree that a suicidal person cannot accept moralizing or a judgmental attitude, hence they do not identify themselves until or unless it seems appropriate. Strangely, callers who have church affiliations often prefer to talk to an unknown minister, especially if their suicidal preoccupation includes religious conflict or involves shame and guilt. It is also true that callers will unburden themselves more freely to a nameless, faceless volunteer who shows sympathy and understanding. No one can estimate how many lives have been saved by these dedicated men and women.

Complete evaluation of the would-be suicide involves a high degree of professional skill, including the study of family, environment, culture, psychological and sociological factors. It may be a shock to realize that sometimes a suicide is reacting to a subtle and unspoken wish of others, and the difficult question, "Does anyone *want* this person to live?" must be answered. The hidden attitudes of the "significant others"[11] as well as those of the disturbed, suicidal person must be fully understood. There may well be unconscious and subtle efforts to eliminate him. If material gain is involved, such as insurance or inheritance, the suggestion of suicide may be more overt, but one would wonder then if this could be construed as a form of murder.

In studying suicide prevention from various aspects, climate and the season of the year must be considered. For example, the month of April consistently shows the highest incidence of suicide and has been estimated to be 12 percent above the average for the rest of the year. The bleakest season, winter, has the lowest rate. This may seem to be a reverse of the rational order, however, psychologists suggest that the depression of a suicide-prone person may deepen when spring returns and he contrasts his own misery with the reawakening of the land and the joy of other people. It is well known that weather conditions, seasonal changes, barometric pressure and humidity all influence mood. Autumn is often associated with dying, and the month of October also shows a higher than average incidence of suicide.

The more comprehensive form of suicide prevention centers, crisis control centers, offer a broader scope in helping troubled persons who call for help. They reason if people are encouraged to call a center and receive positive suggestions concerning helpful community resources, smoldering problems may be handled before they reach the critical stage. This may be an over-simplified view, but when one considers that more than half of all suicides have been seen by a physician within six months of their deaths, and many of them had seen a doctor during the last week of their lives, it indicates that these people *are* looking for help, and sometimes more than medical evaluation is needed. Many patients come to a physician with vague complaints, and unless the physician is specially trained to detect danger signals, or is exceptionally alert to his patient's problems, he may fail to recognize suicidal tendencies. Psychiatrists used to avoid mention of suicide in discussing problems with their patients. Now the direct approach is preferred and patients are asked point-blank if they are contemplating suicide. Often patients welcome this frank approach and show relief in being permitted to bring their tortured thoughts into the open. Volunteers staffing suicide prevention or crisis control centers are taught to use this direct approach. The caller, having admitted his preoccupation with death, is glad to let the volunteer share his burden and may be more amenable to suggestions for help.

In some communities the crisis control centers have sponsored community education programs, which served the dual function of alerting the community to the problem of suicide and announcing the helpful services available to combat it. Education is the only way to dispel misconceptions and superstitions concerning suicide. Whatever is done to promote better mental health in the community will contribute to the reduction of suicide.

APOLOGIA

Much consideration has been given to the right of a person to live and to enjoy adequate health care. In addition to the right to live, there is also the right to die. Scientists and theologians have long debated if any useful purpose is served in prolonging the life of an aged, terminally ill person suffering almost unbearable pain. Heroic measures to sustain life under these circumstances would seem to be rarely justified. Do we have the right to condemn the individual if he commits suicide under such circumstances?

Another example is the case of a young physician who developed multiple sclerosis while still in his teens, and the disease progressed during his college and medical school years. In his mid-thirties he had established himself in practice, but by that time he had lost control of his bladder and bowels and he was convinced that he would be a nursing problem for the remainder of his life. He chose to commit suicide. Are we justified in criticism of this act? Although it is seldom discussed, society has probably become more tolerant of suicide under such conditions. Some cynics might wonder if we have become more callous or more humane.

The question of life versus death, of survival in the face of overwhelming odds versus suicide, will not be resolved here. It is not our province to condemn or condone. It is difficult to argue successfully with someone who is suicidally depressed, and Santayana expressed it well when he stated, "That life is worth living is the most necessary of assumptions, and, were it not assumed, the most impossible of conclusions." Perhaps it is not always the suicide itself which may be considered the greatest tragedy. Sometimes the life that led to this final act of self-destruction was an even greater tragedy.

A suicide note written by an old man said in part, "When you are no longer useful to yourself and others, it's time to go." A wise professor in medical school admonished his students, "As long as you live you should continue to function. When you cease to function, you should cease to live."

REFERENCES

1. Shneidman, Edwin S., and Mandelkorn, Philip: *How to Prevent Suicide*. Public Affairs Pamphlet No. 406.
2. Farberow, Norman L., and Shneidman, Edwin S.: *Today's Health*, December, 1963.
3. Dizmang, Larry H.: Suicide among the Cheyenne Indians. *Bull. Suicidology*, July, 1967.
4. Durkheim, Emile: *Suicide: a Study in Sociology*. (Originally published in 1897.)
5. Farberow, Norman L., and Shneidman, Edwin S. (Eds.): *The Cry for Help*. New York, McGraw-Hill, 1961.
6. Shneidman, Edwin S., and Farberow, Norman L. (Eds.): *Clues to Suicide*. New York, McGraw-Hill, 1957.
7. Garrard, Robert L.: The role of the physician in suicide prevention. *N. C. Med. J.*, vol. 30, No. 12, December, 1969.
8. Schrut, Albert, and Michels, Toni: Adolescent girls who attempt suicide—comments on treatment. *Am. J. Psychiatry*, vol 23, No. 2, April, 1969.
9. Ross, Mathew: The presuicidal patient: recognition and manageMent. *South. Med. J.*, vol. 60, No. 10, October, 1967.
10. Training manual for volunteers. Crisis Control Center, Inc., Greensboro, N. C.
11. Havens, Leston L.: Recognition of suicidal risks. *Current Medical Digest*, June, 1967.

BIBLIOGRAPHY

Benson, M.: Doctors' wives tackle the suicide problem. *Today's Health*, May 1964.
By one's own hand, medicine at work—Special Issue: *Anatomy of Suicide*, June, 1963.

Crisis Control Center, Inc.: Training Manual for Volunteers, Greensboro, N. C., 1968.

Dublin, L. I.: *Suicide: A Sociological and Statistical Study*. New York, Ronald Press, 1963.

Farberow, N. L. and Shneidman, E. S.: *The Cry for Help*. New York, McGraw-Hill, 1961.

Farberow, N. L.: *Taboo Topics*. New York, Prentice-Hall, 1963.

Farberow, N. L., Shneidman, E. S., and Litman, R. E.: The suicidal patient and the physician. *Mind, 1:69,* March, 1963.

Litman, R. E., Curphey, T., Shneidman, E. S., Farberow, N. L., and Tabachnick, N.: Investigations of equivocal suicides. *J.A.M.A., 184*: 924-929, June, 1963.

Litman, R. E., Farberow, N. L., Shneidman, E. S., Heilig, S. M., and Kramer, J. A.: Suicide-prevention telephone service. *J.A.M.A. 192*: 21-25, April, 1965.

Mathews, R. A. and Rowland, L. A.: *How to Recognize and Handle Abnormal People*. New York, National Association for Mental Health.

Menninger, K. A.: *Man Against Himself*. New York, Harcourt Brace, 1938.

Milt, H.: The roots of suicide. *Trends in Psychiatry,* vol. 3.

Physicians may play an important role in suicide prevention. Reprinted from *J.A.M.A.,* Nov. 29, 1965.

Pokorny, A. D.: Characteristics of forty-four patients who subsequently committed suicide. *Arch. Gen. Psychiatry,* 2:31-323, March, 1960.

Resnik, H. L.: *Suicidal Behavior: Diagnosis and Management*. Boston, Little, Brown, 1968.

Shneidman, E. S. and Farberow, N. L.: *Clues to Suicide*. New York, McGraw-Hill, 1957.

Shneidman, E. S. and Mandelkorn, P.: *How to Prevent Suicide*. Public Affairs Pamphlet, No. 406, 381 Park Avenue South, New York.

Shneidman, E. S. and Dizmang, L. H.: How the family physician can prevent suicide. The Physician's Panorama, June, 1967.

Yolles, S. F.: *The Tragedy of Suicide in the U.S.,* Public Health Service Publication No. 1558.

Chapter 9

SUICIDE—A CHRISTIAN PERSPECTIVE

Suicide Prevention—Where There's Hope There Is Life

MERVILLE O. VINCENT, M.D.

From the position of one who is both a Christian and a psychiatrist, what is the major ethical question that confronts Christians, and the Christian physician particularly, in relation to suicide? Two basic ethical principles in most medical-ethical codes are the sanctity of human life and the alleviation of suffering.[1]

The basic ethical question is then "what role, if any, does Christianity have in alleviating the kind of suffering that results in self-destructive behavior?" Does Christianity have anything to offer except . . . "Thou shalt not"?

This is an extremely important question due to the magnitude of the problem. Suicide is the tenth most frequent cause of death in America, it is fourth with teen-agers, and is second among college students. Several recent studies indicates that there are about 100 definite suicides among U. S. physicians annually.[2-4]

Suicide is mentioned several times in the Old Testament. Scripture at no point condones suicide. The whole emphasis of Scripture is on the value of human life and that one's life belongs to God. The corollary is . . . "Thou shalt not kill". The basis for the sanctity of human life for Jews and Christians is that man is created in the image of God. This special nature distinguishes him from the rest of the animal kingdom. However, Scripture records a number of suicides with virtually no moralizing.

> Samson took his life so as to avenge his enemies in the process. Yet Samson made the list (Hebrews 11:32) of those "who had by faith obtained an excellent repute." Saul too (1st Samuel 31)

took his life in preference to being tortured and killed by his enemies. Likewise his armour-bearer killed himself. Abimelch (Judges 9) committed suicide because he assumed he was mortally wounded. He did not wish it said that he had been killed by a woman. Ahithophel (2nd Sam. 17) committed suicide in a rather orderly fashion after his counsel had been rejected by Absalom. In the New Testament, we find Judas Iscariot overcome with guilt taking his life (Matt. 27; Acts 1). The very center of Christian faith is the one who said . . . "Greater love has no man than this, that a man lay down his life for his friends." Christ permitted his own death that He might abolish death and bring life to His followers.[5]

Paul prevented a suicide.* I do not believe we should become bogged down in discussions about the type of funeral of the suicide victim, his place of burial or idle speculation about his eternal destiny. God is omniscient, God is love; I am content to let Him deal with the dead. Our concern is with the living.

From my perspective, the greatest problem relating to suicide today is that a Christian faith is the strongest preventive factor against suicide. Nonetheless, this fact is not recognized or accepted by most behavioral scientists dealing with the problem. Because of this blind spot, its significance is rarely investigated. I am convinced that among people with a vital, personal Christian faith, the incidence of suicide is much lower than among non-Christians or among those nominal Christians who are only related to a Church structure.

MYTHS ABOUT SUICIDE

Before proceeding, it is essential to clear away certain myths that still persist about suicide.

1. *The rate of suicide is steadily rising in the United States.*

The truth is that there has been little overall change in the rate during this century. However, there has been a marked increase in concern about preventing suicide in the last ten to fifteen years. In 1958, only two Suicide Prevention Centers existed in the U.S.A.[6] In 1970, Suicide Prevention and Crisis Intervention Centers[7] number more than 130. The focal point of scientific

*Acts 16:27,ff.

efforts in suicide prevention has been the Los Angeles Suicide Prevention Center, founded in 1958.

2. *Suicide and attempted suicides are the same class of behavior.*

Attempted suicide and actual suicide represent two different, though overlapping, populations. Typically, suicides are committed by those who want to die. Attempted suicide is often a cry for help. Rather than being considered two completely distinct categories, it is preferable to think of the differences on a spectrum of self-destructive behavior.

3. *Suicide is a problem of a specific class of people.*

Suicide is sometimes referred to as "the curse of the poor" or "the disease of the rich". In reality, suicide is much more democratic and affects all levels of society.

4. *In the United States, suicide is more common among Protestants than among Catholics.*

Studies in this area are not conclusive, and some have shown the reverse.[8] Most studies tell nothing about the degree of religious commitment of either Protestants or Catholics involved and therefore have little meaning.

5. *People who talk about suicide don't commit suicide.*

Approximately 80 percent of those who take their own lives have communicated this intention prior to the act. Suicides do not usually occur without warning, though the actual attempt may be quite impulsive, and threats must be taken seriously.[9]

6. *Once a person is suicidal, he is suicidal forever.*

If the reasons for the person's suicide attempt are remedied, he will no longer remain suicidal.

7. *Suicide is inherited and runs in families.*

It is an individual matter that can be prevented.

8. *All suicidal persons are mentally ill. Suicide is always the action of a psychotic person.*

There is much evidence that a sane person can commit suicide. A person with no moral objection to suicide may rationally do just that to avoid suffering. The hari-kiri indoctrinated Japanese on their kamikaze flights in World War II, as well as the Hindu custom of suttee in which widows cremated themselves on their husband's funeral pyres are examples of culturally condoned suicides. Few argue that all involved are psychotic.

9. *If a person is a Christian he will not commit suicide (The Christian Myth).*

This is not true. Nor should this fact surprise us. Many suicides are related to impaired mental health; the Christian faith has an influence on our mental health, but is not a mental health panacea. Many factors have a bearing on one's mental health, including genetics, possible intrauterine damage, early childhood experiences, biochemistry, physical health, the organic functioning of the brain and the vicissitudes of life, as well as a Christian faith. Christians do develop depressions, schizophrenia and organic brain conditions, all of which carry some danger of suicide.

10. *The Christian faith cannot be expected to influence self-destructive behavior (The Secular Myth).*

One's outlook on life determines one's outlook on suicide. Note what Paul wrote while in "enforced retirement" in a Roman prison:

> For me to live is Christ, and death gain; but what if my living on in the body may serve some good purpose? Which then am I to choose? I cannot tell. I am torn two ways: what I should like is to depart and be with Christ; that is better by far; but for your sake there is greater need for me to stay on in the body. This indeed I know for certain: I shall stay, and stand by you all to help you forward and to add joy to your faith.[10]

Contrast this with the statement by Hemingway's biographer:

> I remember Ernest once telling me, the worse death for anyone is to lose the center of his being, the thing he really is. Retirement is the filthiest word in the language. Whether by chance, or by fate, to retire from what you do—and what you do makes you what you are—is to back up into the grave.[11]

I am not suggesting that Hemingway's philosophy of life was the only contributing factor in his self-destructive course, but I suggest it was a significant factor, perhaps the vital factor.

Whalley notes the decreasing influence of the Protestant ethic among young Americans and states: "Clearly, a self-centered value system in which the gratification of personal desires is salient and inward self-development has a low status, leaves the person susceptible to intense frustration by the outer world which is seen as the source of supply"[12]

From a small series of patients studied at a Suicide Center, Whalley noted:

> . . . There was consensus that it was desirable to have a philosophy of life and try to live by it. However, all said they had not found such a satisfying philosophy themselves. They were "still looking"—with different degrees of zeal and hope. Most were uncertain if they would find a satisfying view but had some slight hope. The one patient who said that she was no longer looking for a philosophy of life because she had no hope of finding it, . . . was the only one who committed suicide.[13]

Pepper tackled the question, "Can a philosophy make one philosophical?"[14] He notes that this is a refined application of the broader question, "What control, if any, does a person's thought have over his emotions or actions?" He says that while a philosophy does not necessarily guarantee a particular action, it generally has an efficacious effect. Pepper noted among a group of six suicide-prone patients:

> This sort of vagueness about a philosophy of life, perception, tests of truth, and cause and effect ran through the answers of all the subjects except one. She, along with two of the others, was an agnostic (who stated) "life is purposeless, it just happened."[15]

In discussing rehabilitation in attempted suicides, Pepper states: "It would be beneficial to provide him with an adequate philosophy of life for long-term guidance of his emotional impulses."[16] Christianity does provide such a philosophy, as well as a personal relationship to Christ, and with the Christian community. Interestingly, the Russians comment on this Western weakness in the Great Medical Encyclopedia (Moscow, 1963, vol. 29).

> Suicide is an important social problem that cannot be solved in the capitalist society. . . . In those capitalist countries where the standard of living is high, as in Switzerland, Denmark and Sweden, the causes are different. There, the absence of broad social concerns and the crisis of the bourgeois ideology, culture and moral vacuum, lead to the loss of perspectives, and goals of life, the disappearance of ideals, and thus to suicide.[17]

11. *People have a right to commit suicide.*

The question being, what *right* do we have in interfering with a person who *wants* to take his own life. This question is most often asked by theorists with little practical experience with suicide. Shneidman comments:

> A mature understanding of this issue devolves on understanding the words "wants" and "rights." There is no question that individuals who want to kill themselves are in this mood for relatively brief periods of time. Individuals typically are acutely self-destructive only for a matter of hours, not weeks or months. . . . The question, then, is: "why would anyone limit his attention to a tiny part of a man's life and disregard the greater part of his non-suicidal existence?" Further, practically everyone who is self-destructive is ambivalent about his self-destruction. . . . The typical suicidal person cuts his throat and cries for help at the same time. A benign society must resonate to the cry and respond with sympathetic aid.
> . . . While it is undoubtedly true that an individual may have the right to kill himself, it is equally true that his survivors have their rights. Especially the spouse or the child has a right not to have to live with the memory of the stigmatizing death. . . . We now see this "right" to commit suicide in the same context as the right of the individual to yell "fire" in a crowded theatre.[18]

In short, suicide is not a purely personal event. It has an effect on the survivors including the general community.

12. *The decision to commit suicide is a black-and-white matter, precipitated by a single cause.*

In fact, suicidal behavior is almost always ambivalent behavior, the result of complex and mixed motivations.[19]
Havens states:

> Pathological processes that lead to suicide travel on many roads. Like the diseases of every-day concern to the Internist, Surgeon and Pediatrician, the event itself is seldom simply determined. . . . Similarly, suicide is the final common pathway of diverse circumstances, of an inter-independent network rather than an isolated cause, a knot of circumstances tightening around a single time and place with the result, sign, symptom, trait or act.[20]

13. *Suicide can only be understood and prevented by a scientific approach.*

In preventing suicide, every possible help is necessary. The scientific approach to suicide is both valid and valuable. However, each one interprets the "scientific facts" according to some value system that he brings to the facts in order to put the facts in a framework of meaning. To deny (a priori) that a Christian perspective can have validity in understanding and preventing suicide is to claim that all truth can be reached only by the scientific method. Such a statement is a philosophical statement rather than a scientific one. Useful information about suicide can be found from many sources. The scientific study of suicide is a relative newcomer. Philosophers of all ages, such as Socrates, the Epicureans, the Stoics, Pythagoras, Aristotle, the philosophers of the Enlightenment, and recent Existentialists, have all contributed to our understanding of suicide. Further, insight has come from the world of literature where men such as Shakespeare have made no small contribution.[21]

Rational prevention of suicide necessitates an understanding of its causes. One of the problems in studying suicide is that the person of our concern is put out of our reach by the very act that makes us wish to know and study him.

Factors that have shown a statistical correlation with a high rate of suicide include being divorced, to a lesser extent being widowed or single. . . . There are approximately three male suicides for every female suicide. Attempted suicide presents a different picture; here women outnumber men about 3-to-1. High rates in America are also associated with being white, elderly, or mentally ill, coming from a broken home, or having an alcoholic parent. Periods of economic depression are associated with high suicide rates. So are cultures such as the Japanese that take a permissive attitude toward suicide.

Low rates in America are associated with being married, being black,[22] and having good mental health. Low rates are also associated with war-time and with countries that have a strong prohibitory attitude toward suicide, such as Spain and Italy.[23]

Traditionally, sociologists have followed in the footsteps of Durkheim and have elaborated his view that suicide is a product of certain kinds of societies. His central concept was that "social integration" was inversely related to suicide rates. Thus, sociologists have emphasized social disorganization, social mobility and social isolation as factors increasing the suicide rates. Psychologists and psychiatrists, on the other hand, have tended to concentrate more on the intrapsychic dynamics of the individual— how he developed from childhood and how he adapts to stress from his environment. However, in between these two extremes is the large area of social psychology which is receiving increasing attention from everyone. Hence, sociologist Breed studied the kinds of interpersonal social relationships that were experienced by people who had suicided. He studied intensively 250 suicides.[24] He noted the significance of *Loss* preceding suicide. In particular he noted three kinds of loss: loss of position, loss of a person, loss of mutuality.

He found loss, or threatened loss of position (e.g. unemployment, demotion, failure to be promoted) with the resultant loss in prestige and self-esteem was particularly common among male suicides. The loss of a significant person was most common among female suicides. The loss might be the death of a husband or "social distance"; the feeling that her husband has been lost to her. Loss of mutuality refers to a weakening of mutual social relationships in general. "The individual lacks bonds and ties to other persons and does not share a community of sentiments with others. . . . The common characteristic, as seen in these suicides, resides in the inability of the individual to maintain satisfactory social relationships with others."[25] Those who committed suicide following a loss did so because of the particular kind of meaning given to the loss that led to the conclusion, "I am better off dead than alive." Breed's study strongly suggests that the loss is so important to the individual that it produced a marked depreciation in his own self-esteem. Because suicide victims depended on a favorable evaluation by others to maintain their self-esteem, their loss added to their humiliation. Their opinions of themselves were largely related to the opinions that they felt others had about them.

Frequent themes in psychiatric theories of suicide are shame, guilt, inferiority, alienation, anxiety, loss and hopelessness. Shame is the feeling that one has not reached his own or others' standards. Guilt is the feeling of having done something wrong, and on both the conscious and unconscious level, shame and guilt produce feelings of inferiority. A closely related concept is alienation.

> Feeling inferior alienates one not only from others, but also when there is a gross discrepancy between the person one would like to be and the person one really is—from one's self. These feelings contribute to the development of loneliness and isolation so that life may come to seem more horrible than death.
>
> It is often said that suicidal people are very self-centered and very angry with themselves and others. For many people, self-esteem depends upon a continuous flow of success of various kinds. Personal failures result in the loss of self-esteem. Furthermore, suicidal people may have experienced frustration of their dependency needs; that is, over and over they have found that people let them down, all these experiences generate hostility and lead a person to conclude he is not very important; a low feeling of self-worth, if not outright self-hatred follows.[26]

Kurt Lewin was one of the first researchers to turn his attention on the subject of hope and hopelessness.[27] Farber recently proposed a general theory of suicide, an attempt to integrate the individual and social dynamics.[28] He presents cogent evidence that the varying individual and social dynamics can be combined into a theory that the probability of suicide varies inversely with the person's hope. Hope is defined as, "A confident expectation that a desired outcome will occur." The common factor in all suicides is a despairing hopelessness, frequently the consequence of a psychiatric breakdown, but also occurring in sane but psychologically vulnerable individuals. He suggests the basic feeling within the person who commits suicide is an impaired feeling of competence. Feelings of incompetence contribute to occupational failures, marital breakdowns as well as nervous breakdowns and alcoholism, all common accompaniments of suicide.

Turning to society, Farber finds suicidal-producing forces in every culture. Suicide rates are an expression of the culture; the unifying principle determining the rate within a culture is the degree of hope that the culture engenders in its members. He believes a society that has a low suicide rate will be one where individual members provide support for one another, and that gives reason for a good degree of hope in the future.

A feeling of hopelessness (and increased suicide) is encouraged by a society that places high demands on the individual to be competent at all times in a very competitive, unforgiving milieu or demands a great deal of interpersonal giving. A person who lacks a feeling of competence may need to be dependent and may find himself unable to meet the demands to give.

CHRISTIAN FAITH—AN OUNCE OF PREVENTION
Primary Prevention

Psychiatry distinguishes between primary prevention, secondary prevention and tertiary prevention. In relation to suicide, primary prevention would be anything that would prevent the development of suicidal thinking. Secondary prevention aims at early detection and intensive treatment of those who already have self-destructive impulses. It is at this level that the Suicide Prevention Center plays its significant role. Tertiary prevention aims at diminishing the adverse consequences of those people associated with a person who has suicided.

Meaning and Purpose

Christian faith provides life with purpose and meaning. Recently a physician I knew developed cancer. He could see no point in continuing his existence so in an orderly fashion he arranged his legal documents then hung himself in his basement. Many physicians commented that under the circumstances it was a very reasonable act. Another physician of my acquaintance is still living. He too has cancer and probably he will not be alive when you read this. He has lived a life committed to Christ, motivated by the desire to communicate Christ's love to all those he met. He finds he still has the same purpose in life. He is neither euphoric nor self-pitying, but continues to be very helpful to many people. Recently he addressed our chapter of the Christian Medical Society. Always an active, vigorous man, he told how he had always believed in heaven but was not particularly interested "in depth" in the subject of heaven. He described how this has changed in recent months. He is enjoying his new discovery and this new hope. In the meantime, he was able to convey to the physicians present a greater understanding of the experiences and feelings of a person who knows death is imminent. Though he had had two blood transfusions the day of his address, he was still able to educate, inspire and enrich those who heard him.

Eric Fromm emphasizes that our day-to-day aim in life is to find "meaning." The less meaning we see in our daily lives, the more anxious we are. In a similar vein, Victor Franklin's, *Man's Search for Meaning* informs us that man is fundamentally in search for a meaning, and if he finds a meaning in life, then this binds the self together. He notes we can find meaning at different levels. The vicissitudes of life will either convince you that life has no meaning or it will drive you beyond people and circumstance to find life's real meaning.

> For me, life's meaning is found in the commitment to the God of creation who has revealed Himself in Jesus Christ. I have become involved with and committed to the person of Jesus Christ through faith. This means both that life takes on meaning and that certain priorities are established. With training in science, the tendency is always to stand back and demand that the meaning of a thing be rigorously demonstrated. Yet, it is evident that such assurance can come only after commitment, not before. In a way, it can be compared to becoming a physician. It is impossible to do so without a commitment to go to medical school.
>
> To be committed to Jesus Christ is to try to understand life as He did. It means trying to see people and their problems as He did. It means trying to see myself, my family, and my role in life through His eyes. When we see the world, become involved in it with Christ, life is exciting and full of meaning.
>
> The alternative may be to see life as merely a series of unrelated happenings, and therefore meaningless. Meaning is never resident in the facts themselves, for everyone brings his own meanings to the facts of experience. The study of science will give us facts, but it cannot tell us their meaning.[29]

Christianity gives us a purpose in life individually and in our relationships with others. Our purpose is to "glorify God".[30] I suspect this sounds like a mere cliché to those who are not in a personal relationship with God, but it is the meaning of authentic existence for many who are in relationship with Him. The Christian loves God because God first loved him and expressed His love tangibly in the life and death of Christ. Love experienced demands expression. His love in us must find expression in our love and concern for others which is inevitably accompanied by a decrease in self-centeredness.

Many view life as a practical joke, the price of having been born, a vale of suffering and tears made all the more absurd because of the inevitability of death. Its true that we live in a time of much depersonalization. Problems abound with racial and social strife, war, civil disobedience, materialistic establishments, inequality of the law, extremes of far right and new left, poverty, exploding population, violence, alcoholism and a drugged existence. If anyone has any "good news", surely he can find some meaning in distributing it. The "good news" is that there is a personal God who loves and cares about each individual with his problems and anxieties, this God has revealed Himself to mankind through the Bible and through the person of Jesus Christ.

Because of our relationship to Christ, our relationships with others are valuable. Our responsibility includes anyone with a need, as Christ indicated in the parable of the Good Samaritan. When we tire of helping those around us and are about to feel that love's labour is lost, Christ reminds us, "Truly I say to you as you did it to one of the least of these my brethren, you did it to me".

Previous Shortcomings

People become depressed and discouraged to the point of self-destruction because they are overwhelmed by shame; they have not lived up to the expectations of themselves or of others. We all experience some unrealistic guilt and all of us carry some realistic guilt. Many try to rationalize away their objective guilt. Christ says to us, face guilt, admit guilt and turn from guilt-producing ways. Further, He offers unconditional forgiveness so that we do not have to go on living guilt-ridden lives. The universality of guilt (sin) is made clear by Christ's reinterpretation of the com-

mandments about murder and adultery. Christ is not a behavior-
ist. He does not judge us just by what we do. He sees the drives,
urges and motives within us. He sees that adultery is the child
of lustful thoughts. Murder is the child of anger and hatred. He
sees lust and hatred in all men. All have weak areas; we give in
to things even when we don't want to.

> Those who are weak in these particular areas may have com-
> mitted adultery or murder, but Christ says that in God's eyes
> we are all guilty of these offenses because we all have had
> lustful feelings and felt hatred. Paul concurs when he says
> "All have sinned and come short of the glory of God". There-
> fore all mankind stands condemned before a Holy God and
> needs forgiveness.
>
> Many who don't know of this forgiveness, or who have heard
> of it but rejected it, feel anxious and guilty over wrongs in their
> lives. Psychiatry can help with unrealistic guilt, with the over-
> developed conscience and so on. But only God can forgive the
> wrongs for which we so desperately need forgiveness.[31]

Relief from shame, guilt and remorse adds to one's feeling of
competence. A feeling of competence has been recognized as a
preventive to feelings of self-destruction. A relationship with
Jesus Christ promises the individual forgiveness. It takes away
shame and guilt, offers an ultimate promise to wipe out all the
differences between the ideal self and the real self. One is related
not only to the Heavenly Father in a mutual love relationship
from which obedience follows readily but also, as a result, to all
mankind. Fellowmen are seen in a different light. They are no
longer just threats to one's hopes and securities in the battle for
survival; they are those for whom Christ came to earth and gave
up His life in love. A relationship with Christ offers a new sense
of personal worth. Feelings of incompetence and hopelessness
are countered by the awareness of God's love and concern.

In this new relationship one finds true identity, meaning,
value and purpose.

> Man lost something of his humanity, something of his identity,
> in his separation from God, in whose image he was created. As
> a result, he may see himself as a product of chance. He sees
> others as things to be exploited for the gratification of his own
> needs. Such impersonal attitudes must result in an impersonal

society that permits and enhances all kinds of slavery; whether
in industry, politics or personal relationships. Ultimately, man's
alienation problem has its roots in his alienation from God.

Man's estrangement from God results in friction between
men individually and collectively. Christ took our alienation
upon Himself to the cross, that we might by faith be reconciled
to the Creator—and to our fellow creatures. Christ offers us
a place in God's family, being filled with His spirit and assigned
to do His will.[32]

Security

Where is it? Many would tell us there is no security, or security
is found in money, position, status or human relationships. But
all of these let us down. Thus, "loss" is a precursor to many
suicides. But loss is inevitable in life. Whether or not a particular
loss brings us to the point of suicide depends on the meaning
placed on that loss. If one loses all there is to live for, then they
may conclude they are better dead than alive. Thus, the unique
meaning of the loss is more important than the loss itself. When
the loss is interpreted as evidence of incompetence, it brings one
closer to self-destructive thoughts. Breed noted that loss or threat
of loss of a significant position or person led to suicide, especially
where the persons experiencing the loss were greatly concerned
about other peoples' evaluation of them. In short, those greatly
dependent upon continual admiration of others not only experienced the initial loss but also much humiliation. Three
variables led to suicide. First, the original feelings of incompetence; second, the loss; and third, the anticipated unfavorable
reactions (humiliation) of other persons. Positively, experiencing
a loss, a person is less likely to commit suicide if he has a reasonable conviction of his competence; the loss is not of primary importance and his self-esteem is not too dependent on other peoples'
opinions of him (in David Reisman's terminology, he is inner
directed rather than outer directed). We have noted how Christian faith raises self-esteem. Loss in the material world is less
significant to the Christian than to the materialist, for his ultimate
security is not bound to material things. The threats in the external world are put in a new perspective, for when a person
comes into a relationship with Christ his whole value system

changes. No longer are his primary concerns those things that moths can get at and rust can ruin; no longer are the fragile status symbols necessary.

The Christian finds his primary security in his relationship to God through Christ. Other losses will affect him only peripherally and not in his most vital area—his relationship to God. This relationship puts threats to material existence such as financial loss, loss of reputation, loss of loved ones, suffering, and tragedy into a totally new frame of reference. As Christ expressed it, "For wherever your treasure is, you may be certain that your heart will be there too". If security is wrapped up in people or things, it can be lost. If security is wrapped up in reputation, we are vulnerable to humiliation.

Youthfulness and life itself are two losses we all anticipate with some ambivalence. However, aging and death are positive experiences for those who increasingly value their relationship with Christ, and who increasingly are less concerned about their material well-being and possessions. For them, death is freedom from the physical limitations of this world and brings them into a new closeness with their primary love object. The most important loss that the Christian could experience would be his relationship to Christ. Therefore we are secure as Paul states:

> Then what can separate us from the love of Christ? Can affliction or hardship? Can persecution, hunger, nakedness, peril, or the sword? . . . For I am convinced that there is nothing in death or life . . . nothing in all creation that can separate us from the love of God in Christ Jesus our Lord.[33]

If hope is the best preventive for suicide, I find more reason for hope in the convictions of Paul than in the convictions of Nietzche who said that the thought of suicide is sometimes "a great consolation; by means of it one gets successfully through many a bad night". Our God is called by Paul the "God of Hope" and "may the God of Hope fill you with all joy and peace by your faith in Him, until by the power of the Holy Spirit, you overflow with hope.[34]

> Christian faith offers a view of life and history based on faith in the sovereign God of the Universe; this results in an attitude

neither paralyzed by the pessimism of a modern existentialist, nor headed for the later discouragement of the modern utopian. Christians see a reasonable hope in this world and a perfect hope in the world to come. Within this framework, they are free—indeed compelled to work for the betterment of mankind in the relief of human suffering.[35]

Dependency Needs

Suicidal people are often self-centered and angry with themselves and others. Their self-esteem is dependent upon a continuous flow of success of various kinds. Personal failures result in a loss of self-esteem. Furthermore, suicidal people may have experienced frustration of their dependency needs; that is, over and over they have found that people let them down just when they need them. All these experiences generate hostility, sometimes directed outwards, sometimes inward. The conviction develops that they are not very important to anyone, low self-esteem if not outright self-hatred follows.

Christians are often accused of being afraid to stand alone in the universe, therefore, they have created God in their own image. Or at least Freud would say "in the image of their omnipotent father". But if man was meant to be dependent on God, then such a dependency is quite appropriate. People who deny their dependency on God only substitute other dependencies. Some of these dependencies are quite destructive. Many a person has ignored his needs for dependency on God, only to find himself totally dependent on alcohol, drugs, achievements, status or public opinion. Addiction to food, alcohol and drugs obviously fill dependency needs. Perhaps this is why approximately 25 percent of North American suicides are alcoholics. Others develop self-destructive work habits to feed their faltering self-esteem, and when even this fails often depression and suicide result.

Society

I have emphasized the effect of the Christian faith on the individual. As Christian individuals, we must seek to change society in such a manner as to provide hope for the hopeless. This means individually we must show increased concern for those round about us, particularly the lonely, the isolated, the aged, the mentally ill, those dependent on alcohol and drugs and those from socially disorganized areas and broken homes. The role of Christianity in the community was recognized by Durkheim who felt that religious devoutness irrespective of denomination provided protection against suicide.

> He did not, however, attribute this effect primarily to religious inculcations and prohibitions, but to the fact that religion integrated the individual with a social group. He regarded suicide as a symptom of a social disease. To cure it—society had to be reformed. . . . Prevention of social isolation and integration of the individual with a group were in Durkheim's opinion the most important tasks for suicide prophylaxis. . . . Ministers of religion have played a leading part in these efforts and medical men have acted as advisors.[36]

The Challenge of Suicide

Dublin concluded a Sociological Study by stating: "The remedy then is to make the social group more consistent and more coherent; to make its members realize their mutual interdependence, and to aim toward creating a society that fulfills the needs of each member in it."[37] Similarly, Farber states: "Suicide will be reduced by the introduction into society of sources of hope, of institutions that foster the sense of competence, that supplies something of succorance and even love."[38]

This is a challenge! Farber also states the problem however, "The established religions provide hope for some, but in the main they no longer engage the emotions sufficiently deeply to provide a nourishing, anti-suicidal hope."[39]

> As Christians, we cannot condone suicide. We believe in the sanctity of every human life, a sanctity derived from the fact that man is created in the image of God. However, as Christians we must relate to others in a manner that shows that our opposition to suicide does not mean that we lack sympathy for those who have committed suicide or are contemplating it, or for those who are left behind after suicide. The problem of suicide is a challenge to us as individual Christians to exhibit an increased concern for those about us. As the Church seeks to meet those needs in society that play a part in the chain of

events leading to suicide, so must the individuals who are the Church meet these needs in other individuals. Dare we let the Christ-like life take over in us? Have we caught the significance of the fact that in serving and helping others, we are serving Christ? Do we really live as if Christ is present for us in suffering humanity? Are we as closely identified with the poor, the hungry, the sick, the imprisoned, the outcast—that is, those without hope—as Christ was? Do we want our indifference healed?[40]

While there is hope, there is life!

REFERENCES

1. For a more detailed discussion of these two principles see: Bird, Lewis P., S.T.M.: *Tao Principles of Medical Ethics,* p. 7 and 8 (author's manuscript).
2. Vincent, Merville O.: Doctor and Mrs.—their mental health. *Can. Psychiat. Assoc. J., 14*:509-515, Oct., 1969.
3. Vincent, Merville O.: Physicians as patients. *Can. Med. Assoc. J.,* vol. 100, March 1, 1969.
4. Simon, W. and Lumbry, G.: Suicide among physicians. *J. Nerv. Ment. Dis.,* vol. 147, no. 2, pp. 105-112.
5. Vincent, Merville O.: Suicide and how to prevent it. *Christianity Today, 14* (8):10-12, Jan. 16, 1970.
6. Acts 16:27, ff.
7. Shneidman, Edwin, S.: Some current developments in suicide prevention. *Bull. Suicidiology,* National Institute of Mental Health, Dec. 1967, p. 32.
8. Resnik, H. L. P.: Center comments. *Bull. Suicidology,* National Institute of Mental Health, No. 6, Spring, 1970.
9. Pokorny, A. D.: Myths about suicide. In Resnik, H. L. P.: *Suicidal Behaviors.* Boston, Little Brown, 1968, pp. 61-62.
10. For more details, see The communication of suicidal ideas. In Resnik, H. L. P. (Ed.): *Suicidal Behaviors.* Boston, Little Brown, 1968, pp. 163-170.
11. *Phil. 1*:21-26, N.E.B.
12. Hotchner, A. E.: *Poppa Hemingway.* New York, Random House, 1966, p. 251.
13. Whalley, Elsa A.: Values and value-conflict in self destruction. In Shneidman, Edwin S. (Ed): *Essays in Self Destruction,* New York, Science House, 1967, p. 101.
14. Whalley, Elsa A.: *Ibid.,* p. 125.
15. Pepper, Steven C.: Can a philosophy make one philosophical? In

Shneidman, Edwin S. (Ed.): *Essays in Self Destruction.* New York, Science House, 1967.

16. Pepper, Steven C.: *Ibid.,* p. 125.
17. Pepper, Steven C.: *Ibid.,* p. 127.
18. Choron, Jacques: Concerning suicide in Soviet Russia. *Bull. Suicidiology,* National Institute of Mental Health, Dec. 1968, p. 31.
19. Shneidman, Edwin S.: Some current developments in suicide prevention. *Bull. Suicidiology,* National Institute of Mental Health, Dec. 1967, p. 32.
20. See Stengel, Erwin.: The complexity of motivations to suicide attempts. *Br. J. Psychiatry, 106* (445):1388-1393, Oct., 1960.
21. Havens, L. L.: The anatomy of suicide. *N. Eng. J. Med.,* p. 401, Feb. 25, 1965.
22. See Faber, M. D.: Shakespear's suicides: some historic dramatic and psychological reflections. *Essays in Self Destruction,* pp. 30-59.
23. Hendlin, H.: Black suicide. *Arch Gen. Psychiatry,* pp. 407-422, Oct. 1969. This paper shows a much higher rate of suicide among blacks than whites in the age group fifteen to thirty-five in New York City for the period between 1920 and 1960.
24. Vincent, Merville O.: Suicide and how to prevent it. *Christianity Today, 14* (8):10, Jan. 16, 1970.
25. Breed, Warren: Suicide and loss in social inter-action. In Shneidman, Edwin S. (Ed.): *Essays in Self Destruction.* New York, Science House, 1967, pp. 188-202.
26. Breed, Warren, *op. cit.,* pp. 195-197.
27. Vincent, Merville O.: Suicide and how to prevent it. *Christianity Today, 14* (8):11, Jan. 16, 1970.
28. Lewin, Kurt: Time, perspective and morale. In Watson, G. (Ed.): *Civilian Morale.* New York, Reynal & Hitchcock, 1942, pp. 48-70.
29. Farber, Maurice, L.: *The Theory of Suicide.* New York, Funk & Wagnalls, 1968.
30. Vincent, Merville O.: Look at life with Virginia Woolf; Alfie and Charlie Brown. *Christian Medical Society Journal,* Spring 1970, p. 2-3.
31. 1 Cor. 6:20.
32. Vincent, Merville O.: Some help for the anxious. *Christian Medical Society Journal,* Winter 1965, p. 19.
33. Vincent, Merville, O.: Look at life with Virginia Woolf; Alfie and Charlie Brown. *op. cit.,* p. 5.
34. Romans, Chapter 8:35-39; N.E.B.
35. Romans, Chapter 15:13, N.E.B.

36. Vincent, Merville O.: Suicide and how to prevent it. *Ibid.*
37. Stengel, Erwin: *Suicide and Attempted Suicide.* Baltimore, Penquin Books, 1964, pp. 117-118.
38. Dublin, Louis I.: *Suicide: A Sociological and Statistical Study.*
39. Farber, Morris L.: *Ibid.,* p. 91.
40. Farber, Morris L.: *Ibid.*
41. Vincent, Merville O.: Suicide and how to prevent it. *Christianity Today, 14* (8):12, Jan. 16, 1970.

BIBLIOGRAPHY

Bible, The New English Bible.
Bird, Lewis P.: *Tao Principles of Medical Ethics.*
Breed, Warren: Suicide and loss in social inter-action. In Shneidman, E. S. (Ed.): *Essays in Self Destruction.* New York, Science House, 1967.
Choron, Jacques: Concerning suicide in Soviet Russia. In *Bulletin of Suicidiology,* National Institute of Mental Health, Dec. 1968.
Dublin, Louis I.: *Suicide: A Sociological and Statistical Study.* New York, Ronald Press, 1963.
Faber, M. D.: Shakespear's suicides: some historic, dramatic and psychological reflections. In *Essays in Self Destruction.* New York, Science House, 1967.
Farber, Maurice L.: *The Theory of Suicide.* New York, Funk & Wagnalls, 1968.
Havens, L. L.: The anatomy of suicide. *N. Eng. J. Med.,* Feb. 25, 1965.
Hendlin, H.: Black suicide. *Arch. Gen. Psychiatry,* Oct. 1969.
Hotchner, A. E.: *Poppa Hemingway.* New York, Random House, 1966.
Lewin, Kurt: Time, perspective and morale. In Watson, G. (Ed): *Civil Morale.* New York, Reynal & Hitchcock, 1942.
Murphy, George and Robins, Eli: The communication of suicidal ideas. *Suicidal Behaviors.* Boston, Little Brown.
Pepper, Steven C.: Can a philosophy make one philosophical? *Essays in Self Destruction.* New York, Science House, 1967.
Pokorny, A. D.: Myths about suicide. In Resnik, H. L. P. (Ed.): *Suicidal Behaviors.* Boston, Little Brown & Co., 1968.
Resnik, H. L. P.: Center comments. *Bulletin of Suicidiology,* National Institute of Mental Health, No. 6, Spring 1970.
Shneidman, Edwin S.: Some current developments in suicide prevention. *Bulletin of Suicidiology,* National Institute of Mental Health, Dec. 1967.
Simon, W. and Lumbry, G.: Suicide among physicians. *J. Nerv. Ment. Dis.,* vol. 147, no. 2.

Stengel, Erwin: The complexity of motivations to suicide attempts. *Br. J. Psychiatry,* vol. 106, no. 445, Oct., 1960.

Stengel, Erwin: *Suicide and Attempted Suicide.* Baltimore, Penquin Books, 1964.

Vincent, Merville O.: Doctor and Mrs.—their mental health. *Canadian Psychiat. Assoc. J.,* vol. 14, Oct. 1969.

Vincent, Merville O.: Look at life with Virginia Woolf; Alfie and Charlie Brown. *Christian Medical Society Journal,* Spring 1970.

Vincent, Merville O.: Physicians as patients. *Canadian Med. Assoc. J.,* No. 100, March 1, 1969.

Vincent, Merville O.: Some help for the anxious. *Christian Med. Soc. J.,* Winter 1965.

Vincent, Merville O.: Suicide and how to prevent it. *Christianity Today,* vol. 14, no. 8, Jan. 16, 1970.

Whalley, Elsa A.: Values and value-conflict in self destruction. *Essays in Self Destruction.* New York, Science House, 1967.

Chapter 10

HUMAN HEART TRANSPLANTATION

CHRISTIAAN BARNARD, M.D.

INTRODUCTION

For the past thirty years surgeons have been exploring the possibility of correcting various defects which afflict the human heart. Rapid advances have been made and, eventually incorporating the use of the heart-lung machine, they have been able to correct a wide variety of defects which can be grouped as follows:

1. Lesions of the pericardial sac.
2. Repair of certain congenital abnormalities.
3. Correction of valvular defects.
4. Ischaemic lesions of the myocardium.

Despite the tremendous advances recently in revascularization of the myocardium, little can be offered for patients suffering from generalized disease of the heart muscle, usually as the result of diffuse coronary arterial disease or inflammatory processes.

This is at present a great challenge to the cardiac surgeon, as disease of the myocardium is the most common cause of death from heart disease. As generalized myocardial damage results in failure of the human pump, the only logical method of treatment would be in replacing the heart function. As a mechanical heart has not been perfected to the stage where it can take over cardiac function completely for any length of time, and as the problems of acute rejection in xenografts are still unsolved, human-to-human heart transplantation is the only method of treatment for patients in the terminal stages of heart disease as a result of myocardial involvement.

Heart transplantation is, therefore, an operation developed to replace the failing human heart with a normal heart removed from a cadaver who has died from some other form of disease.

INDICATIONS FOR HEART TRANSPLANTATION

Owing to our present limited knowledge of immunosuppression, heart transplantation must be considered a palliative measure and not a cure and should be reserved for specially selected cases. These are patients who suffer from an irreversible disease of the heart, for whom conventional forms of therapy are of no further help, and who have progressed to the terminal stages of the disease. Having these prerequisites of recipient selection in mind, heart transplantation must be considered the only treatment available and a justifiable and ethical measure for the palliation of symptoms and the prolongation of life.

HOW IS HEART TRANSPLANTATION DIFFERENT FROM OTHER ORGAN TRANSPLANTATION?

Heart transplantation is similar in many ways to any other organ transplantation, in that it is the treatment offered for an irreversible disease of a life-sustaining organ where all other forms of treatment have failed. However, unlike the kidney or liver, the heart must immediately support the recipient's circulation following cessation of extracorporeal cardio-pulmonary bypass. In addition, should graft failure or rejection occur, no recourse can be made to any artificial means of taking over (or supporting) the heart's function for any length of time.

DONOR ACQUISITION

For successful human cardiac homografts, the following criteria must be fulfilled:

1. All the requirements of the law must be observed.
2. Care must be taken that a normal heart is transplanted.
3. The heart transplanted must be genetically as close as possible to the recipient's tissue.
4. No disease must be present that can be transferred from donor to recipient.

Keeping these criteria in mind, the following steps are taken by the transplant team as soon as a prospective donor is found:

1. The ABO compatibility is done. This takes only a few minutes and further preparation for transplant continues only if this is favorable.

2. The consent of the relatives is now obtained. It is our experience that this will not be withheld if the circumstances are explained sympathetically and carefully.

3. Further histocompatibility tests are then performed. At this center, leucocyte typing is done but is not considered to be of great help.

4. The normality of the heart is established by a careful history of past or present illnesses of the donor (obtained from the relatives) and a thorough physical, x-ray and electrocardiographic examination of the potential donor.

5. Evidence of communicable disease is also sought and excluded by careful history and physical examination of the donor.

SURGICAL TECHNIQUE

This should be planned with the following aims in mind:

First, ischaemic and surgical trauma to the donor heart should be avoided.

Second, great care should be taken regarding haemostasis to avoid postoperative bleeding, especially from the multiple anastomoses, and

Third, the milieu interior of the patient must be maintained as near normal as possible, by careful preoperative preparation and adequate total body perfusion during the transplantation.

In order to avoid ischaemic damage to the donor heart, the organ can either be cooled to reduce the metabolic demands, perfused with oxygenated blood to provide for the metabolic demands, or a combination of these two. We selected to use myocardial perfusion with a moderate degree of cooling.

THE TECHNIQUE OF PERFUSION AND REMOVAL OF THE DONOR HEART

Apparatus

The extracorporeal system is diagrammatically depicted in Figure 10-1.

LEGENDS

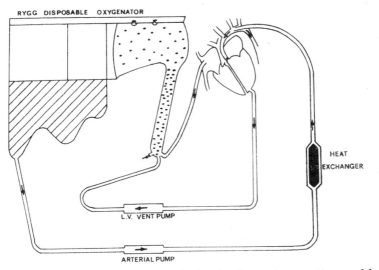

Figure 10-1. Extracorporeal circulation in donor heart. Venous blood drained directly from right atrium into Rygg bag and then pumped through heat exchanger back into aorta. Blood from left ventricular sump pumped into Rygg bag.

Immediately prior to death the donor is heparinized by injecting heparin (2.5 mg/kg body weight) intravenously. The chest is prepared with an antiseptic solution and the operative field isolated with sterile drapes. The heart is exposed by means of a median sternotomy and a vertical incision in the pericardium.

Perfusion of the Donor Heart

Total body perfusion is performed using a single 5/16 inch diameter cannula in the right atrium, introduced through the right atrial appendage for venous drainage—the arterialized blood being returned by means of a cannula inserted in the ascending aorta. A vent is also placed in the left ventricle through its apex for continuous decompression of the left heart. Bypass and cooling are commenced. Total body perfusion at a flow rate of 2.4 1/m²/min of body surface is maintained until the mid-esophageal temperature has reached 25°C when other organs such as the kidney or liver are to be used from the same donor. Providing that only the heart is being transplanted, then as soon as the ascending aorta is isolated, the flow rate is reduced to 300 to 400 ml/min and the aorta is cross-clamped, thereby perfusing only the heart muscle. After about fifteen minutes of perfusion the heart-lung machine is stopped and preparations now begin for removal of the heart.

Removal of Donor Heart

The venous cannula is removed from the right atrium, the arterial catheter and vent are disconnected, but left in position in the heart (Fig. 10-2). The heart is excised by dividing the superior vena cava at the entrance of the azygos vein, the inferior vena cava on the diaphragm, the aorta distal to the innominate artery, the right and left pulmonary arteries and lastly the four pulmonary veins. The heart is now placed in a sterile bowl and transferred to the operating room of the patient, where the recipient is already on total cardiopulmonary bypass, as will be described.

Perfusion of the Donor Heart after Removal

The arterial catheter in the ascending aorta of the donor heart is connected to a coronary perfusion pump fed by the oxygenator of the recipient (Fig. 10-3). This pump is started slowly to expel the air from the ascending aorta and, when all the air is displaced, a clamp is applied distally and coronary perfusion commenced at a flow rate of between 300 and 400 ml/min. The vent is reconnected to suction to prevent over-distension of the left heart, and this also serves to remove air when the anastomoses are completed. The conorary sinus return is sucked back to the recipient's oxygenator.

TECHNIQUE OF TRANSPLANTATION OF HEART

Total Body Perfusion of the Recipient

The extracorporeal circuit is depicted in Figure 10-4. Venous drainage is effected by inserting two 5/16 inch diameter metal-tipped plastic catheters into the inferior and superior venae cavae

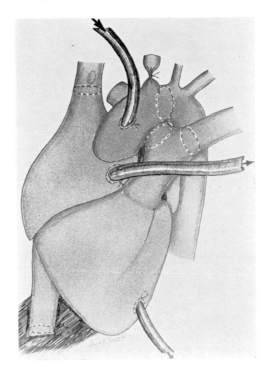

Figure 10-2. Link-up between donor heart and oxygenator and level of division of superior and inferior venae cavae, pulmonary arteries and aorta.

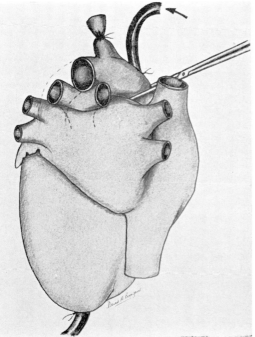

Figure 10-3. Heart of donor after removal, showing total removal of left and right atria, the pulmonary artery with its bifurcation and a good length of ascending aorta and the aortic arch. Perfusion of the heart is then continued by means of the arterial catheter in the ascending aorta and a clamp distal to this.

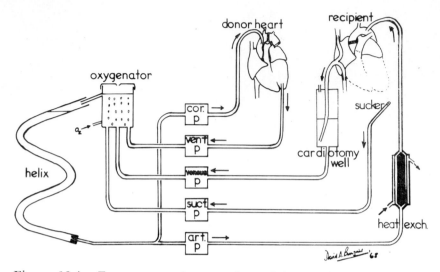

Figure 10-4. Extracorporeal system in recipient. The venous blood is drained through catheters in the inferior and superior venae cavae, introduced through the right atrium. This is drained by suction in the venous well, where it is pumped into the mixing chambers of the bubble oxygenator. It is debubbled and then accumulates in the helix. From the helix it is pumped by the arterial pump through two heat exchangers into the arterial system of the patient. The second line draws arterialized blood to supply the donor heart. Three pump heads provide the necessary suction for the removal of coronary sinus return and bronchial collateral return.

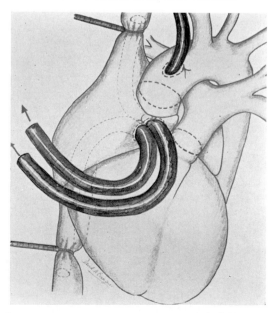

Figure 10-5. Connection between recipient heart and heart-lung machine. Note that the venous catheters pass through the right atrial appendage, but it is suggested that they should pass through the right atrial wall close to the entrance of the venae cavae so that the right atrial appendage can be removed.

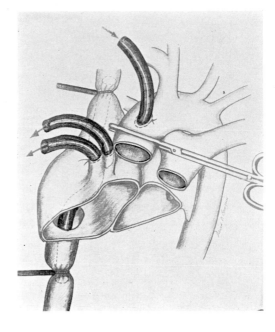

Figure 10-6. The remains of the atria, aorta and pulmonary artery in recipient after the heart has been removed.

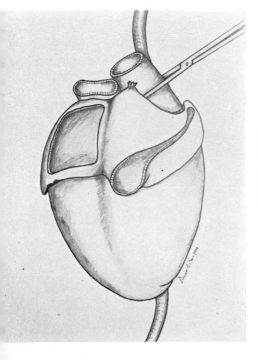

Figure 10-7. The back cuts, the opening into the left and right atria in the donor heart in preparation for anastomosis to the remnants of the atria in the recipient.

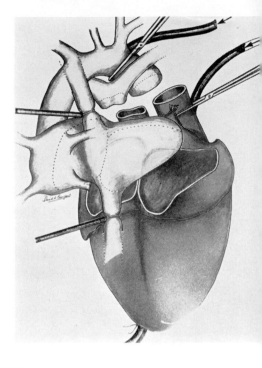

Figure 10-8. The donor heart being placed in position in the pericardial sac of the recipient.

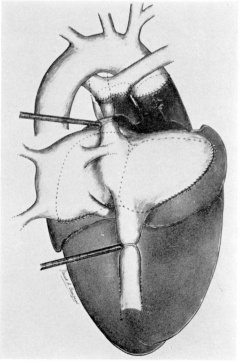

Figure 10-9. The completion of the transplant, indicating the various suture lines.

through the lateral wall of the right atrium so that most of the right atrium and the right atrial appendage can be excised. For arterial return a 5.4 mm ID catheter is placed in the distal portion of the ascending aorta. Total body perfusion is commenced at a flow rate of 2.4 $1/m^2$ body surface area/min, and the patient is cooled down to a mid-esophageal temperature of 30° to 32°C. The venous tapes around the superior and inferior venae cavae are tightened and the heart excised (Fig. 10-5). During bypass, 1 gm potassium chloride per hour is administered to the patient and sodium bicarbonate on doses estimated on the base excess as determined by the Astrup method.

Excision of the Recipient's Heart

The aorta is cross-clamped immediately proximal to the arterial catheter and the aorta divided on the coronary ostia. The pulmonary artery is divided on the pulmonary valve. The base of the heart is retracted anteriorly and the right atrium, interatrial septum and left atrium detached from the ventricles close to the interatrial groove (Fig. 10-6).

Technique of Anastomoses of Donor Heart into the Recipient

An opening is made in the back of the left atrium of the donor heart, by excising the back wall at the entrance of the four pulmonary veins. The stump of the superior vena cava is ligated and the back wall of the right atrium is opened by an incision running from the orifice of the inferior vena cava superiorly and slightly lateral, avoiding the area of the junction of the superior vena cava to the right atrium, and thus also the site of the sinoatrial node (Fig. 10-7).

The connection of the donor heart to the circulation of the recipient is begun by anastomosing the opening in the back wall of the left atrium to the remnants of the patient's left atrium and interatrial septum. This is best done by the surgeon standing on the right side of the patient and commencing the suture line in the middle of the left atrial wall using a continuous 4-0 silk suture (Fig. 10-8). After completion of the left atrial anastomosis, the opening in the donor's right atrium is then anastomosed to the interatrial septum and remnants of the patient's right atrial wall. This is again performed using a continuous 4-0 silk suture. The donor and recipient's pulmonary arteries and aortas are now trimmed to the correct length and diameter. The pulmonary arteries are next connected with a continuous 5-0 silk suture and then the aortas in a similar manner (Fig. 10-9). The coronary perfusion is discontinued, and the clamp on the ascending aorta removed, and rewarming commenced. Whilst rewarming is continuing, great care is taken to remove air both from the right heart by a vent in the pulmonary artery and from the left heart by means of the vent in the left ventricle. If the heart beat does not start spontaneously, it is defibrillated by means of a direct current shock. Intravenous isoprenaline drip of 1 in 450,000 at the rate of 0.4 ml/min is instituted to provide a vigorous cardiac action. The vena caval tapes are released and the catheters in the right atrial cavity are withdrawn into the atrial cavity. The patient is perfused to raise the central venous pressure to approximately 100 mm/Hg and, as soon as the body temperature has returned to normal, bypass is discontinued.

At the completion of the bypass a close watch is kept on the arterial and venous pressures and on the cardiac action. If there is evidence of failure or distension of the heart, partial bypass is immediately reinstituted. This procedure may have to be repeated a few times, until the heart takes over without becoming distended while also providing adequate circulation. The vena caval catheters are now removed along with the catheter in the ascending aorta. Protamine is given to neutralize the heparin in a dose ratio of $1\frac{1}{4}$ mg protamine for each mg heparin, and the heart is inspected very carefully to detect any area of abnormal bleeding.

Once the surgeon is satisfied that hemostasis is adequate, a drain is placed in the pericardial cavity—brought out through the skin of the abdominal walls and connected to suction. The pericardium is then closed. A second drain is placed in a similar manner in the anterior mediastinum and also connected to suction. The sternum is then approximated with wire sutures and the wound closed.

TISSUE MATCHING

Complications which arise from immunological reaction to the graft remain as the most serious obstacle to clinical transplantation. Apart from immunosuppressive treatment, there are several possible ways in which rejection of a graft may be avoided or minimized. Induction of immunological tolerance and enhancement of the graft has been achieved in animal experiments, but has not yet become part of treatment in clinical transplantation. Experience with human kidney allografts indicates that immunological adaptation to incompatible grafts has occurred by chance in a few instances. There are patients on record who have required immunosuppressive treatment for clinically evident rejection during the early posttransplant period, but who have later maintained their graft over considerable periods without any further treatment whatever. At present, rejection can most successfully be minimized by selecting donors whose transplantation antigens are identical to those of the recipient. This is achieved in transplantation between identical twins. With other genetic classes of donor histocompatible identity is seldom possible to achieve. Particularly when cadaver donors are used, histocompatibility matching has its own problems. There are several reasons for this. Firstly, by present serological methods not all transplantation antigens are detectable. Furthermore, the relatively large number of antigens which can be determined give rise to so many different phenotypes that a degree of close correspondence between unrelated donors and recipients becomes an unreasonably small arithmetic probability, unless a large pool of recipients and a large number of donors are available.

It may be accepted as mandatory at present that a donor and recipient should be compatible for the ABO blood groups (these being clearly recognized as strong transplantation antigens) and that the recipient must not possess lymphocytotoxic antibodies which react with leucocytes from the donor. Such a direct incompatibility is associated with early rejection of the graft in a very high proportion of cases.

Several or many antigens which occur on human leucocytes correspond to transplantation antigens, because they occur also on the cells of other tissues. There are several serological methods for recognizing these antigens. Clinical tissue typing consists mainly on detecting leucocyte antigens. Monospecific leucocyte typing sera are obtained from some pregnant women (who form antibodies to histocompatibility antigens inherited from the father, and therefore present in the fetus but not in the mother), from patients who have had many blood transfusions and from volunteers who are deliberately immunized. Leuco-agglutination, lymphocytotoxic tests and complement fixation tests are carried out on the leucocytes of the donor and recipient respectively, and the donor is selected to give the best possible match with the recipient.

There is not complete certainty yet as to the exact degree of histocompatibility which must exist to ensure success of the graft. Because identical matching is difficult to achieve in clinical practice, various schemes have been designed whereby degrees of incompatibility can be graded. The two schemes in widest use at present are those of Terasaki and of van Rood.

Their terminology is as follows:

	Terms used by Terasaki et al.
Symbol	*Meaning*
A	Identical
	A+ = sib-to-sib
	A = Parent-to-child
	A— = unrelated
B	Matched D to R (mismatched R to D)
	B+ = R-D mismatched in 1 group
	B = R-D mismatched in 2 groups
	B— = R-D mismatched in 3 or more groups
C	Mismatched D to R in 1 group
	C = R to D further mismatched in 0-2 groups
	C — = R to D further mismatched in 3 or more groups
D	Mismatched D to R in 2 groups
	D = R to D further mismatched in 0-2 groups
	D— = R to D further mismatched in 3 or more groups
F	Positive crossmatch: R serum reacts positively in cytotoxic test with D lymphocytes

	Terms used by van Rood
Term	*Meaning*
Identity	Leucocyte groups of donor and recipient are identical for the HL-A antigens
Near Identity	Leucocyte groups of donor and recipient are identical for the HL-A antigens, except for one antigen
Not Identical 2-3	Leucocyte groups of donor and recipient are different for 2 to 3 of the HL-A antigens
Not Identical 4 or more	Leucocyte groups of donor and recipient are different for 4 or more of the HL-A antigens

Current experience is that a D grade match according to Terasaki, or a mismatch where four or more antigens are not identical, according to van Rood, is associated with graft failure in a very high proportion of transplants. One of our patients, however, with a D grade match is still alive nineteen months after transplantation.

Leucocyte antigen matching is limited at present by serological techniques which are not yet entirely satisfactory and by incomplete knowledge of the immunogenetics of the human leucocyte antigens. Furthermore, even with the inexact degree of antigen typing which can be performed today, the great variety of phenotypes which appear in the general population make identical or very close matching impracticable in the majority of transplants involving unrelated donors. Nevertheless, leucocyte typing has a great deal to offer. It should be possible in the majority of instances to choose a donor which is better matched than would be obtained on the average by random selection and to avoid altogether the gross mismatches which will occur in a high proportion of unselected transplants. With the best of present-day methods of immunosuppression, relatively lesser degrees of histoincompatibility will offer a greater chance of success to a larger number of recipients.

IMMUNOSUPPRESSION

Treatment of Rejection

As has been pointed out by other workers, the patient who receives a cardiac transplantation has probably a more active immunological system compared to that of a kidney transplant patient who has been chronically immunosuppressed by the chronic uremic state. It therefore appears essential in the patient receiving a heart to initially use high doses of immunosuppression. We commence with 500 mg prednisolone on the day of operation, reducing it by 100 mg every day until the fifth day. For the following two weeks a dose of 100 mg per day is maintained and then it is slowly lowered to 50 mg per day. This dosage is continued for the first month, after which it is again gradually reduced to 30 mg daily and this dose is maintained for one year. Imuran is prescribed at the highest tolerated dose, observing carefully the white cell count and the liver function tests. Antilymphocyte globulin is given for three months. Doses of 5 ml to 10 ml intravenously every twelve hours for the first month. The same dosage is given once a day for the second month and for the third month is administered three times a week. If at anytime rejection becomes clinically recognizable, e.g. by a drop in the electrocardiograph voltage, the prednisolone dosage must be increased immediately to 200 mg per day and even up to 1000 mg per day to obtain an immediate diminution in the immunological attack. The steroid dosage is gradually decreased to the maintenance dose once the clinical rejection is controlled.

Unfortunately when rejection is well established in the transplanted heart it may be difficult to reverse and as to date, an artificial heart has not been developed to take over cardiac function during this period; there is thus a great danger to the patient's life. Even if rejection is reversed it has been our experience that the patient never improves to the state he was in before the rejection episode. It therefore appears to be of utmost importance to prevent rejection, and we feel that this can be done by treating the patients weekly with a single high dose of steroids, once maintenance immunosuppression has been reached. We administer 200 mg prednisolone per week as a booster.

PREVENTION OF INFECTION

A patient chosen for cardiac transplantation is a desperately sick man. Because of his failing heart and circulation he is prone to pulmonary and renal disease, with a consequent greater risk of postoperative infection. This risk of infection is increased by the necessity of having to receive immunosuppressive drugs and large doses of steroids. For these reasons it is considered mandatory to provide such a patient with an environment as free from bacteria as possible. In the case of a recent patient the following preventative measures were recommended and introduced.

Preoperative Period
1. Patient. The patient is washed daily with hexachlorophene soap. Swabs are taken from the skin, nose, throat, mouth and

rectum and are examined for the possible presence of potential pathogens, especially yeasts, Pseudomonas aeruginosa, Klebsiella species, beta-hemolytic streptococci and staphylococci. Antibiotic sensitivities of these organisms are determined where possible. Any obvious septic lesion is treated vigorously.

2. Staff. Nurses and medical staff who are to handle the patient postoperatively have swabs taken from the nose, mouth, throat and rectum for bacteriological examination to determine if they are carriers of any potential pathogens.

3. Room. A room is set aside in the unit, which is then thoroughly cleaned in the following manner:
   a. Gaseous disinfection under bacteriological control.
   b. Thorough washing of all walls and floor with a phenolic disinfectant, using boiled cleaning utensils.
   c. Thorough washing of the bed with liberal amounts of the correctly diluted phenolic disinfectant.
   d. Autoclaving of the mattress which is then covered in plastic, and autoclaving of the pillows.
   e. Flushing of the washbasin three times daily with a suitably diluted phenolic disinfectant.

4. Apparatus. Any apparatus to be used near or on the patient is carefully checked for cleanliness. This applies particularly to the oxygen tent, the suction apparatus and the Bird respirator. This apparatus is dismantled as completely as possible and thoroughly cleaned mechanically, and then all parts which can be autoclaved or boiled are so treated. Parts which cannot be boiled or autoclaved are treated by gaseous disinfection or a phenolic disinfectant. Particular attention is given to any humidifying unit. The water in this unit is changed daily and the water container is boiled at the end of each day, pre and post-operatively.

Postoperative Period

The patient is transferred to the specially prepared unit. All staff attending the patient wear caps, masks, canvas overshoes and sterile gown and gloves, as for any sterile procedure. After any form of attention to the patient, the gloved hands are rinsed in the idopher disinfectant and dried on disposable paper towels.

The patient's sheets and cotton blanket are changed twice daily, taking due care not to disturb the air excessively while doing this. The floors are mopped twice daily with a phenolic disinfectant. The bedpan and urinal are stored in a phenolic disinfectant. They are rinsed in hot water and dried before use. In addition, the following measures are taken:

1. Patient. Every second day, swabs for bacteriological examination are taken from the nose, throat, mouth and anus to assess the presence of potential pathogens or a change in bacterial flora. All venepunctures, intravenous therapy sites and injection sites are treated as for a sterile surgical procedure. Daily blood cultures are performed. Careful attention is given to the perineum and scrotal region. These areas are dusted daily with hexachlorophene and Mycostatin® powder. The minimal number of personnel attend the patient.

2. Staff. Nose, throat, mouth and rectal swabs are taken for bacteriological investigations every week to assess the presence of any potential pathogens. Antibiotic treatment was introduced as required.

WORLD EXPERIENCE WITH HEART TRANSPLANTATION

Up until October, 1970, 165 cardiac grafts were performed in 162 recipients. These operations were carried out in twenty different countires by fifty-nine teams.* The chronology is interesting. The sharp decline in the number of operations performed towards the end of 1969 is most likely due to the disappointing results obtained (Fig. 10-10). This pessimism is mainly due to a lack of understanding of what heart transplantation has to offer dying patients—not a new healthy life, but only a prolongation of life and alleviation of suffering. Thirty-five percent of patients survived beyond the three months period. Death was caused mainly by rejection or the toxic effect of immunosuppressive drugs. The etiology of the cardiac disease is not known in all the recipients, but the information available so far is set out in Figure 10-11.

Our experience with our five patients is that three of them

*ACS/NIH Organ Transplant Registry. Spring Newsletter.

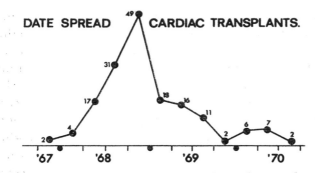

Figure 10-10. Chronology of heart transplantation to date, showing decline in number of operations towards the end of 1969.

survived for more than eighteen months after transplantation. By performing cardiac transplants on these three patients we achieved exactly what we set out to do, in that we have definitely prolonged their lives and alleviated their suffering.

ETHICAL PROBLEMS

Organ transplantation has evoked such mixed and even violent reaction that it would seem worthwhile to explore the ethics governing it—and to do this by examining the three major areas of contention: the act itself, the recipient and the donor.

Is Transplantation Ethical?

News coverage of transplantation in the popular mass media has been widespread, enthusiastic and, unfortunately, too often

PRINCIPAL CARDIAC DIAGNOSIS	No. of Cases
Arteriosclerotic Heart Disease	75
Cardiomyopathy	30
Valvular Disease	10
Congenital	9
Other	6
	130

Figure 10-11. Available information on the etiology of heart transplant patients to date.

sensational and misleading. It has been misconceived in certain sections of the public both as a panacea and as an unethical and unjustified form of treatment. Neither assertion is accurate.

Within our currently limited understanding of immunological attack on an allograft and our inability to prevent such an onslaught, the transplantation of any organ must be accepted as palliative therapy, not a final cure. It achieves palliation which equals, if it does not surpass, some forms of palliation which have been accepted for many years as the only way to deal with malignant diseases. This being established, one cannot accept as unjustifiable or unethical the palliation of symptoms and extension of life itself.

A frequent criticism is that the manpower and the financial expenditure involved in transplant programs far outweigh the results obtained, and that other medical services have a more urgent and real claim to the financial and intellectual effort needed for transplants. This sort of criticism is extremely conservative and dangerously shortsighted. Similar attacks were once levelled by similar critics at open-heart surgery using cardiopulmonary bypass. This happened in the early days of this new technique, but as the surgeons and scientists learned more about heart-lung machines and the management of patients seriously ill from heart disease, methods and apparatuses were simplified and the techniques became more widely applicable.

To curb transplantation at this stage would be to strangle one of the most promising and exciting fronts of medical endeavour of this century. From the experience gained in the problems of rejection, methods of immunological control will be improved and vital organ replacements will become a routine and life-saving procedure. To deny medicine its full thrust in this direction would be irresponsibly short-sighted. Indeed, it is difficult not to conclude that any withdrawal from this new frontier would be professionally unethical. We have only to continue transplantation on a most active scale.

Does the Recipient Receive an Ethical Treatment?

It is currently accepted that a patient should not be submitted for organ transplantation unless he suffers from an irreversible disease of the organ to be transplanted; that conventional therapy is of no further avail; and that the patient has progressed to the terminal stages of the disease—in blunter terms, he should be dying. Allograft replacement of such an affected organ may offer the patient a significant extension of life. Renal recipients may look forward to several years of extended life.

It is still premature to evaluate heart and liver transplants, but we should note that there are recipients of heart and liver grafts who are in their second posttransplant year, and not without dramatic relief. Not only is there extension of life but also a significant palliation of life-crippling symptoms. The cardiac recipient exchanges the horror of terminal cardiac failure for a life similar to that of a vigilantly controlled diabetic; the distress of uremia and frequent hemodialysis is exchanged for daily drug control and a full life.

Is Our Acquisition of Donor Organs Ethically Acceptable?

For many years both medical and lay public have accepted that after the certification of death by three well-known criteria—brain death, no spontaneous respiration, and absence of cardiac activity—a postmortem is performed and the heart, instead of being placed in a bottle, is transplanted in another body in an attempt to save a life or alleviate suffering. There is no ethical principle which establishes this act as unacceptable or immoral. Inevitably, one can only conclude that it is unethical to allow such organs to putrefy with the cadaver, thus denying a potential recipient an extension of life.

There are people who accept this argument and yet voice real mistrust of the management of the donor before the certification of death. These misgivings are entirely unfounded. Years before surgeons embarked upon the transplantation of cadaver organs, neurologists and neurosurgeons concluded it was futile to keep patients alive once there is undeniable and irreversible brain death. In short, it has been universally acceptable that at this stage artificial maintenance of life may be terminated. Moreover, throughout the world responsible medical and legislative groups have defined the moment of death and the handling of a potential donor. Further, with heart transplants even greater care is taken to handle this problem most ethically.

Certain fundamental principles of donor organ acquisition should be emphasized. All patients in need of resuscitation and special care must receive this with the utmost skill and efficiency available today, and potential donors should be admitted under the care of doctors who are not involved in transplantation. This separate group of doctors must decide when treatment is of no further use or avail and should therefore be discontinued or not instituted. They may then discontinue or withhold treatment when they decide that gross loss of cerebral function has occurred and is permanently irrecoverable. Before coming to this decision there must be a positive clinical diagnosis which will permit prognosis. Also, there should be instituted all appropriate clinical investigations which might indicate a remediable or reversible condition.

Cerebral death should be diagnosed on neurological, electro-encephalographic, circulatory and respiratory criteria, using the best available apparatus and skill. If these criteria are fulfilled, the patient is declared dead and only then is it possible to take measures to obtain viability of desired organs. At that stage, a donor may be transferred to the transplant intermediary or referee. There seems little doubt that this is the morally and ethically acceptable sequence of events for this crucial point in the transplantation of an organ.

Because it is desirable that the result of animal and laboratory experiments be applied to human beings to further scientific knowledge and to help the suffering of humanity, the World Medical Association has prepared recommendations as a guide to each doctor engaged in clinical research. One of these recommendations is that in the treatment of the sick person, the doctor must be free to use a new therapeutic measure if, in his judgement, it offers hope of saving life, reestablishing health or alleviating suffering. There is no doubt in my mind that we had reached this point in organ transplantation.

Chapter 11

ETHICAL ISSUES IN KIDNEY TRANSPLANTATION

ROBERTA G. SIMMONS, PH.D. AND JULIE FULTON, M.A.

As a new medical procedure, organ transplantation has attracted public attention to a virtually unprecedented extent. Each heart transplant has received extensive local and national coverage, and many kidney transplants have also had considerable news attention. In the wake of such publicity, many serious ethical issues have been raised: what are the criteria by which some potential recipients should be selected for transplantation and others refused this life-saving treatment? how can a potential organ donor be protected against premature termination of his life? what is an acceptable definition of death? should living donors be used? should the society allocate large sums of money to support transplantation, or should transplantation receive little encouragement in the face of other societal needs?

This chapter will address itself to these and other ethical problems inherent in the burgeoning field of organ transplantation and will focus specifically on the area of kidney transplantation. The kidney is the only organ that has been transplanted successfully enough for the operation to be considered a viable cure rather than an experiment. Many of the problems now being experienced within the field of kidney transplantation will undoubtedly be relevant to other types of transplant programs in the future, as these programs attain greater success.

Before we discuss the ethical issues surrounding kidney trans-

The authors wish to express gratitute to Dr. Robert Fulton for help with this chapter.

The research for this study was supported by Grant MH-AM 1835-01 and 5 K1 MH 41, 688-02 from the Public Health Service.

plantation, a brief explanation of kidney dialysis and transplantation is in order.

HEMODIALYSIS

Hemodialysis, or the purification of a kidney patient's blood by means of an artificial kidney machine, was the first major advance in the treatment of kidney disease. It is used today on a short-term basis by patients awaiting transplantation and on a long-term, relatively permanent basis by those patients who have no transplant operation in sight.

In a hospital, clinic, or even a home setting, the kidney patient is "hooked-up" to the dialysis machine by means of a shunt, or U-shaped tube, one end of which is inserted into a vein and the other into an artery. (The shunt is usually inserted permanently in the patient's forearm.) Approximately twice a week, for a period of from seven to fifteen hours each time, the patient's blood is cycled through the machine, where it is purified, and then returned to his body.

The shunt is, quite literally, the patient's lifeline. Unfortunately, however, the area in which the shunt is inserted is subject to infection and the vessels are subject to clotting. When this happens, the patient must be hospitalized. If the shunt connection should tear apart, emergency measures are required to prevent hemorrhage. This becomes a very serious problem given the limited number of locations that a shunt may be inserted in the patient's body. It should be noted that the alternatives for patients who are sick enough to require long-term dialysis are very few. They must either (1) remain on dialysis treatments, (2) undergo a kidney transplant operation, or (3) face certain death.

KIDNEY TRANSPLANTATION

Kidney transplantation attempts to remove the patient from the status of being "sick" altogether. In this operation, the diseased kidney is surgically replaced with a healthy organ from either a cadaver donor or a living donor. The kidney was the first organ to be transplanted successfully in humans. As mentioned earlier, it is also the only one of the various types of organ transplantation (heart, lung, liver) that is no longer experimental; its success has been medically demonstrated.

According to the Registry of Kidney Transplant statistics, 81 percent of those patients who received a kidney from a living brother or sister and 40 percent of those who received cadaver kidneys have survived two years posttransplant with functioning kidneys. (Two years is the arbitrarily designated period beyond which the patient is felt to be cured.) In many medical transplant centers today, therefore, patients are receiving kidneys with the hope that this operation will give them a normal lifespan as well as an essentially normal life. In fact, kidney transplantation with related donors is more successful in providing a cure than is any operation designed to cure cancer.

WHO SHOULD BE SELECTED FOR TREATMENT? WHO SHOULD BE REJECTED?

It was estimated, in 1967, that some 50,000 persons a year die of uremia, or poisoning of the blood due to kidney failure. Of that group, it was believed that 7,000 to 8,000 would have been ideally suited for either maintenance therapy by means of hemodialysis or for kidney transplantation. In that year, however, treatment was available to less than 2,000 kidney patients due to the undeveloped nature of the dialysis and transplant programs. In the past three years, hospital facilities and medical and economic resources have been greatly expanded, yet, as of this writing, many patients die from what is potentially a curable disease. Who, then, is likely to be rejected for treatment? Who should be allowed to live, and who must die?

The fact that dialysis and transplantation require large, highly trained professional staffs, and expensive, highly specialized facilities means that such centers are likely to be limited to urban areas or to university research hospitals. An ethical issue raised by this fact—particularly when the medical facility is in part federally supported—is the difficulty of providing to all citizens the same opportunities for treatment. Patients living in small communities at some distances from these centers and lower-class patients from all areas would seem to suffer most from this concentration of facilities and staff.

Persons from outlying areas and their local doctors are often unaware of the existence of the kidney center or, if they are aware, might possibly be discouraged by the cost of travel and by the adverse reports of patients being denied treatment at these centers for various reasons.

Many factors seem to work against the lower-class patient in particular. It has been shown that lower-class persons are less likely than others to seek medical care at all. In the urban areas, however, this is mitigated somewhat by the existence of large, general hospitals or clinics specifically designed to serve lower-income families from which referral to a transplant center is likely. Nevertheless, many low-income patients do not attend these clinics but see neighborhood physicians. It is very possible that the physician who the lower-class patient consults will not feel that he would be a likely candidate to be accepted for kidney treatment, or that he and his family will be able to make the sacrifices of time and money required by this procedure. As a result, the physician may not even refer this patient to the center to be considered for treatment.

If, however, going one step further, the physician does refer a lower-class patient, there are further, more subtle obstacles for him to overcome. Some centers select patients for treatment only on the basis of medical criteria; in such programs, persons with the best chances for a medical recovery or perhaps patients with a particular combination of diseases will be chosen over patients who have less promising medical prognoses. Other centers, however, select patients not only on the basis of medical criteria but also may employ social factors in their decisions, and here again, the lower-class persons face heavy odds against them.

At the time of the first dialysis treatments in Seattle, an anonymous committee of primarily lay persons selected the patients for treatment. A major criterion in their decision, over and above the medical considerations, was their judgment of the social value of the patient's life. They decided, in other words, which persons were the most "worth" saving. Such committees would be expected to reject the unemployed, the worker with an "unimportant" job, the person with few family ties, and the person with a history of deviance of any sort. The Seattle board has since been dissolved and the burden of selection, there as elsewhere, now falls largely onto the physicians themselves.

In the treatment of certain other types of patients, physicians have been shown, however, to exhibit a bias toward middle- and upper-middle-class patients—patients, that is, who are more like themselves.[1] There is some evidence of a similar bias in the selection of dialysis patients. Ninety-one percent of dialysis patients are white, 45 percent have at least one year of college education (in comparison to only 18 percent of the adult population of the United States) and 60 percent had incomes (before dialysis) at, or above, the United States median income.[2] Other studies have also suggested a slight middle-class bias in the selection of patients for heart transplantation. There is no systematic study, unfortunately, of the social origins of kidney transplant patients, but it is likely that they would not differ too greatly from those of dialysis patients.

In a study of 87 dialysis centers, it was found that nearly all of the centers (96 percent) use at least one social or psychological criterion in their selection of patients in addition to their assessment of his medical suitability.[3] Ninety-seven percent of the centers believe that willingness to cooperate with the treatment is an important criterion for selection, and 82 percent usually use intelligence as an indicator for such cooperation. Approximately three-quarters of the centers believe that the likelihood of vocational rehabilitation is a valuable means of selecting patients for treatment, and half of the centers utilize a psychiatric evaluation as a selection device.

It would be an oversimplification, however, to say that the disproportionate number of middle and upper-middle class patients who are receiving kidney treatment is due simply to the physicians' prejudice. Rather, the physicians feel that they face an ethical dilemma in the selection of patients for treatment. Many of them believe that a willingness to cooperate with the strenuous requirements of the dialysis program is vital for the success of the patient in dialysis. The dialysis patient must be able to take directions and to understand the necessity for complying with the most minute details of his medical program. Intelligence and education, many physicians feel, play a part in the patient's ability to see the need for such a program and to execute it. To use intelligence and education as selection criteria, however, once again serves to insure that the more privileged, better-educated, middle- and upper-middle class kidney patient will have an advantage over the lower-class patient in need of treatment.

There are some safeguards, and, in effect, "advantages," for lower-class patients, but such measures do not apply uniformly to all.

For instance, under the federally financed Medicaid program, there is a provision (Title 19) which pays for some hospital bills of patients whose incomes are low enough. In some states, kidney patients can receive assistance only if they pass a means test or if they are on welfare. For example, in one state a prospective patient cannot be earning more than $2200 a year (with an additional allowance of $500 for each child), his cash assets must not be greater than $1000, and his property assets must not exceed $15,000. If his assets are greater than these amounts, he will be expected to contribute toward the transplant. In a case of nonpayment, moreover, the hospital can put a lien on all of his property except his home in an attempt to collect the bill. (Obviously, although these requirements may assist some of the very poor, they may put the lower-middle class individual in a financial bind.)

The availability of treatment and finances is determined not only by the patient's income level but also by the locale in which he happens to live. Certain states have interpreted Title 19 of Medicaid to exclude dialysis and transplant patients completely. Frequently one transplant center must service many surrounding states, states which may have a less liberal interpretation of Title 19 than does the state in which the center is located. Hospitals cannot long stand the strain of unpaid bills and it is possible that some kidney centers may be forced to reject all but the wealthy out-of-state applicants.

The discrepancy between states is further widened by the fact that eight states have set aside additional special monies to contribute to a kidney patient's care and treatment. It is clearly better to be sick in some states than in others.

Even the county of a patient's origin may be important. In

some states, the county decides on the patient's eligibility for Medicaid funds and may also contribute to the benefits. One expensive transplant operation, however, can exhaust a county's entire annual medical welfare budget and render it incapable of aiding a second transplant case.

At the present time, therefore, given the lack of national financial planning, it is likely that patients are being denied treatment on an arbitrary basis, such as their financial status or their state or even county of origin.

There is an additional ethical problem in the selection of patients for dialysis or transplantation: that is, whether or not to use psychological or psychiatric evaluations in the decision-making process. Psychiatric prediction is always difficult to make with certainty and, more important, kidney disease itself can cause intellectual impairment.

There appear to be psycho-physical effects of severe kidney disease that are partly chemical in origin and that are improved but not eliminated by dialysis. Among these are apathy, inability to concentrate, irritability, depression, and intellectual impairment—as revealed in slow speech, erratic memory, confusion, and lower performance on intelligence tests and other psychological tests. In severe cases, a psychosis with paranoic hallucinations can develop.

Whereas a successful transplant operation can eliminate some, if not all of these symptoms, the question for the medical judges is whether a psychiatrist can predict the reaction of a severely ill patient to the medical therapy accurately enough to grant him, or to refuse him, life-saving treatment.

Whatever the answer, some centers attempt to do just this. One center refused a young man a transplant operation on the grounds that his operation would be extraordinarily expensive and that such funds should not be wasted on someone of his moral character. (The young man had a history of glue-sniffing.) Another center accepted him, performed a successful transplant on him, and found that he responded by a dramatic physical as well as psychological improvement. He has since obtained a full-time job.

THE DONOR: WHO SHOULD BE USED AND HOW SHOULD HIS WELFARE BE PROTECTED?

The patient's opportunity to receive an organ transplant is limited not only by the selection procedures for obtaining access to the scarce medical and financial resources; his chances are limited also by the fact that in every operation a second person, a donor, is required.

Transplant operations are performed using either living, related donors or cadaver donors. As mentioned earlier, patients who receive a kidney from a living relative do twice as well as do those patients who receive a cadaver kidney from a person unrelated to them. With these facts in mind, two contradictory ethical questions arise: (1) Is it ethical to use a cadaver donor and give the recipient a diminished chance of a successful transplant? and (2) Is it ethical to utilize a living donor and possibly jeopardize one life in order to try to save another?

Several articles have been written about the ethical dangers of transplantation and in many of these, a major concern has been that the poor and powerless will be exploited as donors for more advantaged citizens. The concern has also been expressed that dying patients or their families will be under pressure to donate and that the potential donor will be given less good medical care.

It is reasonable to expect that a physician would feel caught on the horns of a dilemma, caught, that is, between his need to protect the patient who might be a potential donor and his obligation to the prospective transplant recipient to obtain for him as useful an organ as possible.

Living Related Donors

Physicians are aware of the fact that almost all patients with kidneys from living related donors do well, whereas more than half of the cadaver recipients return, sooner or later, with irreversible kidney rejection. There is considerable uncertainty and controversy among physicians, however, with regard to the use of living donors. Some physicians argue that it is unethical to allow the sacrifice of a normal organ with the chance of jeopardizing a normal life. In a fundamental sense, the situation is contrary to medical norms and expectations. *Primum non nocere,* "first of all, do no harm," is a traditional medical rule. The doctor's task is to help cure patients. Asking a relative to donate a kidney can be stressful for the physician and virtually unparalleled in his experience. In this situation, he is placed in the situation of having to ask a person to assume a surgical risk and to undergo a major operation with no physical benefit to himself. The surgical risk, although small, is nonetheless a factor to consider. It has been estimated that there is a 1-out-of-2000 chance that the donor will lose his life during the operation and a 1-out-of-1500 chance that the donor's life will be endangered on a long-term basis.

Although no deaths or major complications have as yet been reported because of organ donation, the physicians fully realize that as more living donors are used, donor deaths or medical complications can be expected to occur. This dilemma has been widely discussed but no clear rules have emerged to guide the physician except for the necessity of "informed consent". It is agreed that the prospective donor must be informed about the degree of risk and the inconveniences that will occur. There is no agreement, however, concerning the degree of effort a doctor should exert to secure a family donor, nor about the method he should use.

It has been found, in many instances, that there is a positive effect on the donor as a result of donation: he often experiences feelings of greater self-esteem and, in fact, may think of himself as something of a hero. Psychiatrists Fellner and Marshall, in their study of donor reactions, found that donors, in speaking of their feelings about the donation, often used such phrases as: "I feel better, kind of noble. I am changed. I have passed a milestone in my life, more confidence, more self-esteem," or "my whole life is different. I've done something with my life."[4] If kidney donation enhances the donor's self-esteem, then some of the ethical concerns about the morality of taking from one living individual to give to another might be less urgent. Intensive investigation is needed, however, of the donor's reactions when the transplant is unsuccessful and the kidney is rejected. In such an instance, the initial rise in self-esteem might possibly be replaced with feelings of intense depression over the fact that the sacrifice was for "nothing".

The question of who within the family should be a donor for a relative with kidney failure sometimes presents ethical and emotional problems for the entire family. In most cases, the decision to donate appears to be a relatively smooth, satisfying procedure. Sometimes it is difficult, however, to find a medically acceptable and willing donor.

Parents seem to feel a great obligation to donate for their children, if possible—an obligation which, incidentally, is not often felt in reverse. The National Kidney Registry statistics show that few recipients have received kidneys from their children. This fact, however, is due both to the general unwillingness of children to donate to a parent as well as to the fact that most kidney recipients have been too young to have children of a legal age. Siblings also seem to be less willing to donate to their ill brother or sister than are the parents.

Many questions arise with respect to who should be allowed to donate. Some critics of the use of living, related donors fear that undue family pressure may be applied in order to force the donation. For instance, should minors be allowed to donate? Or, should relatives institutionalized due to retardation or mental illness be allowed to be used as donors? There is, of course, a very great danger that the use of such persons may be more a result of coercion than of willingness on their part. Hospitals have been unwilling to make these decisions themselves and, in several instances, have placed the matter in the hands of the court. In some cases, minors and institutionalized relatives have been approved as donors, after the court concluded that the death of the recipient would be psychologically disadvantageous for the potential donor in question. These decisions are controversial, however, and it is unclear how a general precedent will be established.

In several cases, "black sheep" members of the family have been known to donate with the hope that this act on their part will, once and for all, prove their worth to the family. Many members of the family may be affected by the need to find a related donor. Nondonors, that is, members of the family who could have donated but do not, may feel great feelings of ambivalence and sometimes experience feelings of guilt.

Conflicts which appear prior to the transplant, however, may be resolved by a successful transplantation; the nondonor's guilt may be eased, the donor's self-esteem may be enhanced, as the patient is enabled to assume something other than a dependent, invalided status within the family.

The Cadaver Donor

Many kidney transplant operations performed today, however, rely upon a cadaver donor. There are two major reasons for this. First, some centers do not encourage the use of living donors, and second, in certain cases it proves to be impossible to find a medically suitable related donor. In these instances, the kidney patient must rely upon a cadaver donor and hope that a suitable kidney will be made available in time to help him. Inasmuch as the organs of elderly patients are not useful, a suitable donor is almost always a young person who is the victim of an accident or who is suffering from brain disease.

The potential "cadaver" donor when first seen is usually a comatose patient whose own life chances are felt to be hopeless and whose brain has ceased to function almost entirely, if not entirely.

Because of the widespread ethical concern about the medical treatment of the dying donor, new rules and guidelines have emerged. For instance, to prevent a conflict of interest on the part of the physician between the donor and the recipient, it has been agreed generally that the prospective donor should be cared for by one group of physicians and the prospective recipient by another. The transplant team, therefore, is not involved in the declaration of the donor's death and it is easier for everyone involved to avoid the accusation of having in any way hastened it.

Another ethical problem arises over whether the two teams of physicians should consult with each other at all in the treatment of the dying donor. For example, if the fluid balance of the potential donor is neglected, as occurs sometimes with patients who are considered hopeless, their kidneys will be useless at the time of their death. Should the transplant team therefore be allowed to intervene in his care and suggest a change in treatment? There is no question that a donor's own chance for life must be protected, and usually what is good for the kidney—or for the heart, or liver, or lungs—is also good for the patient. In fact, there have been instances in which patients who were expected to die recovered because of just such intervention and advice on the part of the recipient's physician concerning the care and treatment of the donor's kidney. Yet some have questioned the ethics of instituting certain treatments or procedures which are designed primarily to benefit the needed organ.

The medical treatment of a cadaver donor raises a larger issue and one that has been a problem for physicians for some time, namely, how long should any apparently hopeless patient be kept alive by extraordinary medical means? In the case of organ transplantation, contrary to certain fears, an unconscious, brain-damaged donor frequently is kept alive longer than normally would be the case, because of the anticipated donation. Had such a patient not been selected as a donor, much of the extraordinary treatment intended to keep his body "alive" after his brain has ceased funtioning would have been stopped. For instance, the respirator machine would have been turned off, corrective fluids and blood transfusions would not have been given, and cardiac massage would not have been administered if the heart had stopped. For the potential transplant donor, all such emergency procedures are instituted. Of course, such measures may prolong the agony of the family for a few days. They are told that although death has not been pronounced, their relative is essentially dead. During this waiting period, it is possible that the family alternates between feelings of hope and despair, and they may even question their decision to donate the organs of the dying patient.

The question of exactly when death occurs is a vital one for transplant surgery. The original definition of death which depended upon the cecession of the heart, and with it, a cecession of the circulation of blood to the parts of the body, posed a great problem for transplant surgery. It is technically possible with new machines to maintain a patient's heartbeat and respiration long after his brain has ceased all function. A new definition of death was needed for the new technology, a definition which would allow for the maintenance of the circulatory system of the body until the time of transplantation but one which would not imply that the organs were being taken from a still-living individual. The concept of "brain death" promoted by Beecher, at Harvard, seemed to fulfill both of these requirements. According to his definition, death occurs when the brain is dead, whether or not the heartbeat is being maintained.

Although Beecher's definition of death has been accepted by most, there was, and still is, some conflict over the measurement of brain death. Some physicians use some of Beecher's guidelines but do not use brainwaves at all in determining when death has occurred. Other physicians believe that a period of three to four hours without brain waves is sufficient to declare the patient dead. Still others insist that 24 to 48 hours must pass without brain waves before *they* are willing to pronounce the death.

Essentially the issue is not so much one of when a death has occurred as much as it is one of which criteria to use in determining it. In other words, most physicians feel fully capable of being able to diagnose brain death and of being able to decide when a patient is dead. But because they are anxious to avoid criticism, they feel bound—in the face of so much publicity about the issue —to utilize one set of criteria or another so as to be able to point to some objective sign of the death.

It is likely that the question of when death occurs will remain an issue among medical practitioners for some time—as will the question of whether a definition of death should be formulated specifically to serve the needs of a new medical technology.

These ethical issues are aggravated further by the limited number of cadaver donor organs that are available at any particular time. Given the total number of kidney patients who could benefit from a transplant operation, there is always a serious shortage of organs available. At the present time, although many persons have signed donor cards willing their organs for transplantation in the event of their untimely death, cadaver organ donation still depends largely upon the willingness of the next-of-kin to donate the organs of a dying relative. The physician must approach the family with the proposal to donate the organs at a tragic moment for the family: frequently just after they have learned that their relative has been the victim of a fatal accident. Many physicians find this exceedingly difficult to do, particularly when they must press the family to make a decision as quickly as possible in order to facilitate the medical procedures that must be followed.

It has been suggested that one way to secure cadaver organs and to avoid the problems of "time" and family trauma would be to utilize the organs of persons whose bodies would be unclaimed after their death. For example, under a law which exists now in Virginia, the medical examiner can give permission for the use of organs for transplantation without the consent of the kin or prior consent of the individual if the case falls under his jurisdiction, if no kin can be located, and if there are no known objections. It has been suggested that this type of law be extended to give the state the right to use the organs from any individual who has not indicated prior disapproval. At this point in time it is unclear whether the removal of organs without the consent of the family or the donor would be acceptable to the American public. The fear that this type of law might be extended into as yet unknown but potentially dangerous or unethical practices might militate against its general adoption. On the other hand, its general adoption would assure a more adequate supply of organs for all types of organ transplant operations.

Living, Unrelated Donors

Many of the problems associated with both cadaver donors and living related donors would be eliminated, or at least greatly reduced, if living, unrelated donors were to be used as volunteers. There is a very serious question, however, as to whether such persons should be used at all. The medical problems which apply to the living related donor apply as well to the living unrelated donor: he will have to undergo the surgical procedure with its associated short-term and long-term risks to his life with no physical benefit to himself. There could, of course, be a derivative psychological benefit; like the related donor, the unrelated living donor could experience a boost in his self-esteem as a result of his willingness to save the life of another individual. One center in California has experimented with living unrelated donors and has found such a response among them.

It has been the hope of surgeons who have conducted these operations that the added time allowed to match living unrelated donors and potential recipients would produce results better than those obtained by using cadaver donors. It is the feeling of many physicians, however, that living unrelated donors will not give results that are significantly better than cadaver donors and that it is unethical, therefore, to utilize this source.

At one time, inmates of penal institutions were used as volunteer donors. This practice has since been discontinued on the grounds that however equitably it may have been handled in particular instances, there was a grave danger that an expansion of such a practice would lead to the abuse of prisoners' rights.

The President of the Transplantation Society, Dr. Hamburger, has pointed to one grave threat that he believes may occur with the use of living unrelated donors, that is, that organs will be sold rather than donated. He notes that if such a system were instituted, other dangers could follow, particularly the dangers of blackmail, of exploitation of the poor, and of the possible use of coercion in certain societies to obtain organs. There are those who are less opposed to the sale of organs for transplantation than is Dr. Hamburger. They argue that there should be no legal proscription now against the purchase of an organ since such a law might be unnecessarily restrictive in the future. Still others see little objection to the buying of an organ at the present time if that is the only way a kidney patient can obtain one. Payment for an organ, they argue, moreover, would possibly relieve the recipient of his feelings of obligation toward the donor —a feeling which has been noted in several instances involving living related donors.

It should be noted, however, that at present most transplant facilities are heavily supported by public funds. If the limited facilities for organ transplant operations are to be used by recipients who can afford to purchase an organ, there will be even less opportunity for the poor to secure treatment. Not only would the poor be unable to compete with the rich for the purchase of an organ (it is possible that the price of an organ would involve thousands of dollars) but also, it is likely that such an opportunity for donor remuneration would sharply cut down the supply of freely donated organs from relatives and cadaver families.

The Transplantation Society has passed a resolution forbidding the sale of organs, and while this resolution does not have the force of law, the compliance of the transplant centers is reflected in the fact that at the present time no center permits the sale or purchase of an organ. Nonetheless, this issue is not entirely settled, particularly with the prospect of more living unrelated donors in the future.

SHOULD TRANSPLANTATION BE ENCOURAGED AT ALL?

Technological advances in medicine are extremely expensive and often require governmental support, particularly in the initial stages. It has been estimated that the cost of a kidney transplant operation now averages about $13,300. In addition, the yearly cost of follow-up medical care can run anywhere from 200 to $1000. If the operation is not successful, the patient may be faced with the need for a second transplant or perpetual hemodialysis. Such dialysis at a hospital center costs approximately $14,000 a year. If it is possible for the patient to obtain a home dialysis machine, which costs between 10,000 and 12,000 dollars, there will still be a yearly cost to him of approximately $4,000.

The costs of heart transplant operations are even higher. One study has estimated that the average heart transplant now costs $18,777, although charges as high as $102,500 have been reported. It has been estimated, moreover, that between 7,000 and 8,000 persons per year could benefit from dialysis or kidney transplant operations and that perhaps as many as 22,000 patients per year might be able to benefit from heart transplantation. If heart transplant technology improves enough to treat all of these patients annually, the cost might reach $200 million a year.

As additional medical technologies develop, the government increasingly will be confronted with a fundamental decision: is it possible and/or reasonable for this society to allocate major sums of money in order to save the lives of the previously incurable? It was recommended by the Committee of Chronic Kidney Disease that the Bureau of the Budget expend $800 million to $1 billion during the years 1969 to 1975 for the training of transplant personnel, for needed facilities, and for the actual care of kidney patients. Such funds have not as yet been allocated.

The decision must be made as to whether the potential benefits of the new technology will justify the costs and, moreover, whether this expenditure is as important as, or more important than, other critical needs of our society. Some physicians object to enormous sums of money being spent on transplantation to the exclusion of other health needs, particularly the basic health and nutritional needs of the poor. On the other hand, there are those who argue that if defense costs were cut and medical aid was increased, our society could afford to pay for all of its medical needs.

The high cost of heart transplantation, coupled with its infrequent success, has made this area particularly subject to attack both by leading medical persons and others. Some have, in fact, suggested a moratorium on all heart transplant operations.

An editorial in a well-known public health journal questions the expenditure of large sums of money on organ transplant operations in general, claiming that other medical programs contribute to the health of more persons for less cost. The editorial goes on to point, critically, to the adverse psychological and physical consequences for the recipient of a transplant operation. Evidence of adverse psychological consequences for kidney recipients is, however, not clear enough to warrant restricting this life-saving operation, although some patients do suffer physical side-effects from the drugs they must take following the operation. These drugs are necessary to prevent their body from rejecting the new kidney. In particular, the face and body may swell, acne may occur, there may be hair loss, and a bone damage may occur which can impair the recipient's ability to walk. Most of the serious problems, however, seem to occur shortly after transplantation or in patients whose body constantly threatens to reject the new kidney. There is certainly no evidence to suggest that patients who have undergone a successful transplantation are any worse off, psychologically or physically, than they were prior to the operation, or, for that matter, that they are any worse off than are patients on perpetual hemodialysis. In fact, the evidence seems to suggest that following a successful transplant they, like the donor, experience a boost in self-esteem and a feeling of having been given a second chance in life. Their vocational rehabilitation, moreover, seems excellent. It has been reported by one transplant center, for instance, that for those patients who have not rejected their kidneys six months or more after the operation, 88 percent (56/64) were working full-time, or were fully active as housewives, or had returned to school.

The fact that such rehabilitation is possible would seem to argue for the continuation of organ transplantation and for the establishment of a national policy to ensure that all persons, regardless of income, educational level, or geographical origin, can have an equal opportunity to receive this treatment. Even if such a policy is instituted, however, many ethical problems will persist, particularly those concerning the organ donor. Whether the society can effect changes in the needed areas within a short period of time, and in the face of many other compelling demands, remains an open question.

REFERENCES

1. Hollingshead, A. B. and Redlich, F. C.: *Social Class and Mental Illness.* New York, John Wiley and Sons, 1958. Sudnow, D.: *Passing On, The Social Organization of Dying.* Englewood Cliffs, Prentice-Hall, 1967.

2. Katz, A. and Proctor, D.: Social-psychological Characteristics of Patients Receiving Hemodialysis Treatment for Chronic Renal Failure: Report of Questionnaire Survey of Dialysis Centers and Patients during 1967. United States Government Printing Office, July, 1969.

3. Katz, A. and Proctor, D.: *Social-psychological Characteristics of Patients Receiving Hemodialysis Treatment for Chronic Renal Failure.* Report of Questionnaire Survey of Dialysis Centers and Patients during 1967. United States Government Printing Office, July 1969.

4. Fellner, C. H. and Marshall, J. R.: Twelve kidney donors. *J.A.M.A., 206*:2703, 1968.

Chapter 12

LUNG TRANSPLANTATION

Max J. Trummer, M.D.

Experimental transplantation of the lung was first reported by Demikhov at the All Union Thoracic Surgery Congress in Moscow in 1947; however, his work did not become known generally in the western world until the translation of his book appeared in 1962. Meanwhile, independent efforts were reported from France, Italy and Argentina in 1950 and from the United States in 1951. In spite of the fact that nearly twenty-five years have passed since its inception, lung transplantation has not achieved the widespread clinical application that would seem warranted by the need for replacement of lungs which have been destroyed by emphysema, scarring of the lungs, diseases of the blood vessels within the lung, and by cancer. To date (early 1971), only twenty-six transplantations of either whole lungs or lobes have been accomplished in patients throughout the world. Only one of these patients lived for as long as ten months. Why, in this era of organ transplantation, has the lung not yielded to the efforts of hundreds of medical researchers?

Perhaps first and foremost is the immunologic barrier presented by the inherent response of the body to foreign tissue, whereby the body tries to reject it. The problem of rejection in the case of the lung is particularly difficult for several reasons. Antigenically speaking, the lung rates very high in its ability to excite a reaction from its host. Some tissues have the ability to excite a more violent response from the host than do others. If we were to rank tissues in regard to this characteristic, skin would rank at the top and would be followed not too far behind by the lung, whereas the heart and the kidney would place farther down on this scale. To compound the problem, the delicate

189

structure of the lung, which was designed to permit the easy exchange of oxygen and CO_2 between the air in the alveoli and the blood in the adjacent capillaries, is particularly susceptible to the rejection response which is mounted by the host against the donor lung. In order to successfully suppress the rejection reaction, it first must be recognized and its degree of severity must be measured in order to be able to appropriately adjust the treatment schedule. Whereas in the case of the kidney, the state of rejection can be judged fairly accurately from relatively simple tests of the blood and the urine, and in the case of the heart much information can be obtained from the electrocardiogram, there is no reliable or simple test to identify and measure the rejection response to the lung. Unfortunately, the X-ray appearance of the transplanted lung is identical, whether it is involved by pneumonia or by rejection. None of the available pulmonary function tests provide characteristics which are specific for the rejection process. As a matter of fact, clear-cut differentiation between rejection and infection is frequently impossible even at autopsy.

Unfortunately, the present techniques for suppressing the rejection reaction of the host usually act in a nonspecific manner by suppressing the general immune response of the body. Therefore, in order to achieve suppression of the host's immune reaction to the organ graft, one must pay the price of also suppressing his immune responses against infection. The lung, in contrast to other organs, is constantly exposed to the bacteria present in the air that we breathe. Therefore, both the lung graft and the opposite normal lung of the recipient are particularly susceptible to infection while the host is under treatment to suppress the immune response.

A second major obstacle to success in transplanting lungs is the fact that there is not available a satisfactory method for long-term artificial support of respiration. The patient who needs a kidney transplant can be maintained for months by the use of an artificial kidney machine (hemodialysis) while awaiting an appropriate donor. In case he experiences a rejection crisis after receiving a kidney transplant he can be tided over this period while the rejection crisis is being treated and until his kidney graft has an opportunity to recover. Furthermore, hemodialysis is required in this instance only on an intermittent basis. A method for continuous respiration by means of an artificial lung has not been perfected as yet, although great strides have been made in this direction. Indeed, it may be ultimately possible to develop an artificial lung of such efficiency and small size that it can be permanently implanted within the patient's chest, thus obviating the need for an organ transplant.

A third major problem relates to the preservation of organ grafts. For greatest efficiency and availability, the ideal would be to devise a system whereby organs could be stored indefinitely and kept in organ banks from which they could be sent to the patient whose own tissues most closely matched the tissue type of the donor. Great progress has been made in this direction in the case of kidney transplantation, to the point that the graft can be shipped to a distant city in order to match the donor wih the best recipient. The delicate structure of the lung and its susceptibility to damage has once again thwarted most efforts in this direction. The lung is most intolerant to the flushing of its blood vessels with any kind of solution, and the viability of its cells can be only slightly prolonged by recourse to freezing or to subjecting it to storage in oxygen under pressure. To date, of the limited means available for increasing the functional survival of the lung, perhaps the best has been to rhythmically inflate the lung with an atmosphere similar to that which is normally present within the alveoli (air sacs) of the lung.

Even though the lung is a paired organ, as is the kidney, the degree of pulmonary reserve available is not great enough to justify asking for the donation of a lung or lobe from a living donor. This brings us to the fourth major problem, and that is the source from which we are to obtain lung grafts. Because we do not feel justified in requesting a graft from a living donor, and because present storage techniques are unsatisfactory, lung grafts may be obtained only from cadaver donors. The graft must be removed immediately following death, and the donor must be a relatively young person whose lung is not itself damaged by emphysema or involved by cancer. Ideally, the donor should not have been subjected to prolonged respiratory support im-

mediately prior to death because such patient's lungs are frequently heavily involved by pneumonia. The most desirable
donor would be a patient who was young and otherwise healthy
and who died as the result of accidental trauma. However, since
most such patients either have some direct or indirect damage to
the lungs, or in modern medical practice are usually supported
for prolonged periods of time by respiratory assistance, the choice
of donor becomes narrowed to a patient who suffered isolated
head injury or who may have sustained an intracranial hemorrhage. In these situations, it is possible to determine fairly early
that irreversible brain death has occurred, in which case it is
useless to support the patient's respirations and circulation artificially for an indefinite period of time.

The decisions concerning whether to continue to artificially
sustain such patients or whether to accept the fact that irreversible brain death has occurred are obviously fraught with enormous moral, ethical, and legal considerations which are beyond
the scope of this chapter. One of the rules which has been
established in organ transplantation has been that the decisions
concerning the treatment of a patient who is a potential donor
must reside with the team of physicians who is concerned with
that patient's care and that no member of the transplant team
may participate in these decisions.

A fifth major problem is a physiologic one. In the case of
experimental lung transplantation the opposite lung of the experimental animal is normal. However, in the clinical setting, a
patient would not become a candidate for a lung graft if he did
not have extensive lung disease which most likely would involve
both lungs. This means, then, that the lung graft which the host
would receive would be an essentially normal lung, whereas his
opposite own lung which he would retain would continue to
be a diseased lung. The common types of conditions which effect
the lung to such a degree as to warrant consideration for transplantation usually result in two major changes in the architecture
of the lung. First, the elastic properties of the lung which govern
the ease with which it can be ventilated are altered, and secondly,
the resistance to the flow of blood through the blood vessels of the
lung is usually increased. Therefore, if a normal lung is placed

in a parallel circuit with such a diseased lung it may be anticipated that the flow of blood to the lungs would preferentially
go to the transplanted lung because its vascular resistance was
less. Ventilation, on the other hand, would tend to overinflate
the retained diseased lung where the forces of elastic recoil were
less. This latter phenomenom would result in over expansion
of the patient's own diseased lung which eventually would com-
press the opposite transplanted lung. In clinical practice this
situation actually has arisen and has presented an extremely difficult problem in management. In certain instances this problem
has been insuperable and has resulted in the patient's death.
Possible solutions to this dilemna would be to select only those
patients whose disease was characterized by restriction of pulmonary activity by fibrosis or scarring. Or else, in the case of patients
with emphysema, to transplant both lungs. The two lungs might
be transplanted individually or might be installed as an organ
block including the heart. Clinical attempts have been made with
each of these techniques, but thus far there has not been long-
term success.

The sixth major obstacle is infection. This has already been
mentioned above as one of the complications of the techniques
used to suppress the immune reaction of the host. However, the
problem of infection deserves emphasis because thus far in the
clinical experience with lung transplantation infection has represented the single most common cause of death. The patient
who is a potential lung recipient usually has a chronic bronchitis
and has experienced repeated episodes of pneumonia. When the
decision is finally made to recommend a lung graft, the potential
recipient often has reached the point where his respiration requires continuous assistance, usually by way of a tracheotomy.
Therefore, at the time that the recipient receives a lung graft his
own tracheal bronchial tree may be the site of infection with
virulent or resistant organisms. Furthermore, as mentioned above,
the potential donor may also have been on prolonged respiratory
assistance via a tracheostomy and likewise his lungs may have
been subject to pneumonia. In the case of infection by organisms
which are resistant to the available antibiotics, all of the immune
mechanisms of the host would be called upon to overcome such

infection. Yet, at that very time the host immune response has to be suppressed in order to permit survival of the graft. The host is at a further disadvantage because changes may occur in the cough reflex and in the mucous secretion and ciliary activity of the lining of the bronchial tree of the lung graft which render it less able to handle its own secretions. A major thrust of present research in the field of organ transplantation is directed towards the development of specific biologic methods of immune suppression which will permit survival of the grafted organ without interferring with the body's general ability to combat infection.

With these obstacles to the success of lung transplantation, in the present state of the art, lung transplantation is not in the established status which has been achieved already by kidney transplantation. Efforts along the direction of lung transplantation must continue but they must do so in a carefully controlled manner. Criteria which are generally accepted for the selection and identification of a potential candidate for a lung transplant require that the patient must have undergone continuous deterioration of his lung function in spite of the very best care that is available. In spite of the fact that such a patient requires a continuous supplement of oxygen, he nevertheless must have failed to show improvement in the laboratory determinations of his blood oxygen levels or respiratory mechanics. Such a patient must have required frequent and almost continuous hospitalization for respiratory failure. And finally, such a patient must be suitable psychologically for this type of experimental clinical undertaking. The transplantation itself should be performed by a team experienced and skilled in this field who not only can do the best possible operative procedure but afterwards can skillfully manage the rejection reaction and provide the type of isolation atmosphere which the patient might require. In addition, such a team must be trained and equipped to thoroughly study such a patient and to make appropriate observations in order that the problems mentioned above may be solved.

It has been fortunate indeed that the lung, even though it is equally as essential to life as the heart, nevertheless does not share the emotional mysticism of the heart. It has been possible therefore for the research endeavors which will set the stage for successful clinical transplantation of the lung to proceed in an orderly manner. Perhaps this conservatism fails to satisfy the impatience of some individuals, and undoubtedly patients are dying who might live if there were some way to replace their destroyed lungs. In the opinion of the writer, however, this is a situation wherein haste will be made slowly; and if a solid foundation is laid we will ultimately benefit the greatest number of patients while subjecting the fewest number of patients to the least risk.

Chapter 13

DEATH, BEREAVEMENT, AND TRANSPLANTING HEARTS AND LUNGS: SOME PSYCHO-SOCIAL OBSERVATIONS AND SOME CLINICAL COMMENTS

ERIC BERMANN
"After the first death, there is no other."
—Dylan Thomas

INTRODUCTION

The basis for this paper is a modest clinical experience with persons who (1) faced imminent death, and (2) nurtured a wild hope that was ambivalently charged. It consists of a series of observations resulting from interaction with half-a-dozen men who were candidates for organ transplantation.*

My involvement with the six men came about as a result of a two-year participation as a member of the heart transplant team at a major university hospital. My role was that of mental health worker on the team. Initially, my function had been conceived as evaluative. As will be seen, however, the psychologically driven character of these men pressed toward more extensive involvement. It is the nature of this involvement that is detailed in the pages that follow.

First, however, it should be recognized that any paper which seeks to describe a very few of the psychological aspects of organ transplants is bound as well to become a paper about certain features of our contemporary society. Try as one might to con-

---

*Of the six men, five were candidates for heart transplantation and one for lung transplantation. Only four actually underwent transplant surgery. Three men have died following transplantation; one died awaiting surgery; one heart recipient is living, and one man still waits for a heart as of this writing.

scientiously delimit its scope, it becomes perforce a paper that comments on technological advances, cultural values and priorities, family organization and, perhaps most especially, on attitudes toward death, dying and the process of mourning. This is, perhaps, as it should be.

In a very real sense then the results of work with organ transplants to be reported here do not primarily represent contributions to knowledge on how to do better transplants, though they may help in this regard. Neither is this paper concerned with moral or ethical issues related to whether transplants should or should not be done. Rather, the crisis of the transplant patient is viewed as a crucible for learning about the character of routine events, their cultural contexts, their interpersonal meanings, as well as a crucible which provides opportunities for gaining information about the psychological interior of people and the long-standing, unverbalized assumptions they harbor. This paper is as much about people as it is about transplants.

THEMES AND NONTHEMES OF HEART AND LUNG TRANSPLANT CANDIDATES

What does a lonely and frightened man, who is trying to simultaneously prepare himself for death and rebirth, want to talk about? What does he not want to talk about? And, most prominently, why does he choose to talk about some things and not others? The remainder of this chapter is devoted to providing some partial answers to these questions.*

Nontheme Number One: The Transplantation Itself

It might be logically assumed that any man who has recently made the momentous decision to undergo heart transplant surgery would have a predilection for talking about little else. In fact,

---

*The answers are necessarily partial for a number of reasons, as should become apparent as one reads. It should, of course, also be kept in mind that these were seriously, degeneratively ill men who, without the transplant, were not expected to live more than a few weeks. Many had been ill for some time—their illness often involving years of debilitation. Some had been continuously hospitalized for better than the last half year. There was much reason to anticipate psychological upset about the coming transplant and the uncertainties of waiting for a donor, but the impact of general malaise and long hospitalization should not be overlooked.

this is not so. Five of the six candidates did not spontaneously converse about their impending surgery. Three of them out-and-out assiduously avoided it, and two would have avoided it if environmental circumstances had not stimulated them to competitive terror about receiving new hearts and lungs.* Thus, when Mr. M, a heart transplant candidate, in the first ten minutes of the first interview informed me that he and his wife had mutually agreed to his having the transplant, and that he did not consciously wish to consider or debate the matter further, he fully meant it.

It was virtually the last time before his surgery—some two weeks and some half-dozen visits later—that Mr. M spontaneously mentioned the topic. While on occasion I would raise it with him, Mr. M was true to his word. He either quickly moved away from contemplating it, or he used it as a springboard to discussions of other manifestly unrelated matters. He acted in almost every way as if the transplant procedure had no intrinsic interest for him. And, as indicated, he was far from being alone among the heart and lung transplant candidates in this regard.

Thus, details of the approaching surgery itself, as well as its sequelae, the nature of the postsurgical regimen, the physical pain and stress to be anticipated, the expected length of the recuperative process, the odds of rejection, the need for antirejection steroids, the physical and hormonal changes attached to the use of steroids, the likelihood of medically induced diabetes, were

---

*Both these men suffered through unusually long preoperative waits, were given, from day to day, conflicting messages by medical staff regarding whether transplant surgery ought after all to be attempted, and were occasionally housed in rooms so proximal that they could not help but be keenly aware of each other's presence and hopes. Environmental circumstances and hospital staff simply did not permit these men to avoid concern about surgery. Significantly enough, when environmental input of this kind was minimal, these men did not discuss the coming transplant, but whined and complained instead about the inconveniences and discomforts of hospitalization. The single exception among the six candidates was a man who could literally think and talk of nothing else but the transplantation. He read extensively about the procedure, spent considerable amounts of time clipping out relevant newspaper and magazine articles for his scrapbooks, and took almost any opportunity to speculate aloud and with evident counterphobic glee on his chances for survival. He remained, however, the distinctive exception to the rule.

all tuned out and left undiscussed by the candidates. Trying to envision with them, or for them, in the gentlest of ways, the psychological prospects and attendant meanings of giving up their own diseased heart and having it replaced in their chest by the healthy heart of an unknown deceased donor, who for a lifetime had carried it in his chest, proved totally impossible. It was untouchably beyond their pale.

One need not search extensively for reasons which caused these men to so avoid the theme of their transplantation. Some ready explanations abound. One, there is the fear that results from the very real prospect of death before or shortly after heart or lung transplantation.* Newspaper accounts had made the survival rate in these surgeries a matter of public record and knowledge. Less publicized, but no secret, was the reporting of that percentage of candidates who had died awaiting donors. The six men need hardly have been informed of the latter figures. Either way they knew how precipitously close to death they were and what kind of race with time they were in. Some quite literally expressed a terror of separation, of being left alone, reverberating as they were not only to matters of decathexis but to an unrecognized and therefore unarticulated fear that they might suffer a heart arrest or breathing spasm before they could signal for help or reach their oxygen. The presence of another person served to enhance their chance for continued life. Hence, despite the fact that they did not talk about such things, one had every reason to believe that each of these men had an inward subjective, if not objective, awareness of his odds for survival. It could only be expected, then, that they would each indulge denial—a denial of death which while personalized in its particulars would none-

---

*The chances for death are great, and death can come in two ways. First, time may simply run out for the transplant candidate and he dies of the heart or lung malfunction. One of the six candidates in this author's sample died waiting for a donor. This may be compared with the figures reported from Stanford University Medical School as of March 1970. To that date Stanford had had thirty-two heart transplant candidates. Twelve died awaiting surgery. Second, death may occur during or right after surgery. Two of the six candidates in this sample had donors, but, by all practical criteria, failed to survive the surgery. Two lived substantially beyond surgery.

theless bear the stamp of commonly shared and socially encouraged attitudes.

But these men had even further reason to evade overt and explicit consideration of their planned transplantation. They had reason to avoid because their conscious wish for life was inextricably bound to its tabooed counterpart—namely, that another human being should die for them or in their place.

The terror of this wish can be palpably experienced by another. One only has to be with a transplant candidate—in this instance Mr. T—when the cry of an ambulance siren, at first sounding afar, approaches the hospital with ever mounting intensity, only to quit suddenly in deafening silence at the emergency drive. Mr. T's conversation has stopped some moments ago and he is caught in an attitude of sudden quiet. The color has drained from his face, and he looks to the window of his ninth floor room expectantly. Seconds pass. When Mr. T speaks again he is flustered, breathy and by now red-faced. There is some momentary disorganization to his verbalizations. He stumbles through some sentences and then makes a noncontextual, curiously petty and derisive remark about the temperamental behavior of Mr. S, who occupies a room two doors down the hall. Mr. S is also awaiting a heart donor. Mr. T reports that two days earlier Mr. S complained bitterly and loudly in less than polite language to the nurses about having to wait for his dinner. Others he insisted had quite unfairly been served first. By the time he had received his meal it was "ice cold." The competitiveness between he and Mr. S has broken through. But Mr. T only appears puzzled as to why he recalls and relates this incident at this moment in time. He pauses, looking perplexed, but then laughs with a snort and continues. He assures me he has never behaved in such a fashion and that he is shocked at Mr. S—"Imagine a grown man . . . and to nurses." He looks to the door and comments that Dr. B should be by soon. He is expectant. But then he adds with a fair measure of irritation, "Dr. B never explains things anyway . . . never anything new, never any information . . . always the same old 'things will be O.K.'" Later I leave Mr. T's room and as I walk past the nurses' station one of the nurses calls to me. She tells me that Mr. S and Mr. T have been having temper tantrums through the week. The tantrums are over the serving of meals and snacks; both insist others have been served before them and that they are losing out. One does not have to be a clinician to recognize the equation between dinner and heart.

The wish that another should die so that he might live is at a minimum a frightening wish for a heart transplant candidate, for it is but one step removed from the reality of the situation and it calls into ready play not only a forbidden death wish but a host of fantasies and a lifetime of prohibited desires. The reality tempts to the surface of consciousness a set of fantasies and wishes compounded of distressing degrees of omnipotence, martyrdom, human sacrifice, miraculous rescue; and these contend with moralistic, ethical and just plain realistic considerations which, on their side, evoke guilt, questions of justifiability, obligation and deservedness. Who, after all, does one have to be, and what, if anything, good or bad, must one have done to deserve or purchase a second chance at life? These men have, then, some rather substantial reasons for denying their impending transplant surgery. The procedure is for them too overloaded with genetic and intrapsychic freight to be consciously tolerated on a day-to-day basis.

This brings us to yet another reason that the transplant candidate cannot openly face and discuss the transplant surgery. Added to the fear of extinction itself is the existential anxiety accruing from the uncertainty of when, where and how death will come.[30] For the heart or lung transplant candidate this degree of uncertainty reaches what may well be the heights of immoderateness. Surely, a great deal of the uncertainty attaches to the "when"—the "when" of death and the "when" of a donor and potential life. No one can specify a target date, nor can one offer much reassurance regarding goodness of match between donor or recipient, much less goodness of outcome.* Every ambulance siren, every visit from the surgeon, every episode of labored breathing becomes a reminder of both the hope and the dread. So too each visit from a relative or friend. Is the candidate to assume the worst and treat it as the last visit? Should he risk

---

*One does not even hint at certain other possible post-surgical sequelae, such as the one-in-three chance of transient psychosis that accompanies all open heart surgery.[2,22,33]

decathexis? Suppose that surgery were to succeed. What then?

The dangers of anticipatory grief reactions and premature decathexis have been remarked upon by others,[24,28] but perhaps nothing points up the dilemma that gives rise to these dangers better than the situation of the heart or lung transplant patient. Unlike the terminally ill and unlike those who are fairly certain of the when and how of their life crisis, the transplant candidate cannot fully afford to decathect. He may need the support of his objects for some time to come. On the other hand, he cannot comfortably maintain the full measure of his cathexis. He must prepare for the worst eventuality while trusting to the best. Caught betwixt and between, he exists almost literally in a state of suspended object relations. On a day-in day-out basis this proves virtually intolerable. It promotes—indeed requires—evasion of the central but unacknowledged topic and preoccupation, the transplantation itself. It reduces candidate and visiting wife, family or friend to hours of awkward silence or to platitudinous conversations that border on banality and leave the unspoken, covert theme as overt nontheme.

Several other factors come together to prevent these candidates from any conscious contemplation and open discussion of their anticipated transplantation. One of these factors has already been referred to on a couple of occasions and has to do with the social pressures to deny death and dying via courageous, if close-mouthed, stoicism on the part of the dying. Because of these pressures the process of dying is one rife with possibilities for mutual projection of fears, mutual trepidation regarding self-expression, and mutual evasion and withholding. One strange outcome is that it is most frequently the moribund and/or terminally ill who are to protect and comfort the living, sparing them anxiety and pain, not vice versa. The same social assumptions transfer to heart and lung transplant candidates. They do not discuss the procedure with others, partially to protect the others through magnanimous heroism.

Mr. I, a heart transplant candidate, epitomizes the altruistic with his recall of his second coronary—an attack which resulted in his hospitalization and the decision to undergo transplant surgery.

Mr. I states that his second attack occurred almost eighteen months after the first. Mr. I had arrived home and was seated on the living room couch discussing the events of the day with his wife. He then felt the familiar pain in his chest and he became quite "woozy." He commented matter of factly to his wife, "something is not right." She became concerned. He could see through his dizziness that she was getting upset and he tried to conceal his pain from her. She tried to get from Mr. I what specifically seemed to be wrong. Mr. I made every effort not to inform her of how he was actually feeling. He gripped the arm of the couch for "all I was worth" trying to keep himself alert, even smiling, but gradually losing ground. Still forcing a smile and enacting nonchalance, Mr. I felt himself "beginning to fade." Mrs. I kept pressing him for what was wrong and what if anything she could do. At this point in relating his story to me Mr. I began to cry. Amid sobs he stated that he had told his wife that she might remove his shoes. She had come over and untied and removed one shoe. Mr. I said that he never even saw her remove the other shoe. When he awoke he found himself in a hospital bed. Mr. I was now crying uncontrollably as he related these events to me. I discussed his crying with him. He stated that he felt extremely helpless—both then, at the time of his attack, and now in remembering it. To be sure a part of this feeling had to do with his loss of bodily control and consciousness. At one moment he had been feeling fine and in command, and in the next something had happened to his body and he felt powerless and couldn't move. And yet, significantly enough, this was not by his account the source of his terror or the major factor contributing to his sense of impotence. Rather, in his recounting, this terror and sense of helplessness, both in memory and in the present redintegration of the experience, were felt primarily as the wife's and only secondarily as his. The true realization of the gravity of what was occurring to him came from the mounting alarm and fright he discerned in his wife's face. Like a reflected appraisal he could read his plight in her eyes. And, clinging to her presence as a vestige of the real world as he resisted unconsciousness, it was Mrs. I who became the focus of his concern and fear. Afraid for her he was afraid for himself. By protecting and calming her he sought to calm and reassure himself. It was she who quite literally mediated his brush with death; it was very much as if Mr. I could not contemplate his own death subjectively, then or now.* His sense of helpnessness and terror, then, were experienced as concerns about her welfare, and what his death and/or dying would do or was doing to her. He could not conceive of her existing effectively or independently of him. With much expression of tenderness he empathized with, even identified with, her and her fear of impending loneliness.* Mr. I therefore behaved most courageously. He was determined to spare his wife any unnecessary pain. He died before a donor became available.

Only one more point need be mentioned with regard to why these men cannot consciously entertain the prospect of transplantation. This has to do with the very simple but often overlooked circumstances that an event of such miraculous and traumatic proportions, based on a procedure so recently developed, can have no substance, no true reality until after the fact of its occurrence. And even then there is question. The surgery is an intervention which from a humanistic viewpoint transcends, for the time at least, other surgeries. It is more than an extension of prior procedures. It is a departure so radical in nature as to necessitate a qualitative rethinking of self and man. As a consequence, it tends in its newness to remain unassimilated and beyond conscious contemplation for transplant candidates.

Nontheme Number Two: Survivors and Would-be Mourners

Almost as remarkable as the transplant candidates' inability to deal with the prospective surgery was their attendant incapa-

---

*This concept is one frequently recognized in the literature on death and dying. Weisman and Hackett,[32] for example, state, "What can any man imagine of his own death? Is it possible to conceive of his own utter extinction? Whatever attempt he makes to project himself into the time of death, it results only in seeing the other one, and object, not the subjective one, the 'I', of the here and now. A phantasy of absolute subjective death is impossible to imagine." (p. 248.) Mr. I's experience would seem to verify the point, not just with respect to fantasy but even at a moment that is tantamount to extinction.

*One could argue that Mr. I's view of his wife's despair is really a defense against the realization or experience of his own death, a defense founded upon a fantasy of omnipotence, i.e. he is so important, so vital to his wife's existence that she will not be able to survive without him: ergo, he is not expendable. While this interpretation may have in fact been accurate, I really had no clinical basis for assuming Mr. I's concern for his wife's welfare to be pure defense. And, defense or not, the literature on death and dying indicates that Mr. I's fears have some substance.[5,21,37]

city for discussing contemporaneous object relations. They shied from and circumvented this topic in much the same way they evaded discussion of the transplantation. Yet, to imply that one or all candidates failed to *mention* family, friends, business partners or acquaintances would be somewhat misleading. Virtually every candidate did itemize such persons to some extent. But, typically, it was to amplify an aspect of "ego" and not "other," e.g. the object was always secondary, incidental to a more primary concern for self. Or the "other" was acknowledged but not illuminated and mentioned merely as springboard to ruminative accounts of the candidates' past experience.* And, not infrequently, the listings of "others" proved surprisingly and glaringly incomplete. For example, mothers and sisters, who it turned out were alive and well and even visiting the candidate as often as twice daily, went totally unmentioned over the course of weeks; one simply assumed such persons were nonexistent, irrelevant or long since dead. It was somewhat disarming, then, after all those weeks, to be matter-of-factly introduced to them on a day when visits happened to overlap.

What emerged with most constancy was the candidates' penchant for either not mentioning significant living objects or *mentioning* them but not *describing* them. Thus, despite their concern for facing death courageously and for protecting would-be survivors, or perhaps more accurately because of these very motives, the transplant candidates' references to living family, friends, and co-workers were oddly circumscribed, peculiarly perfunctory, and a matter of resounding indifference. Mr. I's self-projected concern for his wife's welfare (described above) was about as dimensionalized and affectively laden a characterization of another living person as the six candidates produced. Hence, to have accepted at face value all they offered would have necessitated the con-

*If mentioned at all, children were ordered by age, education, marriage, occupation, location of residence. They remained without personality, had no engaging or repelling qualities—quite bluntly their father's renderings left them bloodless and featureless. Similarly, wives were said to work or not work, visit regularly or irregularly, spend the night at a daughter's home or at an overpriced motel: the wives too by all accounts remained oddly faceless. In like fashion, marriages were labeled as satisfactory or unsatisfactory, with hardly a clue offered by the candidate as to kinds and sources of marital bond or divergence.

clusion that each had a contemporaneous interpersonal life that was singularly sterile, a current life bizarrely devoid of significant human attachments. Yet, from the rare recountings like Mr. I's and from the reports of wives, families and friends, we know the truth to be quite otherwise. These men had been substantially cathected by contemporaneous others.

The wellsprings of the resolute diffidence that attaches to discussion of contemporaneous objects have already been touched on. The candidate's dilemma is that he cannot fully afford to decathect his objects, while concomitantly he cannot comfortably maintain their full measure. He remains in indefinite limbo. Thus, not only must he avoid discussing the transplant and other emotionally charged topics with wife, family or friends, but in their absence as well as in their presence he cannot permit himself the luxury of contemplating or appreciating the intensity of his many attachments to other persons. Any attempt to step inside the distancing mechanism runs the risk of emotional overload, even severe regression to infantile dependence and egocentric preoccupation. To think about family and friends, to however briefly dwell on their human qualities, personal attributes or affective modes threatens to overwhelm. Such thoughts cannot be tolerated on a day-to-day basis, nor over extended periods of time. They are best extruded from conversation and, if possible, from consciousness. The candidate steadfastly maintains counterdependent attitudes that make him appear unfeeling.

Nontheme Number Three: The Future

When men undergo a novel and high-risk surgical procedure which is calculated to extend their life, it might be presumed that they do so out of a wish to secure future goals. The postsurgical activities of the transplant patients who survived certainly gives one little reason to doubt the premise. One man, for example, saw with pleasure a daughter graduate high school and a son married. Another embarked upon a highly active life of camping, fishing and hunting, the kind of life that the progressive heart degeneration had precluded for years. Yet, whether such outcomes or goals were actively contemplated prior to surgery remains conjectural. Certainly, on the basis of preoperative conversations with the candidates, one could not say that such goals had been reviewed in any measured way. Instead, and quite to the contrary, five of the six transplant candidates discussed the future either not at all or in terms that were pathetically banal. Unable to discuss present-day object relations and unable to discuss the prospective transplant surgery itself with all its hazards and implications, the future was for these men, almost by definition and certainly by extension, a subject to be distanced and obscured. Wives or family who cheerfully tried to talk of future trips or anniversaries were greeted by tension-filled silences or an abrupt shift in topic; occasionally there was response to an invitation to anticipate the future, but then it was singularly plantitudinous and empty and recited with a detached numbness, that in its understatement made it all the more poignant and heartfelt.

> Mr. K intimated that he was really quite ready to die. He asserted that he had had a full life—a "better than average" marriage and four children, most all of whom were now on their own. The children had all "received fairly good educations," and all seemed "fairly well settled." He said he had accomplished what he had set out to do. He reiterated a number of times that he had no regrets but did so with a grimness that was tinged with anxiety. He sounded as if he were trying to resign himself to death but couldn't. Yet, he continued to recount accomplishments with a sense of completeness that sugguested he had no more to live for. I wondered with him why he had agreed to the transplant if he firmly believed all he had told me. At first he acted as if the question had stumped him. He said nothing. Then he said, "It would be nice to have the transplant because it would give me a chance to know my wife better and that would be nice." In the ensuing minutes he reiterated the comment mechanically a number of times and always with the same abject tiredness. He died within hours after transplant surgery.

Some Conclusions Regarding Nonthemes and Themes

Thus far some care has been taken in detailing the kinds of topics the transplant candidates typically did not discuss before surgery. As it turns out these were all topics about which, on an apriori basis, one had reason to expect the candidates would talk at some length. That they failed to do so is possibly surprising. From a clinical perspective, however, their avoidance of these themes ultimately makes considerable and compelling sense. The need for denial proved multifaceted and had numerous sources. And indeed, taken in isolation any one of the contributing factors might have sufficed to produce the better portion of results thus far described.

Yet, when viewed from another perspective, all the factors contributing to denial, even when taken in sum, may finally account for a good deal less than half the story—for less than half the variance. In a word, denial as a mechanism may not only fail to account for *all* that was unsaid by these men, but it most assuredly fails to explain that which *was* said, that which *was,* in fact, discussed.

Certainly, from what has been described to this point the six transplant candidates must impress as extremely frightened, highly taciturn, defensively uncommunicative, emotionally guarded, and affectively unresponsive or vulnerable men. Edgy and petty in their discontents they would seem to have erected an extensive, if fragile, stimulus barrier—a barrier that emits little and admits less. But this is just partially so! It must be emphasized here that we have presented only one side of the picture thus far. We have discussed nonthemes but not the themes. In point of fact, the denial of affect and event does not characterize large chunks of the candidates' early experiences. And it is to this— special pieces of early experience—that at least three of the six candidates were inexorably drawn. Most remarkably, all that these men are when confronted with present and future, they decidedly are not when given an opportunity to indulge facets of their past. The recalcitrant and irritable deniers of current and future circumstances are simultaneously vital, voluble, animated, emotion filled, and eager guides and explorers of historical events and significant antecedents. These men, in fact, seemed unable to rest for the compulsion to pursue and reconstruct elements of their distant past, and not unlike the ancient mariner, they tried hard to fix and hold their audience, insisting that, willingly or not, he listen. Bent on confessing, undoing and justifying, they talked a steady stream about highly personal memories. Their press, their desire had an all consuming, desperate quality, one that dwarfed and made pale all those other concerns which to outsiders seemed so real, immediate and paramount. Hence, these men did not just deny the present and future, they were restive and impatient with such topics—topics that seemed to divert their attentions from more important concerns. The past, at least for a time, sucked all their energies to it, creating a vacuum around present and future matters. Denial alone was not operating. Thus, while there is no doubt they avoided major themes in the here and now and that psychically they had good cause for so doing, there is also little doubt that these men were preoccupied with and compelled to rework other themes and other tasks—themes and tasks that while situated in the past took psychological precedence in the current scheme of things.

It is important, then, to stress that the transplant candidate is not simply defending and retreating before intolerable psychic hardships. To assert that he is doing only this is to push the more superficial of explanations. Defensive denial as the sole interpretation overlooks the restitutive, forward-moving, health-impelled and adaptive qualities of the candidate's struggle. At a minimum, it obscures the realization that the candidate is readying himself for the transplantation as best he can. His approach and method are, perhaps, surprisingly circuitous. His priorities do not coincide with the priorities of professional observers and concerned bystanders. Nevertheless, he is working, and regardless of whether he betrays it outwardly or not the transplantation, the future, his family and friends are very much on his agenda. But all in due course, all in good time.

The Theme: Remembrances of Father and Things Past

For the most part, each nontheme discussed was characteristic of at least four, and often five, of the transplant candidates. The incapacity to verbally contemplate contemporaneous object relationships was a nontheme true of all six. There is, however,

usually better agreement about things omitted or unsaid than
there is about things included or said.*

It seems remarkable that now, in turning to the consideration
of figure rather than ground, agreement among transplant candidates with respect to focal themes remains so high, nearly as
high as with nonthemes. Three of the six men presented consistent and deep preoccupation with a single topic. More remarkable still is that the focal theme and the dynamics attendant it
are not of the kind or quality that one commonly encounters.
Thus, if one had reason for surprise at the topics which, for
these transplant candidates, became nonthemes, then one truly
has reason to marvel at the fact that three of these same men displayed almost identical configurations of preoccupation and concern.

Quite simply stated, the overriding, prepotent theme for Mr.
M, Mr. I and Mr. K was their memory of their fathers. These
memories which emerged with ever accelerating pace appeared
unfaded and imbued with adductive qualities. The three candidates seemed, literally, to have little alternative in the matter
of their rumination. In all three instances their fathers had died
years earlier of coronary ailments.** And now in the swell of
their own rapid decompensation and in the face of the transplantation, the candidates' relationship to and memory of their fathers
became the nucleus of their psychic existence. Energies of present-
day cathexis were withdrawn, and paternal cathexis, long dormant
and subdued, was infused once again with a compaction, fullness,
intensity and realism that was startling to witness. All contemporary experience was seemingly without meaning except as it
dynamically related to the past. And, as it turned out for these

---

*Other things being equal, the chances are greater that two objects will
resemble each other more for attributes they do not possess in common than for
those features they do. Phrased another way, silence will have greater intercoder
reliability than will what is said when the silence is broken.

**At the time I saw each of these men their fathers had been dead anywhere
from twenty-eight to thirty-eight years. I have no information on whether, how or
when, the fathers of the other three candidates died. It did not arise as a topic in
discussions with them. They did not volunteer the information and I did not ask.
By contrast, Messrs. M, I and K had pressed the information on me within minutes
of my meeting them.

men, all elements of the present seemed uncannily to converge on the person of the deceased father and the remembrance of the relationship with him. The theme was discussed with a compelling urgency that made one fearful of interrupting. And it was, for all intents and purposes, the only theme to emerge. Quite literally, upwards of 75 percent of their discussion was father-focused. Virtually all else was crowded out*

Style

Similarities did not end with theme content. Quite as distinctive were resemblances in mode of presentation. All three men—Messrs. M, I and K—used a personalized form of flashback embedded within a rambling, groping and surfacely incoherent communicative style.

There were times when, as Mr. I spoke, he seemed to meander. The point he was endeavoring to make seemingly got lost. He found transitions very difficult and could not navigate them concisely or acutely. His explanations of events would seem to lead him through detours, circumlocutions and into cul-de-sacs. At times I found my attention would wander unless conscientiously checked; he seemed oblivious to my presence or that he was losing me. For my part I was sure he had gone astray and lost the thread of what he was saying. I understood the observations of nurses and doctors who had reported in notes or directly to me that he was "confused" and in a state of mental disarray. But Mr. I seemed on the track of things having emotional import. Despite what sounded to me like tedious verbal wandering, water would well in his eyes and tears would trickle out the corners of his eyes. He would wipe them away without comment, almost as if he were fearful of interrupting himself —as if to do so would cost him the scent of what he was after. And invariably, if allowed to proceed, Mr. I made it back to his point and tellingly so. The verbal stumbling, the false starts, the vagaries ceased. Everything, all he had said, seemed to fall into place and one could follow the thread to the culminating point. Once there, Mr. I brought it to life in elaborate detail

---

*As will be apparent further on, the three candidates concerned with their fathers were ultimately able to return to a consideration of present and future circumstances. But only after some therapeutic effort and the working-through of father material. Father material was, in fact, never out of the picture even at the point where present day topics could be more comfortably and effectively addressed.

and with a charged affect and power of description that bordered on the eloquent.

It turned out that Mr. I seldom, if ever, was lost for long. He seemed to sense the direction, the memory he was seeking; but he had to grope his way through crowded years and numerous events in order to find the precise experience and meaning he sought. He was not unlike a man who could not tell you what he was searching for, other than that when he found it he would know that was it. In this way, all that Mr. I related, all that had seemed like so much associational rambling, proved of course to be well tied to his ultimate objective. The listener perhaps could have done without the detailing, but it is doubtful Mr. I could have psychically managed shorter, more coherent routes to his goals.

The style of these men was remindful of something this author had seen twenty years earlier—Arthur Miller's *Death of a Salesman*.[26] Miller's chief formal device in this play is the flashback, and when Elia Kazan and Jo Mielziner staged the play in 1949 they were faithful to its form, employing a number of theatrical techniques to convey the ruminative, regretful, hallucinatory preoccupations of Willie Loman. Chief among these was the use of lighting. It not only served to reinforce the effects of action, but it revealed in convincing, compelling ways the connectedness of past and present; most especially it conveyed how the small and routine details of the present, the habitual gesture, the unremarkable phrase, an unspoken word, could in the mind's eye become points of departure for past reconstructions—reconstructions swelling to such all-consuming magnitudes that present realities are forced into the half-world of shadows. Mielziner achieved his effects by gradually dimming lights on present action while slowly intensifying spotlights on another portion of the stage. These spotlights were to illuminate the corridors of time and pieces of action from the past. Thus, as Willie Loman crosses the stage he leaves behind him a darkly faded and frozen present —its people suspended unmovingly for the duration of his reverie— and approaches a warm, spirited past that is infused with the greater vigor and optimism. The Kazan-Mielziner staging had a veracity that fit these men to a "T." Like Willie Loman, these men psychologically and emotionally traversed time and space.

The telescoping of decades, the interchange of generations, the receding awareness of the present, the gravitational pull to a luminous past and every trip back again had all the urgent and phantasmagoric sweep of drama. Messrs. M, I and K appeared in the most literal psychological sense to leave the hospital room and surroundings behind, and not infrequently I found myself to be but a part of their forgotten present. Rarely, if ever, are redintegrations of such ferocity encountered in the individual therapy hours of patients.

Why the Past and Why the Father?

Earlier, in discussing nonthemes we were faced with the problem of explaining why some things that one had hardly expected would be ignored were outstanding for being almost totally unmentioned. Now we are faced with the other side of the problem, namely, with accounting for why some things which were relatively unanticipated should have assumed the proportions of all-consuming, commonly shared themes. This matter and the questions implicit in it are best and most meaningfully approached (1) through a further discernment of the psychological meta-themes that permeate the unique situation of these men, and (2) through a contextual analysis of what these men actually say and how they say it—the what and how of their attempts over a period of days to work through, in concrete ways, the reality implications of the meta-themes.

Without pretension to comprehensive or exhaustive statement, let me touch on a few of the meta-themes that, in my view, are particularly salient for these men.

1. These men are facing death and as Fulton[9] has observed, "Death asks us for our identity. Confronted by death, man is compelled to provide in some form a response to the question: Who am I?" (p. 3) The candidates, then, may be expected to engage actively in a summing-up process, one that takes them to their past, and in an achievement-oriented patriarchal society, one that requires them to evaluate the history of their accomplishments or lack of them and the extent of their success along a variety of core dimensions vital to conceptions of masculinity. Disappointments, regrets, lost opportunities, fulfillments, satis-

factions are all the stuff of their ruminations. It is not then, on second brush, very difficult to understand the press of their orientation to the past. Nor, by the same token, is it really so difficult to discern why these men focus so on the memory of their fathers. The nucleus of their identities, whatever they be, derive from the major male models of childhood. Fathers become internalized models and judges.

2. These men are not only precipitiously close to death but they are also in the somewhat unique position of having a second chance at life, a chance that but two years earlier would have been denied them. And a chance denied their fathers, three of whom died of heart ailments. This fact intensifies and complicates the matter of summing up and locating one's identity spatially and in time. It prompts questions of not only "Who am I?" but "How worthy and deserving am I?" and it invites direct comparisons of deservedness between candidate and father. Recollections are undertaken in the interests of making the comparisons and answering these questions. It is to be expected that such remembrances are replete with pain and suffering and suffused with sensations of guilt, shame and worthlessness. The transplant candidates review their past and recount their relationship to father in a desperate effort to confess, invite judgment, ask penance and attain redemption. They need and ask forgiveness. They seek any shred of past evidence or current motive for enhancing their sense of deservedness. Unfortunately, their dilemma is such that when found they are likely to repudiate it. They epitomize man's ambivalence toward his self-created illusions of value, purpose and worthwhileness, and they symbolize the conflict between the biological urge to survive and the requirements of civilized compulsions and social mores.

3. Most intimately related to the foregoing is the meta-psychological absurdity that attaches to the entire struggle. How deserving of renewed life can a man be when his very chance for renewal entails the wish that another die in his stead. The candidates knowingly or not ask themselves this question. And, indeed, it is near impossible to believe, short of paranoia, that one can ever be so deserving. Moreover, of course, the wish for another's death runs counter to all but "nationalistic" social tenet;

since these men are in no position to marshal patriotic fervor, they remain burdened by the self-perceived selfishness of the wish. But what is perhaps most distressing for these men is that their wish that others sacrifice themselves in order that they might live finds no object or focus in the present but adheres instead to the most natural, if impractical, of choices—the long-deceased father. Patricidal wishes, with all their ensuing guilt, are very much called into play. And, theoretically, one can see why. Fathers not only provide male models for identification, while simultaneously serving as judges for son's adequacies, but they also are sources of considerable frustration and competition, oedipal or otherwise, real and/or fantasied. Fathers are to be envied, exalted, emulated and surpassed. They also are objects of hate, consciously or unconsciously experienced. For certainly the failure to consolidate a masculine identity pleasing to father cannot be considered the sole fault of the child. Father must bear some of the blame. And to the extent the son realizes this, the father becomes an object of the son's resentment, scorn and disillusion. For the three transplant candidates whose fathers had already died of heart disease the circumstances vis-a-vis father were nonpareil. They nucleated all threads and themes—oedipal desires, death wishes toward father, envy of him, emulation of him, the ambivalently experienced and used opportunity to be like him and/or surpass him; it is surely no accident that he, the father, was the center of all their attentions and energies. Psychologically they had no alternative, though this is of little solace to men in their predicament. A patient once defined "love" for his inquiring eight-year-old son as "a willingness to sacrifice one's life so that another might live." While there are those who might dispute the definition, the three transplant candidates discussed here were not among them. Side by side with their residual resentment and contempt for father there existed the belief that each father had sacrificed himself for his son.

4. Death is a final biological act and as such is unlearned. Dying is a preparatory act and is socialized. As already indicated, the transplant candidates were very much engaged in psychologically readying themselves for death. To have said this much is to have raised a legitimate but seldom explored question, namely,

how does one learn to die? Perhaps the question has been little studied because of the social taboos related to the topic of death; perhaps it has been a question rarely studied because dying persons are, in Goffman's sense,[12] stigmatized individuals—they must be kept at safe distance and must behave as if their burden were as nothing; this aspect we have touched on in discussion of how the dying must protect the living by dying "courageously" for them. A more cynical view would suggest that how one learns to die is a question of marginal research value; it is so precisely because of the devaluation by our society of learnings that have severely delimited pay off and equally delimited future application for the learner. There is no denying that dying is a prime example of an experience that has minimal future application for the experiencing person and by this criterion is likely to be a neglected topic. But this view callously overlooks the dying person's suffering and is thereby anti-clinical. It is, as well, ascientific in its ultrapragmatism.

The dynamics of the transplant candidates can, I believe, be instructive on the matter of how people learn to die. The dynamics strongly suggest that one prepares himself for approaching death by mourning for the self in anticipatory fashion; but, more significantly, they also suggest that mourning for the self is virtually impossible until one has first properly mourned a significant other. The success of one may be prerequisite to the succes of the second. In this way, mourning can perhaps become the very nexus of learning to die and dying. The three transplant candidates who when young had lost their fathers did not, according to their own reports, properly mourn them. Reared in a culture which increasingly provides less opportunity for contact with natural death, and caught in cultural presses which heighten ambivalences toward fathers, none of the three could recall having any emotional reaction to the death of their fathers, either at the time of its occurrence or subsequently over the years. With the stunned embarrassment of insight they each related how unfeelingly they had managed to exclude thoughts of him since. And now they were equally shocked to find they could think of nothing else. *Faced with the prospect of their own imminent death, they found it necessary to mourn their fathers before they could selfishly mourn themselves.* This meant recognizing and articulating the father's strengths and weaknesses; it meant drawing sustenance and courage from the exaggerated (?) memory of him as exemplar of self-sacrifice and bravery (this was clearly a motive for dwelling on reminiscences of father) as well as acknowledging and reexperiencing with awareness a great deal of the rage harbored toward him over the years, a rage often predicated on these selfsame virtues. It is an emotion-packed, guilt-drenched and painfully difficult task for the dying individual to undertake, but then there is no reason to expect that rectifying a failure to mourn and learning to die should really be otherwise.

The Course of Presurgical Interviews with Transplant Candidates

What follows is an attempt to trace the unfolding and development of themes and attitudes as they emerged sequentially and were worked through, or not worked through, over a number of presurgical interview sessions with transplant candidates.

Early Phases: the Flight from the Present and Some Examples of the Route to the Past and Father

It has already been noted that each of three transplant candidates capitalized on the slightest of present-day concerns as points of departure for reminiscences about father. Typically, each one did so almost from the outset. One hardly got past the protocol —mutual introduction, statement of purpose, candidate protest that his psyche and resolve could not tolerate probing—than occasion was found by the candidate for spontaneously and extensively talking about his history. As a case in point, Mr. K used the polite exchange of pleasantries as springboard.

> I had introduced myself to Mr. K and discussed with him my purpose. Mr. K quickly indicated he did not want to answer personal questions or talk about himself or discuss the decision that he and his family had made about the transplant. As far as he and they were concerned it was a closed matter. Thinking about it, he said, only upset him. I commented little except to reflect his feelings, but I did go so far as to suggest that he feared if he talked with me he might have second thoughts about going through with things. He readily acknowledged

this; I attempted to reassure him that this was far from my intent; as a matter of fact he needn't discuss these matters at all as far as I was concerned. I indicated that I simply would be available to him if there was something he wanted to talk about. I emphasized that talking itself was totally a matter of his choice but that I would stop by periodically to visit if he wished since I knew long hours in the hospital could be tedious.

Some moments of awkward silence followed. Mr. K avoided looking at me directly. He seemed to be struggling with some embarrassment, searching for something to say. He glanced about nervously and finally gazed out the window. Quite predictably, but with an oddly wooden tone, he commented on the weather.

It was a nice day, he said. A perfect day to be out on the golf course. He laughed unenthusiastically. I made no comment and he continued. His love for golf is very great and he has played the game for twenty years, though he acknowledged that in the last couple of years or so his illness had curtailed his golfing a good deal. Mr. K said that he had always thought of golf as "an old man's game," and that he had only taken it up at age thirty. He found it very different from what he had first imagined it would be and in a way regretted not having started playing the game years earlier. He puzzled awhile about why it was he had not taken up the sport before thirty years of age. Finally, he concluded that it was because of baseball. Baseball memories superseded golf memories. When he was a youngster and right on up through his twenties his first love had been baseball. It was the single thing he enjoyed most and he spent all his time at it. He played a lot of sandlot ball and was on his high school and college baseball teams. Golf had come later. It was funny, he said, but his father had been an avid golfer also. Yet he had never really played golf with his father, the father having died when Mr. K was in his teens. Mr. K noted with some genuine surprise that it now must sound strange to me that he and his father should have so loved the same thing and yet never shared its enjoyment together. He remarked that it sure sounded strange to him to hear himself say it and he began to cry. I had been with him maybe twenty-five minutes and he was already well into father material. It was merely the introduction.

Here we not only have an example of the candidates' characteristic leapfrogging back through time, but we have some suggestion of what the preoccupation with father is all about.

Themes of identification and competition are ill concealed. Father and son share the same situations and are alike in preferred activities. But they are out of time and out of phase. They cannot share. Thus, despite his unawareness, Mr. K betrays a quasi-oedipal theme. He and father could not love and enjoy the same thing at the same time. Mr. K maintained his distance; certain territories belonged to the "old man" and Mr. K was careful not to tread on the father's turf, at least not until after the "old man" had died. There is also the intimation that things might, and perhaps rightfully should, have been different. That father and son need not have been such strangers or so alien, and there is a sense of mourning for missed chances. But the rueful, regretful quality that pervades the recall of missed opportunities overrides any awareness, at least for the present, of competitive resentments between father and son. Rather the father is idealized.

The Father as Hero

Mr. M had once again responded to an inquiry of mine about present circumstances by immediately moving to the past. I had asked Mr. M about his son's military status—the son was home on leave from Vietnam and seeking an extension of that leave and Mr. M, seemingly oblivious to my question, proceeded to tell me the following about his father; the time period is 1935 through 1940.

> Mr. M described his father as a highly active, charged individual who had unbounded degrees of energy and who entered situations with a bounce and verve that attracted attention and commanded respect. He was highly popular and a leader of men. A veteran of World War I, the father was a staunch patriot and a vigorous member of the American Legion. In fact, he was an organizing force for the state Legion, holding an executive position and making rounds virtually every weekend to state Legion posts. His charge was to evaluate the posts, collect monies, administrate generally, but most particularly his mission was that of building esprit, motivating men, whipping up patriotic fervor. He was a man widely admired. While Legion activities consumed much the father's time, it was not his occupation. By profession, Mr. M's father was a high school teacher. He taught shop, sheet metal and mathematics, par-

ticularly algebra. He was a highly versatile man according to Mr. M. He could step into any course where a teacher was needed. But the father's first love was athletics. He was himself an athlete and he was athletic director of the school at which he taught, as well as its football coach. And he was dedicated. With awe in his voice Mr. M described the hours his father put in, the fire of his drive and will to win. Mr. M recalled a trip to Los Angeles in 1936 for the Olympic trials. Mr. M's father had spent a year grooming two or three teenagers for the occasion. These boys had practically lived in the M house, and the father had overseen their diets, training, pacing and living habits. He personally footed the bill for their expenses to Los Angeles and drove them with his family across country. Mr. M was sixteen or so at the time and recalled the trip as full of good memories. His pride in his father was evident as he spoke. "He was a maker, a builder of men," Mr. M said, "an American, an educator and an athlete."

Then, virtually in the prime of life, Mr. M describes that his father was "cut down." In the fall of 1939 the father was driving himself at his typical pace—teaching, coaching, administrating and maintaining his active, traveling role in the American Legion. The father contracted bronchial flu or pneumonia that fall. Yet, he did not slow down but carried his activities through the Christmas holiday. He collapsed and was hospitalized. The "flu had settled in his heart." Virtually invalided, Mr. M's father was forced into retirement at age forty-seven. For the next two years, until his death, barely able to hobble about, the father bridled at inactivity. Mr. M marveled at his father's will to live and to stay engaged. The father could not walk any distance or stand for any length of time. He described how his father daily tended his garden, hoeing it, raking and watering it, from a kitchen stool that had to be periodically moved so he could tend a new area. He recalled how the father played cards, talked and enjoyed visitors, and especially how the father maintained a lively interest in world and local affairs via radio, newspaper and telephone. Without complaint and shunning assistance or special attention, Mr. M's father would do all he could for himself, and Mr. M was amazed at his ingenuity and capacity for self-help.

The idealization of father was overwhelming. It is almost impossible to conceive of a more perfect male identification model or a less attainable one. The idolatry suggests belated, defensive identification, and an earlier failure to mourn. But

Mr. M has, at least in his mind's eye, finally achieved a oneness with father, something that understandably had eluded him all his life. He, like father, is closest to death at age forty-nine,* and he, like his father thirty years before him, was first hospitalized in the local VA hospital. It seemed clear that Mr. M was intent on maintaining, enhancing and consolidating an identification with father that would see him through the crisis of his own surgery. His counterdependent attitudes and behaviors in the hospital toward nurses, aides and doctors were reminiscent of his descriptions of the father's invalidism, though Mr. M himself seemed unconscious enough of the connection. His self-imposed and occasionally labored efforts at being like father—the decrying of solicitious concern, the insistence of self-accomplishment though bedridden, the valorous outlook and stiff upper lippedness in the face of adversity—seemed vital sources of sustenance, fortitude and borrowed ego-strength. It was as if Mr. M had to continually remind himself of how father had done it, figuratively feeling his way into father's skin and taking on his characteristics. But there was more to it than borrowed courage. There was, for example, much to indicate that Mr. M's early and major identifications were not fully or satisfactorily those with the idolized father; there had been failure and disappointment on both sides and now the striking parallels between the heart disease of father and son provided Mr. M with an almost welcome circumstance to demonstrate that he had finally made it as father's son, that the ultimate in identification had been achieved.

Equally heroic, and as culturally valid, is the different form of valor displayed by Mr. K's father. It, too, seemed to inspire attitudes of strength and endurance while diminishing grievous self-pity. And it too seemed to derive in good measure from a failure to mourn.

> Mr. K had already outlined his love for baseball. It led him to discuss his father's attitude toward his playing the game. He noted that his parents were immigrants from Eastern Europe, that his father had arrived in this country as a young adult, and that he himself was, as a consequence, a second-generation

---

*Mr. M had outlived his father by only a handful of days at the time I first spoke with him.

American. He said his father had always objected strenuously to his playing the game of baseball. His father had other ambitions for him and would not or, Mr. K assumed, could not understand his devotion to the game. This led Mr. K to a consideration of some of the pressures endured by second-generation children in this country. For example, the fact that they were caught between the pulls of two cultures. He asserted that second-generation children often had to carry out the hopes of their immigrant parents. Such parents came to the United States seeking opportunities for their children and not merely for themselves. What the parents achieved they achieved for their children. All parental hopes and aspirations were transferred to the children, and this placed second-generation children in particularly sensitive, vulnerable and conflictual spots. Their lot was a difficult one. Mr. K noted that in his family there was a tremendous emphasis on cultural growth, education and achievement. He had started playing the piano when he was eight, and he took lessons weekly until he was twenty. Like any child, he used to fight and resist piano as much as possible. He preferred playing baseball. Mr. K now paused. Then he said he wanted to tell me an anecdote about the piano, baseball and his father.

His father, he said, was very devoted to him and to his development, so much so that the father would take him to hear symphony concerts and opera and would sit next to him for hours in the living room listening to his son practicing the piano. For hours the father would sit, even if Mr. K played nothing but scales or some turgid practice piece that his teacher had assigned. Mr. K himself did not see how the father could derive pleasure from the music since the father had neither an ear for music nor an intrinsic like for music. It was his devotion to Mr. K and his future that motivated the father. Mr. K went on to say that one day he had practiced the piano for half an hour. He told his mother he wanted to go out and play baseball while it was still light, asked and received permission to do so for an hour on the proviso that he would then return and practice the piano for another half hour. When an hour was up and he did not return home his father arrived at the sandlot. The father was enraged and physically grabbed Mr. K, twisting his arm behind him and steering him back to the house. He forced Mr. K back to the piano, and sitting down next to his son, listened to him play the scales for the next hour. Mr. K in relating this laughed embarrassedly. He recalled his shame before his baseball teammates and commented that the entire scene sounded as if it might have been lifted from the scenario of a 1930s movie. It wasn't unusual for those times or circumstances. Once he had finished practicing the piano that evening, Mr. K reported that his father's lecturing began anew. Why, his father asked him, would he want to spend his life rummaging around, grubbing in the dirt of the sandlots getting filthy, playing a silly game like baseball when instead he could be playing the piano and learning something that was both worthwhile and of lifelong value. Again, Mr. K noted, almost as an aside, that this kind of lecture coming from a father was not remarkable for its unusualness. What was unusual, however, was his discovery years later, following his father's death, that the father had been a topflight baseball player, indeed, a player of superior caliber to Mr. K himself. His father, despite being an immigrant and despite a belated start, had been sufficiently skilled at baseball to earn a professional baseball contract. In other words, the father must have loved to play the sport and done it often enough on a sandlot and semiprofessional basis to acquire skills of considerable excellence—excellence enough to merit professional offers. Mr. K's father never told him of this, never intimated the slightest interest in baseball. Mr. K learned of it only subsequent to his father's death. The contractual offers were found among the father's effects, and Mr. K's mother filled in the details and background for her son.

Mr. K was obviously still awed by the discovery and all it meant. Mr. K interpreted that his father sacrificed inestimably for his son, that what was good enough for him was not near good enough for his son, that the father wanted things better, different and more for the son, and that via tremendous devotion to the boy he could urge him into arenas of success that the father had never approached or tasted.

Here then is another kind of father whose recounted virtues are of such portentous magnitudes as to defy the achievement of self-satisfactory levels of identification, at least under ordinary circumstances. One owes the man everything, and one cannot begin, throughout a lifetime to emulate his magnanimity. One merely exaults him and treasures the hope. But, as with Messrs. M and I, the prospect of death and transplantation seems to have provided Mr. K with a final, if tortured and contorted, opportunity to solidify and consolidate that identification which was never satisfactorily made, an opportunity to close out some long unfinished business—mourning—and to let go. Hence, with time, but prior to surgery, Mr. K not only began to enumerate the many sacrifices he had made on behalf of his own family, but he came to openly recognize that he construed his possible death as a supreme sacrificial act which would bring untold benefits to his surviving family. What is more, he found in his father's self-denial a model for endurance in the midst of terrors. Self-pity is a luxury that ill behooves the son that aspires to be a man. Thus, like Mr. M, Mr. K drew nourishment for the encounter with death through an effort to feed on every remembered detail of father's style. Mr. K breathes in each facet of father's personality, in order that he might breathe out utter selflessness. And, as in the case of other candidates, all awareness of paternal flaws and any insight into competitive resentments toward father were, for the time being, submerged. This was, however, a status quo that could not long be maintained. These men were in transit, well embarked on a driven psychic hunt that did not permit extended respites. They recognized, in fact, were propelled by the knowledge that they had but limited time to complete their grief work.

The Son as Failure and Disappointment

Adulation of father did not immediately or even quickly abate. But it was soon melded with comparative self-judgments, all disparaging. This was, however, a self-depreciation curiously devoid of bathos, and in its way it culminates in the initial significant and spontaneous, i.e. unprompted by me, insight into the connectedness between all the memories of father *and* future and present happenings. As such it introduced the first real crack in the transplant candidate's psychological armamentarium against overt recognition of contemporaneous circumstances. The simultaneity of descriptions of esteemed father and downgraded son, running side by side as they did, permitted the insight.

> Mr. M omitted from his description of his father any direct reference to how he felt thirty years ago toward the father and the father's illness. That is, Mr. M provided few cues as to what he experienced at the time. But it was not difficult to sense Mr. M felt himself to have been a deep disappointment to his father. Mr. M related, for example, that he was never

an athlete of any note, but at the same time makes it clear that his father had deeply wanted him to be one. He never went out for football in high school or college because he was "too small, . . . no more than 140 pounds." Nonetheless, one gets a glimpse of the father's early and enduring investment in the son, since Mr. M also depicted how his father had built "honest-to-God regulation goal-posts" on the lawn in the front yard of the house. Mr. M recalled working quite hard at learning how to kick. With endless hours of practice he became quite proficient at "drop-kicking" and "place-kicking," and by the time he entered college could kick field goals "from 35 to 40 yards out." Still, he did not go out for the team, and Mr. M stated that it was apparent to him by early high school that he was no athlete. Mr. M made no mention of his father's reactions to his lack of athletic ability, but the aura of disappointment was difficult to conceal, most especially as he described his father's coaching investment in other teenage boys. He was hardest on himself. Mr. M concluded his anecdote about the Olympic trials by summarizing: "I guess not many on that trip (to the Olympic trials) mistook me for my father's son. But it was a great trip anyway."

It was also clear that on the scholastic front Mr. M deemed himself a gross disappointment to his father, though again he could not bring himself to explicitly state that this was his father's perception. The father, of course, was college educated and a high school teacher. Mr. M, though, maintained very marginal grades and throughout the two years of his college career was on probation. When he finally quit college after two years he had not yet attained sophomore status. Saying nothing about father's reaction, Mr. M explained his poor academic performance as a function of his working for money while attending school. He never studied, never read, often cut class and barely scraped by. "Hardly my father's son" was the phrase Mr. M employed on this occasion.

We have, however, some more direct inkling of how Mr. M's father looked upon his son from still another memory that Mr. M relates in a later session. In the spring of 1941, after the father had been invalided nearly eighteen months, the father became highly concerned about Mr. M's draft status. Keenly aware of the international situation, knowing that many young American men were volunteering for service in Europe and Asia, or being drafted under the peace-time draft law of September 1940, and cognizant that the Atlantic Charter had been signed that spring, Mr. M's father began to question why his son, who had such marginal academic records, had not volunteered for service or been drafted. His frequent questions and presssurings were met by silence from Mr. M who explained that he had secretly married some months before and did not want to inform his father of this. Frustrated and dissatisfied with his son's closemouthedness and suspicious on other grounds, the father called Mr. M's draft board in order to ascertain his son's status. He was informed by the local draft board of Mr. M's 3-A classification—a classification meaning the potential inductee had a dependent. Mr. M recalled how an enraged father confronted him with the information that evening, accusing his son of cowardice and draft evasion. What is more, the father had assumed that Mr. M had claimed him, the invalided father, as the dependent. This, according to Mr. M, doubled his father's fury. When Mr. M clarified the situation by telling his father of his secret marriage, the father was not assauged. He took the hasty and secret marriage as an effort on his son's part to circumvent the draft and evade his responsibility to his country. At this point it was possible for me to discuss with Mr. M that he considered himself to have been a relative failure and a source of deep disappointment to his father who had expected so much of him. Mr. M confirmed this impression with tears and emotional self-castigations.

In not very dissimilar fashion Mr. K elaborated the numerous ways in which he had, (1) taken his father for granted and, (2) showed him no gratitude. These included among other things his resistance to playing the piano, his ridicule and defiance of paternal advice offered in his best interests, his failure to do well in school, his negativism toward paternal endeavor, his lack of enthusiasm for, or even interest in, the family business, and his general drivelessness, his ambitionlessness.

Mr. I, in somewhat more abbreviated form, recounted a variety of occasions in which he felt he had let his father down and/or outright insulted him, but it was also he who most tellingly revealed the dynamic of the guilt that seemed to underlay great portions of the repetitive adulation of father and derogation of self. Amidst tears he concluded his comparative history by sobbing:

My father . . . he's the one should have had this chance . . . not me . . . me? I don't deserve it . . . he was the one . . . he deserved everything good and never got it. He did everything for me and I did nothing for him. His time just came too soon . . . too early. Thirty-five years later and I'm lucky . . . I can have a transplant . . . but it really should have been him, you know . . . not me . . . I mean, like what did I do to deserve this chance? Who am I? But my dad? He deserved it every bit . . . He was someone, a deserving man . . . It just doesn't seem fair. Does it?

Mr. I, in registering these sentiments, gave overt expression to the more tacit experiences of the other transplant candidates. And in very real psychological terms he was, as spokesman, quite right, "It does not seem fair." The circumstantial twist is that the injustice referred to was not suffered by father alone, though this is perhaps the way Mr. I has phrased the matter. What is equally or even more unfair is that the transplant candidates should have to bear additional, intensified guilt. It is precisely this that they fear, should their transplantations prove successful. Success portends outliving father's years, surpassing father, and a continued existence dominated by the plaguing belief or realization, justified or not, that they, who did nothing but fail their all-sacrificing fathers, should now enjoy the luxuries of a second life when their more worthy fathers had been denied the opportunity. It is melodrama written in guilt, and it brings the transplant candidate face to face with illusory issues of immortality and omnipotence—after all "why me?" To listen to these men, few persons could be less deserving than themselves. The transplantation itself was, then, oddly twisted in its denotative meaning. It was not merely viewed by these men as a chance for renewed life as a means of surpassing father or attaining identity with him, it was charged as well with punitive implications. Outcomes were construed with ambivalence; they were unfair but fair. Death was a highly feared but an easy out. Second life was welcomed but in large part was so for its very promise of continued and intensified guilt. This was a situational ambivalence that in its acute persistence was virtually unbearable, especially given the ambiguities of a transplant surgery which had no set time, no preknowledge of donor, and so on. As a consequence, there was a healthful press for presurgical resolution. This required an acceptance, even an acknowledgement, of the fact that the transplant candidate was both entitled to and deserving of his severe self-castigations. What he said was accurate in at least one major sense. While his belief that he had failed his father in many ways could be disputed as selected and distorted memory, it was more difficult to dispute the evidence which suggested he had failed his father by never really mourning him. His claim to have "done nothing" for father may actually translate as "I have not even mourned him." Hence, by extension, the candidate was unworthy of the transplant and second life until he did so.

Son as Ingrate: the Death of Father and the Failure to Mourn

Thus far, events of sessions with three of the transplant candidates have been described as if they occurred in logically ordered sequence and coherent manner. This has been done for reasons of organization and in an effort to clarify and illustrate major points and themes. Quite obviously, however, this was not at all the way things proceeded or bouyed to the surface of discussion. The constant flux of emotion, the leapfrogging from present to intermediate past to deep past and back again, and the seeming casualness, even looseness, of ideational flight and associations, all of which characterized the communications of these men, has already been described to great extent. The order, while there, required some piecing together for purposes of articulation. Once the stage of self-castigation was reached, however, imposition of structure became decidedly less problematic. Events now ordered themselves and unfolded rather clearly in almost uniform pace and order. It is as if three men who were all milling about and stumbling, yet gradually moving in the same general direction, had suddenly and finally located their objective. Assured of purpose and direction, they seemingly fell into coordinated step and proceeded in unison over nearly identical courses.

The point of consolidation, the climax, was reached with the vivid, palpable recall of the day the father died, and the subsequent meaningfully charged memory of the near total failure to mourn.* It was here that the three candidates self-inflicted whiplashings reached their crescendo.

Mr. M recalled that his father died in the late summer of 1941. Despite the father's weak and invalided state the death was relatively unexpected at the time. It was another coronary. Mr. M remembered that he was not home at the time although he was nearby and readily located. He was working a number of jobs that summer trying to scrape together tuition monies for college in the fall. Among his jobs was delivering milk; he was out on the milk route the morning his father died. He had been playing cribbage with his father the night before and nothing had seemed to herald his father's death. It was very early in the morning, and sunny, and very quiet—few if any people were up yet—and Mr. M's brother-in-law came and found him in the midst of making his deliveries and told him the news. Mr. M, with an attitude of wonderment that seemed to suggest he was almost transposed to the scene, recalled the moment. He was vividly, indeed terribly aware of every detail about him—the intense early morning summer sunlight, the greenness of the trees, the very dark and long shadows, the fresh, clean scent of the air, the absence of wind, the palpable quietness, the silence of the road. Each detail seemed as real to him now as then, and he marveled for a moment at his ability to absorb so much of his surround then and his capacity for vivid recall of it now. It was seemingly his only remembered reaction to the news of his father's death—a memory of being frozen in one spot, time suspended and unmoving while he intensively drank in every external detail about that moment, registering it indelibly; omitted totally was any experience of emotion, shock, surprise, grief, anger, or otherwise. These did not come then, or upon return to his parents' home that morning, or subsequently. And suddenly, with this realization, Mr. M had new reason for amazement. With something akin to a startle reaction, he seemed to recognize that he had never mourned his father. And, what is more, he seemed for the first time to appreciate the significance of that omission. And slowly, as if implications dawned on him one or two at a time, he seemed to first savour and then comprehend with horror the full meaning of events or the lack of them.

He cried and disparaged himself. How, he wanted to know,

---

*For a rather full description of the mourning process, as well as some clinical examples of the failure to mourn, the reader is referred to Eric Lindemann's 'classic' article on reactions to the Coconut Grove fire.[24]

could he live with a person for almost twenty years and yet have
no reaction to that person's death? He accused himself of being
heartless, cruel and unfeeling. Of having deserted his father.
And yet he seemed genuinely mystified by it, all because he had
so loved his father and could think of nobody but his father at
this time. What must people have thought of him? His mother,
his siblings had been distraught, had cried and wept, had been
virtually incapacitated for days, weeks or more. But he, he
had barely interrupted his routine. For example, he had continued to work his many jobs and he could recall having no
feelings of upset. He did not cry. He just maintained his
routines. Mr. M wondered momentarily if maybe he had not
at the time already resigned himself to his father's death. I
pointed out the intensity of his current reactions and the emotions that seemed so new to him. He concurred readily that this
was the first time he had ever experienced their like and concluded that he had never reacted emotionally to the father's
death. He reiterated the father's many virtues and begged my
forgiveness. He said he had always considered himself senti-
mental and easily moved to tears, and now he realized that there
was a very significant exception. He even speculated some
about the relatedness of his sentimentality to his failure to
"feel" at the time of father's passing.*

Equally painful are the remembrances of Mr. I:

Mr. I recalled his father's warmth and givingness, and crying
he insisted he had badly disappointed his father. Later, he
described the father's sudden death, the result of a thrombosis.
The father had gotten up one morning, was getting ready to
go to work, and keeled over. It was that uncomplicated and fast.
Mr. I, now fifty, noted that he had outlived his father by four
years. He stated he could never understand his reaction to his
father's death. It was a "mystery" to him then and he had
wondered about it since. His mother, he said, was "terribly
broken up." She simply couldn't get used to the fact that the
father was not around. But Mr. I himself had not reacted directly to the sudden death. Despite felt love and admiration,
he did not become upset. Mr. I remembered how he forced
himself to act like a grief-stricken person. He did this, he said,
mainly for his mother and "to save face." "It was the way I was
supposed to behave . . . but I really didn't have the feelings."

---

*Mr. M seemed to have reference here to a mechanism somewhat akin to
Wolfenstein's[34,p.80] notion of "mourning at a distance."

He chastized himself, but then wondered aloud if maybe children didn't react as strongly to death as did grownups. Maybe they simply didn't care as much. Certainly his father's death hadn't hit him hard in the way he thought today it should. He referred to himself as a sham and began to question his worthwhileness once again. It was just a brief step to discussing openly with him his persistent guilt and his residual anger.

Anger at Father

The emergence of anger toward the deceased father followed hard upon the candidate's recognition that he had been unable to mourn.

> Thus, I suggested to Mr. I that I might help him understand why he had not mourned his father. That, in essence, he and I could try and resolve that "mystery" regarding his reaction to his father's death which had puzzled him all these years. I explained the picture was often complicated. I reassured Mr. I as best I could and said I could understand how, despite his many attainments, he could still think of himself as a failure and a disappointment to his father. After all, his father's standards and expectations were very much alive within him. With this much suggestion Mr. I began crying anew. What followed in this and subsequent visits were some vivid recountings of the many frustrations, disappointments and angers experienced by Mr. I as son to his father. In sum, these amounted to a near total inability on the part of the father to accept Mr. I for what he was and, for that matter, what he was not.
>
> Grievances over his incapacity for ever pleasing father, even when he had achieved something with good success, paternal impatience and lack of praise, open displays of competitiveness with the striving son on the part of the father—these often closing off avenues where Mr. I might have attained independent ascendancy—were all among the outpourings of remembered disappointments with a father who at first seemed all-giving but who now, on reflection, was recognized more realistically as a man who failed his son as much as his son had failed him.

Mr. K produced a more intellectual thesis about why he had failed to grieve for his father than that arrived at by Mr. I. Rage at father, while expressed, was distanced some. Nonetheless, the process proved emotionally trying and tear filled in its unfolding, and Mr. K could make use of some of the vital connec-

tions between the past and his present circumstances and fears
—connections that came to light only after anger toward father
had been recognized and found some expression. With Mr. K,
as with Mr. I, the father was seen as a man unable to allow for
the individuality, the separateness of the son. Mr. K was particularly insistent that his father viewed him (Mr. K) as an extension of self. As noted earlier, Mr. K was the son of immigrant
parents, and he elaborated with affect on some of the problems
this created for him personally and for other second-generation
persons in this country. His father he felt had unfairly placed
him in an impossible situation.

> Mr. K asserted that the second-generation child often was ex-
> pected to carry out the hopes of the first-generation immigrant
> parents. The parents, leaving poverty-stricken or persecutory
> areas of the world, came to the United States not so much in
> the hope of achieving for themselves but more with the hope
> of providing something better for their children. Mr. K seemed
> to definitely believe that most emigration of families was under-
> taken for the benefit of children and future generations, and
> that this made it extremely difficult for the children of immi-
> grant parents. Because they were already older and fairly set
> in their ways and traditions, the immigrant parents did not
> have to, or in fact could not, substantially alter their values
> or behaviors. These were established parts of their personality.
> All aspirations were transferred to the children, and the par-
> ents made the children very aware of this fact, that, in effect,
> they as parents had sacrificed personal ambitions, goals and
> opportunities for the children. This, however, Mr. K felt was
> only part of the dilemma. As, if not more, problematic was
> the parents' ambivalence and confusion regarding goals and
> values for their children. They wanted the child "American-
> ized," to adapt to and pursue American values. At the same
> time, they keenly felt the child's rejection of parental and
> ethnological values and traditions. As a consequence, the chil-
> dren could only feel damned for what they did do, and damned
> for what they failed to do. They could not possibly satisfy two
> conflicting sets of expectations. Hence, Mr. K concluded the
> pressures on him were enormous. He felt driven to achieve
> economically, culturally, educationally, socially, and no matter
> what he did or how he did it, it never satisfied his father.
> Baseball, school, the piano, the family business were prime
> examples he used. And each time he failed to satisfy his father's

standards he was made to feel guilty, since the father had sacrificed so much on his behalf. Mr. K was, then, able to recount some of his rage and resentment toward father, though it must be admitted that much of it was not vividly redintegrated, being tempered instead with moderate doses of intellectualization. In all, however, Mr. K did cathart a good deal and he succeeded in venting considerable amounts of anger at his father's saint-like virtuosity.

Finally, it might be noted that Mr. M's rage at his father's open preference for and devotion to other children, who more satisfactorily conformed to his hypermasculine expectations than did his son, was when it came rather undisguisedly expressed. Excruciating and poignant in its vehement and bitter statement, it revealed a long list of accumulated grievances that had long been suppressed. Once again the central theme revolved around a pervasive sense of impotent fury which derived from the explicit realization that father had demanded the impossible. He had, in Mr. M's view, expected his son to be like him, to emulate him, to surpass him, while he simultaneously had communicated the reverse expectation as well, taking every opportunity to competitively outshine, undercut, show up, and ruthlessly defeat or embarrass Mr. M's haltering and hopeful efforts at identification and achievement. Mr. M described himself as the victim of an exquisite "double bind." His anger was unmitigated and white-hot in its intensity, and he all but accused his father of systematically rejecting and emasculating him. And he could not forgive his father's illness nor his death. These were viewed in irrational but not uncertain terms as culminative acts of rejection and desertion, through which the father had expressed his final contempt for wife, family and son.* Nonetheless, Mr. M cried uncontrollably as he recalled how much he would have given to please his father, and how impossible it was to do so even under the most favorable of conditions, and how, even now, he felt admiration, respect and love for the man far in excess to that felt toward any other individual he had ever known.

*For example, Mr. M seemed unforgiving of the fact that his father's illness had impeded and interrupted his education, first by requiring him to work multiple jobs and numerous hours, and second by forcing him to quit college altogether within a month of the father's death.

Connectedness of Past and Present: Working Through and "Letting Go"

If the transplant candidates had come no further than this, one might have concluded that much of significance had been accomplished. Recovered memories, redintegrations, catharsis and the freedom to indulge long-delayed mourning, represent substantial achievements. But they are, in the end, only partial achievements. Because, in sum, and as a continuous process, they are also but prelude to more ultimate confrontations—those with the very nonthemes and nontopics so assiduously avoided by the candidates through this point in time. Thus, the past may be said to have true existence only by virtue of its connectedness with contemporaneous concerns; and, in like fashion, the present may be considered as having real meaning primarily in terms of anticipated and future events. While this view has some obvious and severe cultural and biologic limitations, it seems nonetheless to have social relevance for the transplant candidates. They are free to deal with future possibilities only when able to freely contemplate the present situation, and, as should be apparent, the latter circumstance only obtains when the candidate extricates himself from some tacky past entanglements. Remembering and mourning father not only permits anticipatory mourning of self,* and preparation for the transplant, but it brings to light some

---

*The term "mourning for the self" is understood to mean, (1) sorrow and anticipatory grieving over the loss of one's own life, capacities, skills and functions, and, (2) bereavement, again anticipatory, for the impending loss of loved objects —family, friends, and so on. It is often forgotten that death entails loss at both ends—the living lose the deceased but the deceased, knowing of his approaching death, must reconcile himself to the loss of loved persons too. Since we are typically so concerned with the living we often lose sight of this fact, but the significance of the loss experienced by the dying person should not be underestimated. It may, indeed, in our culture, constitute the most potent source of death anxiety. As Kaufman (1959) has suggested, our feelings about death change drastically if we feel reassured that the world or all human life about which we care would end were we to die. As should by now be clear, the transplant candidates could not mourn themselves, their own demise and their separation from others, until first mourning a prior significant loss that they could not grieve for earlier. Others[8,24,35,36] have noted similar phenomenon and mechanisms; namely, that mourning left undone in the past is undertaken at a later time when new separations and/or losses remind of the old, causing it to surface. This seems very much to be the mechanism involved with the transplant candidates.

unanticipated and astounding parallels in the candidates' perceptions of future, present and past happenings. Drawing out these parallels, clarifying them, and providing the symbolic and emotional linkages between them comprises the final phase of presurgical psychotherapeutic endeavor with those candidates. Once again, three of them prove remarkable for the similarity of their concerns and dynamics.

Some of the mutually experienced themes connecting the candidates' past to their present have already been touched on; others have been hinted at but remain implicit; still others have not even come to light as yet in the discussion. All, however, actively involve the candidate in contemplating the transplantation and death, the potential mourners and survivors, and the future.

Among the commonly encountered themes already mentioned is the relation between the candidate's wish that another human die so that he might survive and the failure to mourn father. The elaboration and clarification of the connectedness between these two psychological phenomena was not especially difficult for them to perceive, though as with other things the candidates differed in their capacities for realizing the full measure of the relatedness involved. In a word, however, the candidates became aware that their failure to mourn father rooted in part on their intense anger at him, that their anger at him had culminated in something vaguely akin to a childlike wish that something untoward happen to him, that his actual death was tantamount to fulfillment of that wish, and that currently their (the candidates') chances for future life resided in a reactivation of that selfsame tabooed wish that others die on their behalf. Even more, the wish that another might die sacrificially and become donor proved intolerably close to the long-sealed-off view of father as self-sacrificing benefactor for son. The parallel forms of the wish arose in the course of the candidates' reviews with a starkness that made it impossible to keep the linkages obscure. Hence, the candidates came to understand that their fear of thinking about the transplantation, the donor, the new heart, the future, in part was related to, rooted in, unresolved conflicts and hostile-destructive wishes toward father. Purged of the latter psychic burdens through cathartic mourning, they were better able to prepare themselves for the imminent future. Quite relatedly, some of the candidates were able to discuss the connection between this wish for the transplant operation and their rivalry with father. Mr. K and Mr. M, for example, saw quite clearly how their physical predicament had psychologically helped them to gain a long sought and legitimized identification with father, and how the success of the surgery would allow them to finally surpass father. And neither was oblivious to the guilt-ridden implications of success nor to that other part of them which wished for failure —and death—so as to preserve the status quo while simultaneously assuring that unbearable guilt would not eventuate. Each man proved able to discuss both sides of the issue, and the total process seemed to have calming effects.

More implicit, at least to this point in work with the candidates, were themes of dread. Unable until now to address the present and future, these themes remained almost obtrusively and oppressively latent in all the recounted memories of past. With the emotional purgation that punctuated the recall of father, however, themes of dread gained preeminence among the candidates' preoccupations. Surprisingly enough, the candidates did not experience the dread with regard to their physical fates. They were increasingly less concerned about the matter of whether they might live or die and concomitantly more interested in what their life or death might mean to their families and/or to the memories of their family members. What emerged with striking clarity now was the candidates' horror that their lives had come full circle and that family situations and outcomes were being recapitulated and replayed in the most eerie, even grotesque, of ways. The candidates, however, were quick to realize that this was no piece of cruel trickery, nor for that matter accident. When they saw it they saw it for what it was—intergenerational contagion of family theme, personal style and attitude toward death. These men were, for example, concerned that they would be treated by their sons with the same "callous neglect" that they had given their own fathers at the time of their deaths.

> Mr. K had already elaborated on his own failure to mourn for his father and his resulting guilt. He had cried a great deal

and had given expression to much of his residual anger toward father. Now, he moved to the contemporary scene. He told me about a close friend of his who had a family, a son of sixteen among its members. His friend had died rather recently and Mr. K remarked that he had watched the sixteen-year-old son's reaction with interest. The boy did not manifest any overt distress over the loss of his father, and Mr. K was reminded of his own reaction to his father's death. He mentioned that people had said of his late friend's son that the boy must have cared little for his father, and that they had looked upon the boy's unperturbed behavior as an embarrassment. Mr. K was privy to these discussions, and he observed that similar things must have been said about him after the death of his father though he, of course, would not have heard them.

I asked Mr. K why he had told me this at this time. He looked puzzled and suggested that since we had been talking about his reactions to his father's death it was natural he remember the more recent reaction of his friend's son. I agreed with Mr. K that this was so, but I pointed out that something more seemed involved too. I wondered with Mr. K if he weren't trying to communicate a concern to me. I wondered if he weren't trying to tell me that history can repeat itself, that events that happened in the past can happen again in the here and now, that other sons can forget and neglect their fathers just as he had. He tumbled immediately into tears. He could not stand to have his own children watch him die a little bit at a time. He was, in fact, glad that he had been hospitalized for a time and kept from their steady view. He could collect himself in their presence when they visited him at the hospital, but it would be impossible to do it around the clock. They were all devoted and they all came to see him. One son, of course, lived some distance, had a family and could not visit as regularly as the others. It turned out he had rarely been by. Mr. K began to elaborate on his worries about this son. He had done poorly in school despite stellar promise and superior intrinsic abilities. He had gotten through college marginally, behaving erratically and spending money liberally. He married prior to finishing school and over Mr. K's objections. Mr. K had found it difficult to "get next to" the boy. Their relationship, it turns out, had been strained.

I now pointed out to Mr. K the striking parallels between his description of his relationship to his own son and his earlier description of his relationship to his father. I said I felt sure he was himself aware at some level of the parallels, and that what he was really telling me was about his fear that his son was sufficiently alienated from him so as to not mourn him should the transplant fail. That precisely because he saw so many similarities between the father-son situations, he felt he knew what his son experienced and what his father had experienced before him. Once again we talked about how his current predicament seemed to officially finalize his identification with father, even to the point of viewing his son as like himself vis-a-vis his father. Ultimately, we were able to discuss Mr. K's central terror—his great fear that if his son failed to mourn him, as he had failed to mourn father, immortality would be denied him. In this eventuality, "My life would have been worth next to nothing." Next to this fear, the possibility that his son might harbor hostile-destructive wishes toward him was almost as nothing.

While Mr. K was certainly most concerned with the possibility of being denied immortality, he was now able to voice other anticipatory concerns as well. Thus, he expressed concern about his wife's welfare should he die. He had seen his mother's distress and suffering in the wake of his father's death, and he cried as he contemplated his wife's potential pain and impotence. He, like Mr. I, came to view his death as an almost hostile act toward the wife and family, and he, like Mr. M, overdrew and possibly embellished the nature and extent of the wife's dependency on him. Knowing Mrs. K and Mrs. M to be devoted but competent, self-sufficient and highly resourceful women, and while not for a moment doubting the depth of their devotion, the strength of their marital bonds and the possibility of some deep-seated dependency on their husbands, one could not be deluded that they would be as totally impoverished and enduringly incapacitated as their husbands made out. It was a highly sensitive and touchy matter to discuss with the transplant candidate and points up one of the many differences between counseling the dying and terminally ill, where appropriate decathexis is the goal, *and* therapeutic work with the transplant candidate, where decathexis must be carefully regulated because of the good prospects for survival. Their concerns were squarely in the context of their reaching for some measure of immortality. If, indeed, their wives were to be permanently incapacitated to the point of malfunction by the candidates' deaths, then the candidates could maintain a belief in their enduring impact on the world. The extent to which they would be missed and the degree to which others could not get along without them seemed to have become for these candidates a measure of the significance of their lives—testimony to the fact that their existence did after all make a difference.

Mr. M introduced in clearest fashion still another, and to this point, obscured parallel between past and present. Once again the relationship to his father was invoked as prototype, and once again the comprehension of the earlier relationship paved the way to articulation and understanding of the present crisis between father and son.

Mr. M had discussed his father as hero, as martyr, as stalwart patriot, and as gallant and unflinching in the face of death. He had also raged at his father's open imputation that Mr. M was unmasculine and/or cowardly. Now, he offhandedly allowed that his illness and his possible death might prove a means of saving his son who was due to see military service in a combat zone. Mr. M stated, "If I die on the operating table, my son will be exempted from duty because he will be the sole support of my wife." Mr. M recognized that he was in part seeking the silver lining by rationalizing the good that would obtain from surgical failure. His death would be near sacrificial and a rebirth for the son. Mr. M then began to wonder about his son's motives: Did, for example, the boy really want exemption and would he claim the father's indigence as a basis for it? Would it in fact be cowardly for the boy to seek exemption? I took this opportunity to point out to Mr. M that he was now simultaneously identified with his father and his son, and that this placed him in considerable conflict, made him wary of his son's motives and, to some extent, threatened to further alienate his boy from him. I suggested that with the intensified sense of identification with his own father, he was drawn to adopt his father's attitude toward his son, Mr. M, and that in this way his son was like a replica of himself, at least as he had remembered himself to be nearly thirty years ago. Thus, while suspicious of his son just as his father had been suspicious of him, he also could feel a keen identification with his boy as well. The anger and resentment he had harbored toward father, he must also assume his son harbored toward him now. Mr. M was quickly intrigued by the parallels and picked up the lead. He wondered aloud if maybe this wasn't the reason for his having dwelled on the past and his father during the past weeks. And he was able to readily advance the idea that a part of his fear was that his son would be unable to mourn for Mr. M, just as Mr. M could not mourn his father. He too was frightened that some measure of immortality would elude him. Finally, Mr. M was able to visualize how his wish to "sacrifice" himself for his son might hurt as much as help the boy. He recalled the painful intensity of the guilt induced in him by his father's self-denying, self-sacrificing attitudes and it filled him with chagrin to recognize that he might similarly want to compromise his son. Rather than a benevolent wish, Mr. M came to regard it as distinctly hostile in intent. With this insight his rage at his son for possibly "using" him, while in the very process of deserting him, abated considerably.

On the whole, there can be little doubt that the major task in this last preoperative phase of work with the transplant candidate was that of assisting him in the reconciliation of the pieces of his past, present and future. If further involved an effort to minimize the candidate's fear that he would be deprived a measure of immortality, i.e. a reduction in his tacit conviction that his life may have counted for naught. Value or meaning seemed to attach, for the transplant candidate, to coherence and integrity of experience. And the reality of the matter was that their lives did have an inescapable thematic unity and continuity and did touch and deeply affect the lives of those around them. Their struggle in the weeks of waiting for surgery was consonant with the process of "summing up" (the stock taking) and is a piece of the quest for identity that death is bound to engender in all of us.

Mr. I was as startled as any of the candidates to find remarkable parallels between his situation vis-a-vis his children and his remembered situation vis-a-vis his father. He too was concerned that he would be unmourned and soon forgotten. He talked about how his family was already pulling away from him. They no longer made efforts to visit him regularly. As we discussed his feelings about loss and being left, Mr. I was able to advance the notion that failure to mourn a deceased did not mean that the deceased had been forgotten, lost or relegated to the past. Based on his own recent experiences, he decided that what the failure to mourn was really about was mixed attitudes toward the deceased. He himself pointed out, however, that many elements of the unmourned father had, in his instance, been retained. He simply had never recognized it as such until now.

He began to describe the many interests and facets of his father's personality that he had taken over and made part of himself. Over the years he had done any number of the things his father had done or had wanted to do. I emphasized that I felt he was very correct in his observation. That, despite his mixed feelings toward his father, he had done these things for his father and for himself. I pointed out that these were almost the same thing, and in a sense he had kept his father alive within him even though he had never thought of it in precisely those terms, but that he was sure his children had already done the same despite their seeming withdrawal at this time. Mr. I speculated about people who had made great contributions to the world—people who had become famous and whose names and reputations lived on after their death. Mr. I acknowledged that he had not achieved anything like this, yet he felt that some measure of immortality had come his way insofar as he had been able to give tangible and intangible things to his children. He commented on the vividness with which he could now remember his father, and he stated that he would be satisfied if thirty years from now his children could call up memories of him with equal vividness. With a rather pensive and speculative attitude, he said that he felt sure they would be able to do so.

SUMMARY AND CONCLUSIONS

I have described in some detail experiences with and impressions of six men who were candidates for heart and lung transplantations. I saw these men at a time when these procedures were highly experimental. As of this writing there has still not been a successful lung transplant performed. I have tried to consider in close view the crisis of the transplant candidate as a curcible for learning about the psychological insides of people as they face imminent death and/or the renewed hope for extended life. Attention has been given only to preoperative findings. Posttransplant events have not been touched on and are left for another time. Also put aside for future consideration are data derived from contacts with the members of the candidate's family.* A number of cautions are in order. First, data are based

*Then, too, only hinted at and not discussed are a number of themes which for purposes of conceptual coherence have been treated as peripheral, i.e. themes such as the candidate's loss of privacy and the assault on his personal dignity, or his enforced hyperdependency and the resultant embarrassment at exposing his infantile helplessness, or among still other unmentioned themes his engrandized sense of self, something steadily inflated by the attentions of a hospital staff which dotes upon the candidate both as potential prize and as public curiosity.

only on the six cases seen by the author, and there is little basis for assessing the generalizability of findings and/or the representativeness of the sample. One cannot say, for example, whether the prominent dynamics of the men reported on here reflect the peculiarities of persons who agree to this kind of surgery, i.e. men who agree to heart transplantation may have unique motives quite different from those who, given the same opportunity for a transplant, refuse it. Nor can it be said whether all men facing death experience the kinds of conflicts sampled here, or if only do those facing transplantations of hearts and lungs. It is simply assumed that the experiences, conflicts and dynamics reported here have in some measure moderate applicability to all dying men and wider applicability to all men agreeing to undergo heart or lung transplant surgery. That is, these findings probably apply to a fair percentage of heart transplant candidates, and one would guess to a substantial, if lesser, percentage of terminally ill patients. Emphasizing the partial and tentative nature of answers, then, is largely a matter of proper caution.

Second, much discussion has concentrated on data derived from but three of the six candidates. The caution regarding generalizability is well taken, therefore, even in this sample.

Third is a point related to the preceding, namely, that a personal need or bias may well have shaped my views of and experience with these men; to the extent this is true, the representativeness of my report may be questioned. For example, all the men were not seen with the same frequency or for the same length of time prior to surgery. One sometimes had little control over this factor. Some candidates awaited donors and surgery longer than others. In another sense, however, the author may have exerted some selective control over the matter of frequency. It was always necessary to keep in mind one's own reactions to death, one's own sources of resistance, fear and need for mastery of the topic, and to continually balance and weigh these against what similar conflicts and defenses were costing a candidate in pain. Not unexpectedly, more success was achieved in relating to some candidates than others. What is reported here may to some extent reflect that differential success.

Fourth, the discussion does not pretend to be exhaustive of topics touched on by all or even any one of the candidates. Time and space prohibited such completeness. Some decision regarding inclusiveness had to be made. It was made in favor of highlighting the themes common to these men—themes considered common either by virtue of their mutual presence or absence; obviously enough, however, the transplant candidates discussed matters other than those reported on in detail here.

Central to all that has been described is the notion that people learn to die and that this learning is a function of cultural inputs, prior experience with death and mourning. Equally central, but perhaps more tacit, is the notion that once a person has truly mourned for a significant other, he is subsequently free to mourn for others who, in the course of time, may die—including the self. Conversely, the failure to mourn a significant other acts to inhibit the mourning of other persons at later dates, including the self.

There are other significant corollaries which have been explicitly discussed in this paper or at least alluded to. One is that mourning is becoming increasingly difficult in our technologically advancing society; in a day and age when people die away from home, in hospitals and among relative strangers, and in a day and culture when natural death is seldom encountered, terror of death is the common experience. Death becomes trauma, and the vulnerability of the mourning process is practically a guaranteed outcome.

If nothing else, the clinical experience with the transplant candidates amplifies these points. But it suggests more as well. First, it suggests that when mourning fails to occur, much pain is incurred and felt over the span of many years. There is a fantastic psychic cost to our society involved here, one which is still relatively undiscovered and one which very much needs recognizing. Second, the clinical experience with the transplant candidates suggests that there exists within the individual, and hopefully within the society, a press toward health and good adaptation. The transplant candidates were working and struggling to find their way to solutions. We ought to create the mechanisms or at least the atmosphere for society to do the same. Third, the material covered suggests that as currently constituted our rapidly advancing technological society creates more problems than it can know, much less tend to. Fourth, it is suggested that thousands of persons approach the end of their life in similar psychic predicaments, i.e. needing to mourn, sum up, and account for an identity, but lacking a notoriety that obtains for them a team of mental health specialists; as a consequence they die silently and painfully, distanced from their closest family. If not for the transplant procedure, one may be sure the six men discussed in this paper would have suffered the same ignominious end and we would be no much the wiser. Fifth, the clinical data with these men strongly suggests the need for a mental health team in medical realms where death and trauma are the order of the day. There are a variety of reasons for this but three main ones will suffice. (1) While surgeons and cardiologists and other medical men should not be insensitive to the psychology of death and their own counterphobic biases toward death—in fact I believe their medical school curriculum should include courses and sensitivity training about such matters—I do not believe that they should be expected to carry the burdens of the psychotherapist as well. It is too time-consuming, too draining and debilitating. (2) The mental health team is also necessitated because, as the experience of these men made clear, the candidate cannot comfortably expose to his wife or family his fears, rage and irrationalities. Not only is a family member generally loathe to accept the supportive-therapeutic role, but the dying person has left sufficient human dignity that he is not willing to suffer that final humiliation, the baring of all the horrors of his present and past to a family that, remembering him as he once was in struggling to decathect and pull away. Instead, the mental health team member provides the ready and needed audience, one that does not press for solution or attention to so-called current crises and immediate realities. By the same token, the candidate can afford to be helplessly dependent and/or "undignified" and "despisable" in the mental healther's presence; the mental health person has no prior knowledge of the man, and the candidate need not put up or maintain the brave facade. (3) Finally, the mental healther remains interested in the candidate and not in his heart or lungs. This is no small item in a setting where all attentions are likely to go to an internal organ *other than* the candidate's embroiled mind itself.

In sum, this paper has been an effort to gain leverage on the pattern and inner meaning of what it feels like to face death, die, in present-day America. And if there is any point to be taken from this paper it is this: Dying has historically, and especially in our culture, been an extremely lonely act. It has, by consequence, also been very painful. Technological advances threaten to make it even more so, yet more lonely and more painful. I would like to think that the work with these six transplant candidates is a strong indication that this eventuality need no longer be the inevitable one.

REFERENCES

1. Abram, H. S.: Adaptation to open heart surgery: A psychiatric study of response to the threat of death. *Am. J. Psychiatry, 122*: 659-668, 1965.
2. Abram, H. S.: Psychological problems of patients after open heart surgery. *Hosp. Top.*, pp. 111-113, Jan. 1966.
3. Bermann, E.: Death, the family and some social taboos. Unpublished Manuscript. University of Michigan, 1970.
4. Cleveland, S.: Proceedings of the First International Symposium on the Socio-Medical Aspects of Organ Transplantation in Human Beings. Houston, March 1970.
5. Cox, P. R. and Ford, J. R.: The mortality of widows shortly after widowhood. *Lancet, 1*:163, 1964.
6. Cramond, W. A., Knight, P. R., and Lawrence, J. R.: The psychiatric contribution to a renal unit undertaking chronic hemodialysis and renal homotransplantation. *Br. J. Psychiatry, 113*: 1201-1212, 1967a.
7. Cramond, W. A.: Renal homotransplantation: some observations on recipients and donors. *Br. J. Psychiatry, 113*:1223-1230, 1967b.
8. Deutsch, Helene: Absence of grief. *Neuroses and Character types,* New York, International Universities Press, pp. 226-236, 1965.
9. Fulton, R. L.: *Death and Identity.* New York, John Wiley and Sons, 1965.
10. Geiken, P.: Proceedings of the First International Symposium on the Socio-Medical Aspects of Organ Transplantation in Human Beings. Houston, March 1970.
11. Glaser, B. G. and Strauss, A. L.: *Awareness of Dying.* Chicago, Aldine, 1965.

12. Goffman, E.: *Stigma: Notes on the Management of Spoiled Identity.* New Jersey, Prentice-Hall, 1963.
13. Goldman, E.: *The Tragedy of Lyndon Johnson.* New York, Dell, 1968.
14. Hebb, D. O.: The mammal and his environments. *Am. J. Psychiatry, 111*(1):826-831, 1954.
15. Hinton, J.: *Dying.* Middlesex, Penguin Books, 1967.
16. Husek, Jacqueline M.: Psychological aspects of chronic hemodialysis: a summary and review of the literature; suggestions for further research. Unpublished manuscript, School of Public Health, University of California, Los Angeles, 1967.
17. Kemph, J. P.: Renal failure, artificial kidney and kidney transplant. *Am. J. Psychiatry, 122*:1270-1274, 1966.
18. Kemph, J. P.: The role of the psychiatrist on the kidney transplant team. In the *Proceedings of the Academy of Psychosomatic Medicine.* International Congress Series No. 134. New York, Excerpta Medica Foundation, pp. 95-97, 1966.
19. Kemph, J. P.: Psychotherapy with patients receiving kidney transplant. *Am. J. Psychiatry, 124*:623-629, 1967.
20. Kemph, J. P., Berman, E. A., and Coppolillo, H. P.: Kidney transplant and shifts in family dynamics. *Am. J. Psychiatry, 125*(11):1485-1490, 1969.
21. Kraus, A. S. and Lilienfeld, A. M.: Some epidemiological aspects of the high mortality rate in the young widowed group. *J. Chronic Dis., 10*:207, 1959.
22. Lazarus, H. R. and Hagens, J. H.: Prevention of psychosis following open heart surgery. *Am. J. Psychiatry, 124*(9):1190-1195, 1968.
23. Lifton, R. J.: Psychological effects of the atomic bomb in Hiroshima: the theme of death. *Deadalus, 92*:462-497, 1963.
24. Lindemann, E.: Symptomatology and management of acute grief. *Am. J. Psychiatry, 101*:141, 1944,
25. Lydgate, J.: Where is thy sting? *Spectator, 206*:308, 1961.
26. Miller, A.: Death of a salesman. In Gassner, J. (Ed.): *A Treasury of the Theatre.* New York, Simon and Schuster, 1950.
27. Molish, B.: Proceedings of the First International Symposium on the Socio-Medical Aspects of Organ Transplantation in Human Beings. Houston, March 1970.
28. Rosner, A.: Mourning before the fact. *J. Am. Psychoanal. Assoc., 10*:564-570, 1962.
29. Ross, Elisabeth Kubler: *On Death and Dying.* New York, Macmillan, 1969.
30. Sartre, J. P.: *Existentialism and Human Emotions.* New York, Philosophical Library, 1957.

31. Thomas D.: A refusal to mourn the death, by fire, of a child in London. In *Collected Poems*. New York, New Directions, 1953.
32. Weisman, A. D., and Hackett, T. P.: Predilection to death. *Psychosom. Med., 23*:232-256, 1961.
33. Welkind, A.: Psychiatric complications of cardiac surgery. *J. Med. Soc. N. J., 65*(3):112-116, 1968.
34. Wolfenstein, Martha: Death of a parent and death of a president: children's reactions to two kinds of loss. In Wolfenstein, M. and Klimen, A. (Eds.): *Children and the Death of a President.* New York, Doubleday, 1965.
35. Wolfenstein, Martha: How is mourning possible?, *Phychoanal. Study of the Child.* New York, International Universities Press, *21*:93-123, 1966.
36. Wolfenstein, Martha: Loss, rage and repetition. *Psychoanal. Study of the Child,* New York, International Universities Press, *24*:432-460, 1969.
37. Young, M., Benjamin, B., and Wallis, C.: The mortality of widowers. *Lancet, 2*:454, 1963.

Chapter 14

WHEN DO WE DIE?

Arthur Winter, M.D.

In the past, when the patient stopped breathing and his heart stopped pumping, we pronounced the patient dead. Of course, sometimes these signs were imperceptible and there may even have been a slight mistake in the exact time of death.

But, why is the determination so important now? Is dying any different than before? The reason is that we are now in the age of modern miracles, the age of transplantation of organs. People are alive and contributing to society when, just a few years ago, they would have died without the use of transplanted tissues. There are mothers, fathers, children, doctors, laborers, teachers, writers, who have been given new kidneys, corneas and even hearts.

It is very important that we precisely determine the moment of death so that those tissues that are so necessary can be utilized for others who so desparately need them. There must also be a selection of which people will be donors and a selection of those who will be recipients of these organs. This decision, of course, comes from two sources: (1) from a person's own desire beforehand to donate his organs in a legal manner or from the closest member of his family, and (2) the physically ill recipient who accepts an organ so he may live a more normal life.

The new definition of death is that when the brain is dead, the body is dead! We do know that the brain dies within five minutes. There are factors which will modify this so that we must be very careful when we do pronounce someone dead. We must determine at what point the patient can "return to life" because of our modern devices, with or without neurological deficits, and at what point he has reached the inevitable status of death.

The following cases indicate how difficult the determination of death can be today. In some severe brain damage, the patients were dying and there was no chance whatsoever of their returning to life. In others, patients who had brain trauma, the patients appeared to be dying and, yet, were able to return to life with minimal neurological deficits.

Case One

A nineteen-year-old Marine was admitted to St. Barnabas Medical Center after sustaining severe head injuries in an automobile accident. On admission, he responded briefly but was semi-comatose. His pupils were dilated, fundal vessels were engorged and he had blurring of the discs indicating increased brain pressure. His scalp was almost completely detached from the skull. He was bleeding profusely. At times, there were some spontaneous movements in the lower extremities. Pressure dressings were applied. X-rays disclosed an older occipital wound due to mortar fragments and, superimposed on this, a fracture line from the second injury. Diagnoses were cerebral concussion, laceration of the scalp and mortar fragment injury to the skull. The patient was given antibiotics and tetanus antitoxin, and we took him immediately to the operating room to repair this deep laceration and to see whether he had subdural hematoma. Burr holes disclosed an acute subdural hematoma and the laceration in the scalp was repaired. He never regained consciousness. His pupils showed some reaction to light on the first postoperative day. Vital signs remained stable for twenty-four hours and he was given vigorous treatment which included hypothermia, antibiotics, and steroids. In spite of all this, his condition seemed to deteriorate. That evening the patient had a respiratory arrest and then a transient cardiac arrest. A closed chest massage was carried out and an endotracheal tube was hooked up to the respirator. His pupils did not come fully dilated at that time, but there was a gradual dropping in his blood pressure to hypotensive levels. We gave him Mannitol and intravenous Solu-Cortef®. We took him back to the operating room to determine whether he was rebleeding or whether he had massive brain edema. The flap was turned and it was evident that it was massive brain swelling in spite of all methods that we used. The brain literally started coming out of the defect in the skull. His postoperative course was that of gradual deterioration due to massive brain injury, secondary cardiac arrest and respiratory arrest and, therefore, irreparable brain damage.

This was a case in which there was irreparable damage to the brain, secondary to his severe head injury. A healthy young body with a dead brain, he was a possible donor for organ transplantation. However, there were no recipients for the organs at the time of death.

Case Two

A forty-four-year-old man was admitted to the hospital because of severe frontal headaches for the last two weeks. An ophthalmologist found papilledema and unilateral hemianopsia. He had an equivocal right facial droop, blood pressure was 160/70, pulse was 78. He had some pain on flexion of his head with some question of nuchal guarding. The patient was obtunded and he had some difficulty doing serial sevens. The impression at this time was that he definitely had increased intracranial pressures possibly due to vascular subarachnoid bleeding because of the nuchal guarding or possible brain tumor. At lumbar puncture, pressure was 180, 10 red cells, but no white cells. Protein was 92 mg% and sugar 124 mg%. Left carotid arteriogram, EEG, and brain scan revealed a very large temporoparietal lesion. Postoperatively, he did very well. On radiation therapy, he continued to improve for six months. His headaches disappeared and he wanted to go back to work. Then, there was evidence of recurrence and, in spite of radiation and chemotherapy with Actinomycin D, the patient's course became worse. His wife gave permission for organ transplantation, but as the body was enroute by ambulance to another state, the heart stopped beating and personnel were not available to restart it.

In these two cases, death was predetermined before the heart stopped beating. One death was due to a severe brain injury and the other to a malignant tumor. In the latter case, it would have been senseless to prolong his suffering and use extraordinary means to keep him "alive."

Following are other cases in which the patients approached death but were able to return with varying results.

Case Three

A six-year-old girl was hospitalized after being hit by a car. She had been thrown a distance of fifty feet and was rendered suddenly unconscious. She remained in the hospital for a week where a tracheotomy was performed. She was treated with hypothermia because of a temperature ranging up to 106. She had fractured ribs, fractured right humerus, and was comatose. She looked like a "broken doll." Brain scan, electroencephalogram and other diagnostic studies indicated increased pressure over the right temporal area. At subtemporal decompression, we noted marked swelling of the surface of the brain but no evidence of subdural hematoma. Seven hours postoperatively the child seemed to respond to painful stimuli and became more alert.

There was a gradual decrease in her spasticity and she started to respond to sound. The child became progressively more alert and was given carbon dioxide therapy to increase the vascularity to her brain and hyperbaric oxygen treatment with steroids. As each day went by, she became brighter. Suddenly one day, she smiled. With her eyes she was following the examiner about the room and within three weeks she could obey commands. Then, there was evidence of spontaneous laughter. She could now respond to questions by nodding her head and verbalizing. Then she recognized her mother and improved daily in her vocabulary and conceptual ability. The child finally was taking feedings by mouth, her words increased to sentences, recognition and personality improved and she was discharged. She continues to improve now five months after her initial injury in which she was deeply comatose. The diagnosis here was laceration of the brain, cerebral concussion, multiple fractures of the femur, ribs, and abrasions. Her intelligence was intact but she was left with spasticity. She continues to receive physiotherapy and is attending school.

Case Four

A thirty-seven-year-old female was brought into the emergency room in coma. She had tried to commit suicide by taking an overdose of drugs, locking herself in the bathroom, slashing her wrists, and jumping out of the second-story window. When she arrived in the emergency room, she was in shock. Blood pressure was 70/0, the pulse was thready, and the patient was bleeding from her right ear and scalp and slashed wrists. The pupils were dilated and she was showing decerebrate posturing. The impression was that she had a brain laceration and was in shock from the profuse bleeding from her scalp and wrists. She also had a basilar skull fracture. The patient was given plasma and whole blood to maintain her blood pressure. X-rays revealed a fracture of the skull in the temporo-occipital region on the right. There was the possibility of an epidural hematoma too. Burr holes were made, using the anterior portion of the fracture line as a clue for possible epidural bleeding. There was no epidural hematoma, but as soon as the burr hole was made, it was found that the patient had acute subdural bleeding. Just prior to the operation the patient was on the stretcher and we were shaving her hair. At this point, she had a sudden cardiac arrest. We began immediate cardiac massage and then started to defibrilate her. She had four more arrests. We felt, of course, the patient had expired, but because of her age and the type of injury, a first burr hole was made over the area described. As soon as the dura was open, the subdural hematoma burst, spurted out under pressure, and evacuated itself. Then the patient's cardiac rhythm and heart beat returned to normal and became spontaneous. The brain surface itself was purplish in color, indicating underlying severe brain damage.

She gradually improved to the point where she did recognize her parents. With intensive physiotherapy and care, she learned to walk again but there is a great deal of personality change here. At one time, she had been a pretty, talented young lady and had been a singer on television. The personality had changed since her injury in that she was uninhibited in her language, saying whatever came to mind, and she required constant nursing care because of the suicide attempt. At her last evaluation, in a nursing home, she was walking by herself. She did recognize some people, but there was still evidence of severe brain damage. There was, according to the follow-up history, some continued but slight improvement since her initial injury.

With this type of patient, It was impossible to determine beforehand how much restoration of cerebral function there would be and what the final outcome would have been. Since her heart had stopped five times and had to be restarted, how many times was she really dead? Is she really alive now? If we knew the final outcome, would we still have tried so hard to fight death? Even though someone who wanted to live might have benefited from the organs of a young, physically healthy woman who wanted to die, the new criteria of death did not apply. She was alive, even if she did not want to be.

Case Five

This six-year-old girl was a passenger in her mother's car. The front tire blew out and the car ran into a telephone pole. When she was brought into the hospital, she was comatose, bleeding from her ears and nose. She had dilated pupils, became apneic and then started a convulsive seizure of the left side of the body. She had, at this time, severe swelling over the right side of her face and jaw and it looked as if she were going to die within the next few minues. I immediately gave her intravenous Dilantin®, Solu-Cortef®, and Mannitol. We took her to the operating room. This all took place within a period of about thirty-eight minutes. As soon as the dura was opened the spinal fluid shot out under pressure. It was then evident that this skull was depressed at almost ? cm into her brain. After the Mannitol was administered and the decompression operation completed, the surface of the brain started to pulsate. Her color improved. We then put her on steroids, Chymoral®, Dilantin, and intravenous fluids. Within eight days, she began to verbalize. The tracheotomy cannula was removed. She is now attending school and is doing very well in her school achievement.

Here is a youngster, where it looked as if the moment of death was very close, yet because of the excellent cooperation of the house staff and operating room, we were able to reverse the procedure and bring her back to normal function.

Case Six

A seventy-one-year-old woman was found comatose by the police in her apartment. There was a garage under her apartment, and a driver put his car in and forgot to shut off the ignition. This left the car running. The couple on the second floor above noted severe headaches and nausea and opened the windows, felt better, and notified the police. The couple then remembered that there was a widow on the first floor above the garage. The police broke in and the woman was found in deep coma. The car had been running for hours. The comatose state was due to carbon monoxide poisoning. At the hospital she was treated with medication to reduce brain swelling and with hyperbaric oxygenation. When I saw her in the hospital, she was comatose, completely unresponsive to any stimuli, her pupils were in moderate dilatation and her prognosis was very poor. But then, she responded to treatment and showed a gradual return of cerebral function.

Here is a patient who seemed to be on the verge of death from carbon monoxide poisoning, but she was able to be restored to complete normal functioning.

These cases illustrate the need for a new definition of death. All six could have provided their organs for transplantation. According to the ad hoc committee at Harvard, specific defined conditions are necessary to pronounce a patient dead. They are as follows:

1. Unrecepitivity and unresponsivity. The patient is unaware of any stimuli and does not respond to them.

2. No movements or breathing after it has been stopped for a period of three minutes, it is obvious that he is not breathing by himself.

3. No reflexes. The pupils are dilated and fixed. They do not respond to any source of bright light. Irrigation of the ears does not produce any head turning or ocular movements.

4. A "flat" electronencephalogram is to be checked so that it remains isolectric at double the standard gain which is $5\mu v/mm$. At least ten full minutes of recording are required by the ad hoc committee suggests that they be done for at least twenty minutes. There also should be no response on the electroencephalogram to external stimuli such as noise or skin pinching; these stimuli ordinarily do provoke changes on a normal brain.

All these tests mentioned above should be repeated at least twenty-four hours later. The EEG may be modified, however, by toxic conditions such as hypothermia, or drugs such as barbiturates, and this must be excluded before accepting just the EEG.

In their report, the committee suggests that:

The patient's condition can be determined only by a physician. When the patient is hopelessly damaged, his family and all colleagues who have participated in major decisions concerning the patient, and all nurses involved, should be so informed. Death is to be declared and the respirator turned off. The decision to do this and responsibility for it is to be taken by the physician in charge, in consultation with one or more physicians who have been directly involved in the case. It is unsound and undesirable to force a family to make a decision.

Of course, if the family does not want the doctor to turn the mechanical devices off, he should respect their wishes. The physician who does declare the patient dead and turns off the respirator is not to be connected in any way with any transplantation procedure. This is to avoid any whisper of self-interest by the physicians involved. Personally, I think that the defined twenty-four hours (as suggested by the ad hoc committee) is a long time to wait with patients pronounced dead; that if the brain lives only five to ten minutes, at most, during an anoxic state, that an hour be considered as time sufficient when all the criteria are fulfilled as defined by the Harvard Group.

SUMMARY

Obviously, some people enter the state of coma and are near to the status of death, but yet return. Some who return can come back to a normal life. Others may come back with some or a great deal of neurologic deficit. It is important to determine which of these will come back and how much deficit they will have.

In the first two cases above (irreparable brain damage and a malignant brain tumor), we are able to define death and fulfill the criteria as indicated by the ad hoc committee of Harvard. The definition of death and its new criteria must be considered because of its relationship to newer concepts involving organ transplants. We must say that when the brain has died the patient has died! This cannot be defined as euthanasia because the patient is dead and the physician has not interrupted life!

Chapter 15

THE DWARF AND HIS FUTURE

A. Herbert Schwartz, M.D. and Jane S. Sturges, M.S.W.

Whether out of curiosity, respect, or monetary greediness, throughout history man has shown interest in dwarfs. Portraits of dwarfs can be found in almost all periods of art, with abundant representations in early Egyptian, Greek, Roman, Mayan, and pre-Columbian cultures. In antiquity, hunchback dwarfs were considered ill omens. Norse mythology pictures them as ugly, but powerful creatures. Even in the early Christian era, they were thought to be designated against by the gods. It was much later, in the Middle Ages, that dwarfs became symbols of good luck. Then some of the clever ones, instead of being relegated to the group of deformed beings despised by society, were highly sought after by royalty for pets, court jesters, or companions for their children.

> The appreciation accorded dwarfs in the 17th century is illustrated by an accurate Spanish record which states that Antonio el Inglés, one of the court dwarfs of King Philip IV, received a salary of 72 ducats, only 8 ducats less than that of the most celebrated and highly favored Spanish court painter, Diego Rodriquez y Silva de Velásquez. The paintings of dwarfs by Velásquez were so highly regarded that in the 17th and 18th centuries, many dwarfs, when members of the courts, achieved high social status and were allowed to eat, drink, and hunt with the kings.[1]

Dwarfs eventually passed from popularity, becoming relegated either to socially isolated existences or service as entertainers. However, during the past fifteen years, physiological and psychological research on growth hormone and dwarfism has resulted in recent medical advances which have produced a new interest in and new hope for the dwarfed child.

Dwarfism and giantism are the two extremes of human stature. While other factors are sometimes involved, the usual cause for these abnormalities is the production by the pituitary gland of too little or too much growth hormone. There are actually a number of kinds of dwarfism, and only in recent years has it been possible to distinguish pituitary (hypopituitary) dwarfs from other types. (The pituitary dwarf, while obviously short in stature, is in most other respects a perfectly formed human being.) It was the isolation of human growth hormone (HGH) in 1956 by Dr. Choh Hao Li of the University of California Medical Center that led to the first major breakthrough in the medical treatment of pituitary dwarfism. Since then, hundreds of pituitary dwarfs have been treated, and in many, growth has been successfully stimulated. Increases in stature have ranged from 1.4 to 18 cm in one year.[2] Though it has been observed that the best response to treatment is between the ages of five and ten,[3] the bones of the pituitary dwarf are capable of further growth beyond adolescence and even into early adulthood.

However, because of the scarcity of human growth hormone (HGH), which can only be obtained by extraction from human pituitaries at autopsy, research and clinical application have been impeded. Almost every pituitary, even from aged donors, contains HGH, but only enough for a few days' supply. For example, HGH from 100 to 300 pituitaries is needed to stimulate the growth of one child with pituitary dwarfism for one year. The National Pituitary Agency and a lay organization of parents called Human Growth, Inc. were formed to further the collection of pituitaries. In spite of their efforts, however, there is a far from sufficient supply to treat the estimated 5,000 to 10,000 pituitary dwarfs in our country. Therefore, up to the present, HGH has only been available for research, and then only in limited quantities.

Unfortunately, nothing will do as well therapeutically as human growth hormone. Though GH is secreted by the pituitary gland in all vertebrates, unlike many other hormones, it is exceedingly species specific. A number of researchers have studied the effects in man of growth hormone from pigs, sheep, and cattle, but none can stimulate growth. Monkey growth hormone is the only exception. Its effects closely parallel those of HGH but differ quantitatively.

HGH, in addition to stimulating growth in pituitary dwarfs, can sometimes correct growth disorders in which the role of the pituitary is less clear. Notable among these is dwarfism associated with Turner's syndrome, caused by the absence or abnormality of one of the sex chromosomes. HGH may also be beneficial in correcting growth disturbances resulting from administration of large quantities of corticosteroids, as in the asthmatic child who must be kept on steroids as a lifesaving measure.

For all of its proven growth-promoting activity, the hormone does not (as one might expect) disappear from the body when a person reaches full stature. Evidently it performs varied functions throughout life. For example, there are indications that blood sugar and growth hormone are linked together in a sort of mutual feedback system, but what biological functions such a control system might have is unknown. The most immediate effect of the administration of HGH is an acute fall in blood sugar levels, which is followed by a rise in both diabetic and normal individuals. However, the relationship between the hormone's growth-promoting and blood-sugar-reducing effects is unclear.

HGH also has a marked anabolic effect, stimulating nitrogen retention, though how this occurs is not clear. These anabolic effects obviously help to explain the hormone's growth-producing activity. There is evidence that the hormone's anabolic action may prove valuable in reversing the very severe negative nitrogen balance associated with major trauma, surgery, injury or burns. Experiments with animals suggest that HGH may one day help to heal burns and knit broken bones as well. In addition, present indications are that HGH lowers blood cholesterol, enhances resistance to infection by stimulating antibody productions, and reacts with sex hormones to make them work more effectively.

However, in research on growth hormone, questions outweigh answers, whether we consider its physiological functions or its therapeutic potential. In conditions where there is some evidence that HGH may be beneficial, in none of them is there any hard data on how beneficial, or for how long, or in what patients. Even in pituitary dwarfism, by far the best-documented area of HGH therapy, we cannot now predict which patients will respond to it and which will not, let alone determine precisely the proper timing of dose or optimal dosage.[4]

One must bear in mind, as well, that the assessment of research to date on the biological activity of HGH must be tempered by the knowledge that without using a synthetically produced and therefore more likely pure hormone, the various preparations from human pituitary glands have had varying degrees of purity and of effect. Dr. Choh Hao Li has again made medical history, just recently, by unraveling the hormone's complex chemical structure and producing it synthetically. When this laboratory process can be refined to produce a fully biologically active and commercially available hormone is not yet known.

As for current psychological research, a growing professional interest in growth abnormalities and current social and professional concern for the care of children, especially those who have been emotionally deprived or physically abused, has been noted in the literature. Recent publications suggest new syndromes in which the production, the mechanism of release, or the inhibition of HGH by another substance may be implicated. Several studies have suggested an association between growth failure and the social and emotional environment of the child.

The devastating effects of severe emotional deprivation and institutional life on infants have been recognized for many years.[5] A study in two institutions for homeless children in postwar Germany showed dramatic evidence of the effects of a disturbed emotional climate on the weights and heights of school age children.[6] However, awareness of psychosocial factors within the family as a possible cause of growth failure is of more recent origin. How emotional factors influence growth is not completely understood. Speculations include effects on appetite and food intake, disturbances of intestinal motility and absorption, interference with intermediary metabolism and utilization, and influence on endocrine regulation of growth by the hypothalamus, pituitary, or adrenal cortex.[7]

One study of infants with failure to thrive unexplained by organic disease found in their families multiple stresses plus diminished ability of the parents to meet or master their increasing responsibilities. The reason why one particular infant in a family failed to thrive remained unanswered but may have resulted from some inherent vulnerability in the infant, his special meaning to his family, or added stress associated with his birth. Mothers of these infants were described as failing to thrive as mothers and presenting the need for nurturing themselves in order to promote their capacities to nurture their babies.[8] A similar study of children with clinical findings suggestive of idiopathic hypopituitarism found short stature but one aspect of a continuum of adverse effects of a distorted parent-child relationship and perhaps the first clinical suggestion of such a disturbed relationship. The suggestion was made that historical features, physical and laboratory findings, and rapid growth in an adequate environment should distinguish this syndrome from idiopathic hypopituitarism.[9]

"Deprivation dwarfism" is a term used to describe a clinical condition of children who exhibit extreme short stature and have suffered emotional deprivation. These children show adequate growth for a variable period of time before a diminished rate of growth develops. Other features of this syndrome are an often voracious appetite, a marked delay in skeletal maturation, and persistent sleep disorders. Emotional disorders in the parents and grossly disturbed family relationships are generally found to be present. Changes in the child's environment, such as foster home placement, usually result in significantly improved growth and improvement in personality structure.[10]

On the other hand, some researchers have challenged the primary basis for the concept that there is an emotional control over growth independent of caloric consumption. They conclude that maternally deprived infants are underweight because of undereating which is secondary to not being offered adequate food or not accepting it, and not because of some psychological problem.[11] Others questions the methods, interpretations, and conclusions of these studies, recommending that attention be invested in both psychological factors and caloric intake for any child with unexplained growth retardation or failure to thrive[12]

However, some of these studies of the psychological aspects

of growth have either not measured or not adequately determined the child's production of HGH. It is obvious then that in order to define this interface between the psychological and biological factors in growth, collaborative studies by child psychiatrists, psychologists, social workers, and pediatric endocrinologists are needed.

Relatively little has appeared in the professional literature regarding the emotional development of children who suffer from dwarfism. One study called attention to the use of denial in dwarfed people and a tendency toward psychological infantilism, often augmented by the way dwarfs are treated by others.[13] Some dwarfs have been described as making "poignant attempts" at mastery of the problems posed by their short stature. Aiding the child to face up to his lack of growth and to correct his fantasies about the cause of the problem has been found to be helpful. Some investigators have reported intelligence testing on dwarfed individuals and found a normal distribution. They have commented on the difficulty adults have in treating the children as individuals rather than mascots, pointing out that such children, as they advanced into teens, become more handicapped in their social and psychological adjustment.[14]

Others have confirmed the lack of impairment as measured in intelligence tests but found that school achievement often lagged behind. The degree of psychological maturation achieved tended to parallel the degree to which the dwarf had been treated socially according to his age, not size. Psychopathology, when present, was of the inhibitive, dissociative type with constriction of the cognitive field, and aggression and acting out were conspicuously absent.[15] Other researchers found that in the majority of children with short stature studied, school achievement was satisfactory. The influence of a stable family and the stimulus of the educational system appeared to have provided this group of children with a means to acceptance through social and academic performance.[16] Still another study of children and adolescents with pituitary insufficiency found a lower intelligence quotient for the group as a whole, as well as for a variety of clinical subgroups when compared with the normal population. Also noted was a distinct deficiency in visuomotor functioning.[17]

The evaluation of the validity of research on the psychological aspects of the child of short stature (dwarfism) must be tempered by the absence in many studies of accepted criteria of abnormality in both psychological and physiological functions and by the infrequent confirmation of findings by other researchers using similar research criteria and methods. The following descriptions from a recently completed five-year psychological and physiological study of twenty-five significantly dwarfed cihldren and their families,[18] and from a review of over 100 questionnaries completed by members of Human Growth, Inc. throughout the country, must be seen as observations and speculations rather than hard data.[19]

Many of these children experienced an early distortion and perhaps deprivation in the mother-child relationship secondary either to a death in the family, physical illness of the mother or child, psychological illness in the mother, or a marital separation of the parents occurring around the age of six months to two years. Also, a few of these children experienced physiological difficulty prior to birth or shortly thereafter. How frequently these varied psychological and physiological trauma occur in the overall population of dwarfs and to what extent they affect present or future production of growth hormone is not known. However, the concept of critical periods during which a biological development can and must take place is not foreign to embryological, biological, nor psychological development. Perhaps an early trauma may impair growth hormone not only temporarily but also for life?

A further disruption of the mother-child relationship begins when the mother suspects, despite the delivery of a healthy baby, that something is wrong. A confirmation of this suspicion usually takes place when the physician finds that the child is not growing adequately. This frequently takes place between one and eight years of age. As the parents become more certain that their child will be extremely short, they begin to experience a sense of loss much as the parents of a congenitally deformed child experience at his birth. However, the parents of the potential child of short stature are first confronted with a more prolonged expectation of normality for their child and, then, the loss of this expectation.

They may react with feelings of guilt and depression with further stress on the mother-child relationship. With such a loss, marital stresses are frequently increased, leading to a further decrease in mother's ability to nurture her child.

As for the child, he, too, experiences a loss when he begins to realize that he is markedly shorter than other children and may not be normal. This is not the same as if he had a deformity from birth. Birth abnormalities can sometimes be accepted as something for which one is not responsible and therefore be more readily integrated into the body concept. The loss experienced by the child of short stature is different, too, from a deformity resulting from an accident, illness, or surgery. As there is no such obvious cause for short stature, there is more chance the child may experience guilt for a supposed transgression.[20] This guilt is frequently translated into magical thinking that if only he had eaten more of his "Green Giant peas" or other foods which were good for him, he would have grown. Sometimes the child projects this guilt onto his parents, holding them responsible because he was the last born or born close in time to another sibling. Such a child becomes angry and seems to turn this anger onto himself, producing further guilt and depression.

The final blow to both parents and child is the constant intrafamilial confirmation of his deformity that occurs when a younger sibling grows larger than the child with short stature. Fortunately, when this occurs, most children of short stature are already in school and have begun to utilize obsessive compulsive mechanisms for dealing with anxiety. And if they are at least average in scholastic ability (and most are), the parents' often repeated phrase, "It's brains not brawn that count," does not fall on deaf ears but become a stimulus to overachieve at school. Concomitantly, they frequently find peer acceptance in assuming the role of a mascot. Many of these male children experience difficulty in identifying with their fathers, for they cannot be proud of their physical abilities nor their aggressive prowess, because they learn sooner or later that it doesn't pay. Others can beat them up, and their retribution is too quick and easy. Frequently they develop verbal or intellectual ways of dealing with their aggressive feelings or perhaps rechannel them into school work, gymnastics, or special abilities.

Most of the children examined showed symptoms and signs of depression. However, this psychological diagnosis in childhood is just beginning to be elucidated in the medical literature, and such a diagnosis is not yet clear-cut. But, because of the recent data and theories about the biochemical changes that occur and are perhaps at times etiological in depression, a question must be raised: Does growth hormone play a role in depression?[21] Very preliminary data on growth hormone levels in adults who are depressed does not suggest this, and there is no reported data on children.

However, there are some interesting laboratory findings and speculations to be considered. First, one drug (A) used in humans for treatment of cardiac abnormalities produces a side effect of depression. In certain animals, this same drug blocks the release of growth hormone from the pituitary gland. Second, another drug (B) used in humans for treating depression, in animals will reverse the blockage in growth hormone caused by the first drug (A). But such thinking is speculative.[21]

With the recent remarkable synthesis of human growth hormone, however, a new path has been opened. For now human growth hormone may soon become readily available in a fully biologically active, pure synthetic form, which will provide physicians not only the opportunity to treat all those who we know at present will benefit, but to investigate further therapeutic uses. The door will be opened, as well, to a further definition and confirmation of the functions of human growth hormone and the role it plays in the etiology of various physical, and perhaps psychological, illnesses.

> A great discovery is a fact whose appearance in science gives rise to shining ideas, whose light dispels many obscurities and shows us new paths.[22]

REFERENCES

1. Hodge, Gerald P.: Perkeo, the dwarf-jester of Heidelberg. *J.A.M.A.,* *209*(No. 3):403-404, 1969.

2. Beck, John C.: The growth hormone puzzle. *Hosp. Practice,* May, 1967, p. 36.
3. Making the hormone: *Medical World News,* February 21, 1969, p. 35.
4. Beck, John C.: The growth hormone puzzle. *Hosp. Practice,* May, 1967, pp. 36-44.
5. Leonard, Martha F., Rhymes, Julina P., and Solnit, Albert J.: Failure to thrive in infants. *Am. J. Dis. Child., 3*:600, 1966.
6. Leonard, M. F. *et al.*: From Widdowson, E. M.: Mental contentment and physical growth. *Lancet, 260*:1316-1318, 1951.
7. Leonard, M. F. *et al.*: p. 600.
8. Leonard, M. F. *et al.*: p. 600-612.
9. Powell, G. F., Brasel, J. A., Raiti, S., and Blizzard, R. M.: Emotional deprivation and growth retardation simulating true idiopathic hypopituitarism. *N. Engl. J. Med., 276* (No. 23):1271-1278, 1967.
10. Silver, Henry K. and Finkelstein, Marcia: Deprivation dwarfism. *J. Pediatr., 70* (No. 3):317-324, 1967.
11. Whitten, Charles F., Pettit, Marvin G., and Fischhoff, Joseph: Evidence that growth failure from maternal deprivation is secondary to undereating. *J.A.M.A., 209*(No.11):1675-1682, 1969.
12. Leonard, Martha F. and Solnit, Albert J.: Growth failure from maternal deprivation or undereating. *J.A.M.A.,* Vol. 212, No. 5, 1970.
13. Hampson, J. L. and Money, J.: In Michael-Smith, H. (Ed.): *Management of the Handicapped Child.* New York, Grune and Stratten, 1957.
14. Martin, M. and Wilkins, L.: Pituitary dwarfism in diagnosis and treatment. *J. Clin. Endocrinol., 18*:679, 1958.
15. Pollitt, Ernesto and Money, John: Studies in the psychology of dwarfism. I. *J. Pediatr. 64*(No. 3):415-421, 1964. Money, John and Pollitt, Ernesto: Studies in the psychology of dwarfism. II. *J. Pediatr. 68* (No. 3):381-390, 1966.
16. Rosenbloom, Arlan L., Smith, David W., and Loeb, Dorothy G.: Scholastic performance of short-statured children with hypopituitarism. *J. Pediatr. 69* (No. 6):1131-1133, 1966.
17. Frankel, Jacob J. and Laron, Zvi: Psychological aspects of pituitary insufficiency in children and adolescents with special reference to growth hormone. *Isr. J. Med. Sci., 4*(No. 5):953-961, 1968.
18. Patients were studied in the Yale University Children's Clinical Research Center, supported by a grant (RR-00125) from the General Clinical Research Centers Program of the Division of Research Resources, National Institutes of Health.

19. Schwartz, A. Herbert, Grunt, Jerome A., McCollum, Audrey T. *et al.*: The Child of Short Stature. To be published.
20. Schwartz, A. Herbert and Landwirth, Julius: Birth defects and the psychological development of the child: some implications for management. *Conn. Med.*, *32*(No.6):457-463, 1968.
21. Schwartz, A. Herbert and Sturges, Jane S.: Psychological Effects of Human Growth Hormone in Children of Short Stature. To be published.
22. Bernard, Claude: *An Introduction to the Study of Experimental Medicine*, Pt. I, Ch. 2, Sect. ii, translated by H. C. Greene.

Chapter 16

MORAL AND SOCIAL IMPLICATIONS OF GENETIC MANIPULATION*

Amitai Etzioni, Ph.D.

The acceleration of biological engineering has been urged before Congress by Nobel Laureate Dr. Joshua Lederberg. He has called for the establishment of a National Genetics Task Force to increase the momentum of efforts aimed at unlocking the genetic code of man. Such a breakthrough in biology could lead to the prevention of many illnesses whose origin is wholly or partially in the genetic code.

There is much to be said in favor of such a task force. But it ought to be accompanied by a task force on the social and moral consequences of genetic manipulation. The imminent breakthroughs in biology may affect man as much or more as he was affected by previous revolutions in engineering and physics: the imposition of a new set of capacities, of freedoms, of choices society must make, of evil it can inflict.

Gene manipulation may also allow man to tamper with biological elements which heretofore had to be accepted, including the sex of children to be conceived, their features and color, and ultimately their race, energy levels, and perhaps even their IQs.

> Only 10 or 15 years hence, it could be possible for a housewife to walk into a new kind of commissary, look down a row of packets not unlike flower-seed packages and pick her baby by label. Each packet would contain a frozen one-day-old embryo, and the label would tell the shopper what color of hair and eyes to expect as well as the probable size and I.Q. of the child.[1]

*"An earlier and much shorter version of this article was published in the *New York Times* (September 5, 1970)."

267

While Dr. Hafez's predictions may be on the extreme side in terms of pace of progress expected, many other scientists have called for and predicted genetic control.*

Even now tests are made of the fluid in which the fetus floats to determine if there are any genetic defects *and* if it will be a boy or girl. Those tests are then used, at least in some instances, to order abortions. In conjunction, the tests plus the abortions amount to a very crude mode of genetic control. As the test, so far, cannot be carried out reliably before the fetus is fourteen to sixteen weeks old, the danger to the mother has to be weighed as compared to the benefits of "ordering" the desired child. However, in the near future this procedure may well be carried out when the fetus is two months old and be used routinely with very little danger. Thus, what may start as the biological control of illnesses could become an attempt to breed supermen. While this may appeal to some, think about the agonizing problems if man has to act as the creator and fashion the image of man.

SHOPPING FOR GENES

What supermen will the national task force order? Blond or brown, white or black? Highly charged or low-keyed? More males? And, who will make all these decisions—the parents shopping for genes in the supermarket, again expecting society to pick up the bill for the aggregate effects of individual decisions? Or, a government agency, a task force?

Fortunately, it seems we do not have to stop the genetic combat of illness to prevent genetic engineering for racist purposes. Contrary to widely held beliefs, studies show that the energy of science may be guided into one area to the relative neglect of others. It is generally thought that scientific work requires that the scientist follow any lead his investigating spirit encounters and which may take him any place. The findings of a sub-discipline of a field trickle freely into the others: hence, one kind of genetic manipulation will willy-nilly open the door to others.

Actually, most scientific findings are not readily transferable, and their application is affected by moral taboos. Next to no

---

*See, for instance, Dr. H. J. Muller's article in *Science*, September 8, 1961.

work is carried out in the psychology needed to develop sub-liminal advertising, and those scientists who sought to prove racist theories are starved for funds and academic recognition.

Before such guiding of scientific efforts can be effectively applied to the new genetics, we must have a clearer notion of the moral and social choices involved in the biological revolution and the mechanisms by which science can be guided without being stifled.

EXPLORE THE OPTIONS

Let us not again sail blindly into a storm unleashed by scientists anxious to unlock all of nature's secrets with little concern for who and what will be blown over in the resulting tidal waves.

During a recent meeting of ministers and rabbis in Princeton, I suggested that a board be set up by thoughtful men within the religious field and humanities as well as concerned biologists to examine the moral and social consequences of the imminent biological breakthroughs in the area of genetic control.

Before we go further we should examine the moral and social issues involved. No board of the kind envisioned could rule on these matters. This is not the way our society is run. But it could call to the attention of the public some of the dimensions involved and alert the scientific community to what it is getting into.

REFERENCE

1. Dr. Hafez: Foreseeing the unforeseeable. *Kaiser Aluminum News,* No. 6, 1966, p. 22.

Chapter 17

MORAL ISSUES IN SPORTS

Adrian C. Kanaar, M.D.

INTRODUCTION

Man loves danger, especially when related to competition. It challenges him to achieve beyond previous records. To disallow dangerous sports on a moralistic basis would be to rob him of one of the most exciting facets of his very nature. However, some limits must be defined beyond which we would not really be engaging in a *potentially* dangerous sport, but in a foolhardy and pointless pursuit.

An acceptable sport should necessitate skill, require self-discipline, emphasize sportsmanship, and improve physical and mental development. Examples are competitive ball games and athletics, including boxing, wrestling and gymnastics; individual fitness programs, marathon events, scuba diving and sky diving; racing with wheelchairs, cycles, cars, horses, dogs and planes; shooting rapids, climbing mountains, skiing, tightrope walking, stunts, and long distance journeys in small boats or rafts. Unacceptable "sports" are those which brutalize physically or emotionally, endanger bystanders or imitators needlessly, and produce no physical or mental benefit. Examples are cock-fighting, bullfighting, all-in wrestling with no holds barred,* competitive eating and drinking, marathon dancing, playing "last across," or "chicken" and Russian Roulette.

Some psychologists believe that those who take part in dangerous sports have a death wish. If this were commonly true, there would be far more fatalities. The astonishing skill which the ex-

*As usually practiced in the United States, this is a farce in which the competitors only pretend to hurt each other.

perts develop belies such a death wish, although it might be more common amongst those who are foolish enough to play Russian Roulette or to engage in acceptable dangerous sports but without proper training or protection.

Unfortunately there is of course a tendency for acceptable sports to be made unacceptable by foul play. What goes on under the surface in water polo is sometimes a disgrace. A racing car driver or a jockey may unfairly cut off one who is overtaking him, thereby endangering the life as well as the chances of a victory of his opponent. Violent body blows or deliberate strikes with a stick or ball are common in ball games. Blows below the belt or intentional breaking of bones or dislocating of joints, tripping or needlessly violent tackling are by no means rare. Rather than relying on skill, a boxer may keep reopening a cut on his opponent's face. Precompetition doping of athletes or animals, deliberate maiming of horses or damaging of racing cars to produce accidents also add a quota to the injuries sustained. It is not only extreme competitiveness which leads to such breaches of fair play, but the lure of financial rewards, or actual bribery by gamblers. The temptation is also increased for those who are professionals and have their livelihood at stake. The concept of the amateur who plays for love of the sport and is genuinely happy to see the best man win, even if it is his rival, has been sorely weakened, even for the amateur, because sport has become big business. Even the Olympics have not escaped the taint.

The simplest synonym for sport is fun (Webster). It can cover every type of recreation and diversion, but this chapter will be chiefly concerned with competitive sports, individual and team. What is considered moral or immoral in sports will vary from one country to another and from one period to another, as much as the opinion on sexual mores has done. Therefore an attempt has been made here to use the world moral in a biological sense, as meaning what seems good in the long run for man and his environment, rather than to apply it in a codified religious or philosophical sense. As a Christian, the author sees no conflict in this, however, since he believes that the Judeo-Christian ethic fully supports both competitiveness and sportsmanship, in the classical sense of the latter word.

In order to achieve perspective it is important to trace the development of sport.

HISTORY

The evolution of the Olympic Games in ancient Greece may be traced back as far as 1829 BC,[1] but the actual four yearly Olympiads began in 776 BC and ended in 426 AD.[2] With the decline of Greece and the rise of the Roman Empire, far more sinister "games" took place in Rome. Gone was the concept of sportsmanship. Its place was taken by the most savage blood sports in the history of man. Gladiator killed gladiator, beast killed beast, and 50,000 spectators roared their approval.[3] Gladiators were first used in entertainment in 264 BC. Three hundred years later ninety-three days of games were held annually, reducing the Roman citizens working days to little more than the modern five-day week. The Coliseum served these fearful purposes from 72 AD to 523 AD, though human duels were abolished in 404 AD. As well as the thousands of humans killed, "The empire was stripped of its major fauna forever—North Africa of its elephants, Nubia of its hippos, Mesopotamia of its lions."[4] The lesson of the Coliseum is one for all of us to consider when we find ourselves enjoying cruelty, whether to man or animal. Some of us yell "finish him off" when a dazed boxer is about to receive a KO. The Romans cried "Jugula!"—"Kill!" when rejecting the plea for mercy from a defeated gladiator. What would we have said? If we develop a lust for witnessing or causing death, injury or suffering, rather than admiring skill, strength, and the fellowship of true sportsmen, we are in danger of losing all that we have gained from the Olympics, the Age of Chivalry, and from both Christianity and humanism. In fact, all that makes our own lives far safer than they would be in a totalitarian state.

The modern revival of the Olympic Games began in Athens in 1896, thanks to the vision and organizing genius of Baron Pierre de Coubertin of France. He saw it as a source of better understanding and good will between nations, and so it has often proved, at least for many participants. Wider hopes that it might reduce international tension have been doomed to disappointment. The Games reinforced the concept of amateurism and, most importantly, the ideal of sportsmanship. The founder's concept was that "the important thing is not winning but taking part . . . and fighting well." Webster's dictionary, evidently giving the American view, defines the sportsman as "a person who can take a loss or defeat without complaint, or victory without boasting or gloating, and who treats an opponent with fairness, generosity and courtesy." The Oxford dictionary, perhaps unconsciously, reveals the wider concept, involving the whole of life, with which the British grew up: "One who believes that life is a game in which opponents must be allowed fair play." Such ideals inspired youth in many countries. In the very year that the Olympics were revived, Gilbert Patten, an American short story writer began a series on his fictional character Frank Merriwell who was, with an occasional slip, the embodiment of sportsmanship. Half a million American schoolboys avidly read of his exploits at Yale, to the tune of 20,000 words a week. This lasted for seventeen years and latterly became a radio series. The effects of these stories were profound and are even evident today.[5]

A light shines brightest in the dark, and it was in somber circumstances that the Olympic Games convened in Germany in 1936 under gathering war clouds. On that occasion a young German athlete taught the world a much needed lesson. Here is the graphic story as told to the *Readers Digest*[6] by Jesse Owens, one of America's greatest athletes.

Adolf Hitler, arming his country against the entire world, had perverted the Games into a test between dictatorship and freedom. In a way I was competing against Hitler himself and his myth of "Aryan supremacy." I was entered in four events, and Hitler had been grooming his best athlete, Lutz Long, to beat me in one of them. I held the world broadjump record, and only Long had approached it.

The qualifying jumps came early. On his first try in these preliminaries, that August day in Berlin Stadium, Lutz Long broke the Olympic record. In the trials! When my turn came, Hitler rose from his box and walked out. Mad, hate-mad, I fouled on my first try. On my second, I didn't jump far enough to qualify. With just one try left, panic hit me. Nearby stood Lutz Long, chatting with friends, a tall, perfectly built, sandy haired youth, unconcerned, confident, Aryan. I walked away, shaking. I was back in Oakville again. I was a nigger.

Suddenly I felt a firm hand on my arm. I turned and looked into the sky-blue eyes of Long himself. "You are a better jumper than this," he said. "What has got your goat—what Reichskanzler Hitler did? Look, you must qualify." He steadied me, suggested that I draw a line short of the takeoff board and jump from there—and the panic emptied out of me like a cloudburst. On my third and last try, I qualified by more than a foot.

The next several nights, Lutz and I sat up late and talked eagerly, about ourselves and our world. It was as fine a friendship as I would ever have with a white man, though we were destined never to see each other again. (He was killed in World War II.)

Of my four gold medals, I won three—in the 100-meter and 200-meter dashes, and in the relay—with Lutz cheering me on. In the broad jump we competed hotly. But when I finally won, Lutz, pulling me with him while Hitler glared, held up my hand and shouted to the gigantic crowd, "Jes-se Ow-ens! Jes-se Ow-ens!" The stadium picked it up. "Cha-zee Oh-wenz! Cha-zee Oh-wenz!" My hair stood on end. Thanks to Lutz, I was one step father from blackthink and hate.[7]

The history of sport in the U.S.A. has been written by many authors. Robert H. Boyle traced its significance in the class system[5] and John R. Tunis its influence on education and the American character.[8] These two books are based on an exceedingly wide background of reading and experience and should be studied to substantiate any unreferenced data in this section. In colonial days there was some boxing (pugilism), bowls, fishing, horse racing and cockfighting, but the Puritan influence tended to suppress sport, especially as a Sunday activity. Gymnastics made a modest beginning after the War of Independence, but life was hard, with little time for fun. However, in 1842 the English game of rounders was imported and modified as baseball. By 1850 it had become the national game, and in 1869 professional baseball began. Protestantism encouraged "muscular christianty" both in Britain and the United States, and the YMCA has given magnificent leadership in sports for youth. Two leaders of the YMCA devised basketball in 1891 and volleyball in 1895. Between 1875 and 1900 the flood of newly popular sports included croquet, tennis, archery, golf, roller skating and cycling.[9] The latter had a revolutionary effect, both social and technical, only to be outdone later by the automobile and the aeroplane. In early days the train, with special rates for traveling teams, paved the way for the rapid expansion of competitive sports.

At the turn of the century a remarkable character gave a boost to American sports. Theodore Roosevelt, a rugged athlete himself, became at forty-one the youngest president our country has ever had. He naturally became "a self-conscious patron of youth, sport and the arts."[8] He embodied the "square deal" and could be relied upon to "play the game" and was an opponent of all kinds of skullduggery, regardless of political consequences.

The developments of the nineteenth century were trivial compared with the sports explosion which followed the two world wars, as the now affluent society settled down to enjoying itself. Restrictions of race and class gradually diminished, as the Negro became accepted and the truck driver earned as much as the school principal. Developing its American League, National League and World Series, professional baseball grew steadily in popularity for eighty years, but latterly football began to challenge it for primacy. The American Intercollegiate Football Association was formed in 1876, and the Western Collegiate Conference in 1896. For fifty years football was mainly an amateur game in college circles, before professional teams were formed Professional boxing, basketball and hockey also have a large following.

Many sports organizations make sincere efforts to increase the safety as well as the technical possibilities and popularity of their sport. The author of this chapter was given very competent first aid by the Ski Patrol when he broke his ankle on the slopes. More than fifty sports have national associations. Every year sees new ones, some of which become a tremendous success almost overnight. Some relatively recent ones are skydiving, skin diving, snowmobiles and dune buggies.

Sports has long occupied a central place in the lives of millions of Americans, but live spectator sports have passed their peak. The number of baseball fans fell from 62 million in 1949 to 29 million in 1961 (due almost exclusively to the disappearance of most minor leagues, with major league attendance remaining very high). Boxing has almost suffered a KO with a fall from 2 million in 1950 to ¼ million in 1963, the number of clubs in the same period falling from 350 to six. Television has a major responsibility for these changes. By making the top level competition available to all, it tends to replace the public's willingness to support local events. This narrowing of the base makes it increasingly hard to maintain a high standard of performance and decreases audience interest. Significantly, television did not adversely affect horse racing where betting is the bait. Participants in fact increased from 8.5 million in 1940 to 36.6 million in 1962. It is a healthy sign that, in spite of television, participant sports are booming, with more than 40 million fishermen, 35 million boaters, and half a million skydivers—to mention but a few. With more than 120 days of leisure per year, compared with less than sixty days in 1900, and with far more spare cash, Americans spend over 40 billion dollars a year on recreation, more than 200 dollars for every man, woman and child. For the first time in the world's history, a wide variety of *participant* sports are within the grasp of the working man. And for the working woman, whose modern emancipation has opened innumerable doors .

The physician and the interested layman need to know what competitive sport means to those who work so hard at it.

THE PSYCHOLOGY OF ATHLETICS

Popular attitudes towards sport vary from the adulation of the fan and the scorn of the uninvolved to the downright opposition of those who believe that competitive sport is one of the major defects of modern life. It is hard to ascertain whether personality makes the athlete, or vice versa, or whether both statements are true. One critical evaluation is by a former tennis champion who was also a sportswriter and a fan and is now a psychiatrist. After reviewing his own clinical records and twenty papers on the psychology of sports, Dr. Arnold R. Beisser[10] analyzes the motivations underlying sports, individual and team, amateur and professional, and the fans who support them. He describes patients whom he saw professionally after their sports careers, which had been of inordinate importance to them, had come to an end. One's first reaction is that similar analyses might be made of anyone whose chosen field had suddenly collapsed, whether it was a marriage, a business, an artistic pursuit or some professional ambition. However, he has much to say about sports from many other angles. Beisser records the astonishing importance of sports in American society, as judged by the mass media, the enthusiasm of the fans, and the monetary value of success as a professional.

> Cumulative annual attendance figures for football, basketball and baseball exceed a billion. Regular participants in golf, tennis, and bowling number many millions. Participation in school and club team sports has been a part of almost every American life. Perhaps ours is more nearly the sporting nation than an affluent nation, a capitalist country, a political democracy or anything else.

Support of the local team provides far more than a casual interest for the fan. He becomes a member of the tribe and shares deep emotions with other fans, emotions which give him identity. This is not merely a safety valve, for it may take the place of family, church, ethnic and neighborhood groups. Thus, spectator sports may be therapeutic. Fan and team are symbiotic. "The experience itself is elemental in a way that has been ascribed only to sex, crime, and sports." The emotional needs of the fan may also be met by his fantasy projection of himself in a role in the team, as aggressor or defense man, according to his mood or personality needs. Lacking skills, strength, courage or opportunity to play, he may still be a whole-hearted participant. Like the athlete, he may also go too far in his enthusiasm.

Dr. Beisser's analysis of the meaning of victory is profound. Since strong competitive (aggressive) effort is needed, it is associated with unconscious homicidal and other destructive instincts and hence potential feelings of guilt. Fear of the responsibilities and loneliness of victory are also deterrents. So strong are these hidden impulses that many athletes keep failing to achieve their potential for purely emotional reasons. Hence, individual or group therapy from a strong coach or a well-balanced and psychologically knowledgeable parent, or even from a psychiatrist, is needed to provide protection and strength. If the competitor can resolve these basic conflicts he is likely to experience an integration of his personality which will stand him in good stead in other aspects of life. An analysis of sportsmanship reveals how hard an ideal it is to achieve. Much that passes as a gracious, sporting attitude on the part of a loser may really indicate a lack of competitiveness, arising from an unconscious desire to lose.[11] On the other hand, the strongest competitor (and the coach, team and fans) may feel that he has to generate a grudge, usually groundless, in order to excel. Armed with this he may behave with deliberate violence and hostility towards his opponent. The increment of ability which he obtains from this self-inflicted paranoia is akin to the astonishing strength and cunning of the maniac. It can drive its possessor to incredible feats of endeavor and endurance. Perhaps this fact influenced Beisser's choice of the title of his book, the *Madness in Sports*. The grudge is but one of the number of gimmics which may be used to help oneself and/or hinder one's opponent. Once the game is over, the grudge may be gone—win or lose. A physiologically and psychologically sounder gimmic is used by Jackie Stewart[12] in preparation for car races. He imagines himself as "like a bouncy sort of ball. . . . If the ball remains too hard it has too much bounce and is difficult to control." He therefore "consciously deflates." He goes to bed early before the race and is completely relaxed, fearless and under excellent self-control when the race begins.

Who then is the real sportsman—the poorer competitor or the aggressive one? The author of the present chapter does not believe that either fully fills the role, but that the strong aggressor is more out of line. The ideal sportsman should have so mastered his emotions that he can go all out without the need for overt hostility. He may find this easier to do if his personal ambitions are subjected to some higher allegiance. This may be the honor of his coach, school, college, team, or country. In many cases it has been to honor his Creator, who gave him the ability to compete.[13] This is certainly the goal of members of the Fellowship of Christian Athletes, a group which now has a membership of 100,000. Billy Graham's appointment as Grand Marshal of the Rose Bowl Parade of January 1, 1971, typifies the association between personal faith and Christian ideals in athletics.[14] A strong positive goal is surely better than the purely negative one of beating a competitor. The same is true when one is mainly competing against the elements or the clock, as in downhill ski races, gliding, sailing, crossing the ocean on a raft, or long distance swimming. There must be conviction of one's ability to succeed, devotion, determination, good planning, and continued self-discipline. With these, "a trained mind will long outlast a failing body and seemingly intolerable extremes of privation, pain and horror."[15] We may conclude that self-control is the hallmark of the athlete, in training, in competition, after victory and after losing. His instincts are being focused powerfully upon a chosen goal. However, he is not prepared to sacrifice his self-respect in order to achieve it. He will put aside many desires in order to succeed, but he will not behave uncharitably to an opponent and will not give way to conceitedness as a victor or to self-pity in defeat. Only as individuals and teams approach this ideal can we say that modern sport continues to encourage true sportsmanship.

THE PHYSICIAN'S RESPONSIBILITY

At the dawn of Olympic history, physicians were responsible for the basic training of athletes.[16] A thousand years later the physicians were proving too soft for the lay trainers who favored a more Spartan program, including bathing in cold mountain streams. The two groups were often at odds.

Since the revival of the Olympic Games, physicians have played an increasingly important role.[17] In 1911 at the World Hygiene Exposition in Dresden, Germany, and in 1913 at a meeting in Paris, European physicians emphasized the importance of exercise and sports. In 1928 this concern led to formation of what is now called the Federation Internationale Medico-Sportive (FIMS). This meets every two years and is composed of forty national organizations and four regional groups. Fifteen journals are devoted to sports medicine in almost as many countries. Physicians accompany the Olympic teams and treat their illnesses and accidents. In parts of Europe sports medicine is now a specialty, with professorships, and two to five-year training programs for physicians who wish to enter this field.

At the annual and regional meetings of the American College of Sports Medicine, reports are made on research by physicians and others. Numerous physical tests are carried out on competitors, including champions.[18] Standards of excellence are thus set up. Appropriate reports are collected in the Olympic Medical Archives in the Olympic Museum in Lausanne, Switzerland. In 1964, after repeated representations by the American Medical Association's Committee on the Medical Aspects of Sports, the United States Olympic Committee appointed a physician as chairman of its Medical and Training Services Committee, with the result that the best medical opinions in the country were concentrated on the development of athletes and preparation for the games.[19] This was particularly timely, in view of the high altitude problems[20] associated with the next games held in Mexico in 1968. In September 1968, a whole edition of the Journal of the American Medical Association was devoted to sports medicine and the Olympic Games.

Physicians have played a role at all levels of team games in the schools and in professional sports, and the AMA has provided excellent medical guidance.[21-23] The team physician is nearly always finally responsible for supervision of training, for exclusion of those who are injured or ill, for enforcing the use of proper protective equipment, for being present during competition to give immediate first aid and decide whether the injured player may safely continue.[24,25] Dr. Max Novich states flatly: "No physician should ever use [a local anesthetic] so that an injured player can continue in action." The physician has to exercise good medical judgment, using only such medication as is essential for health. However, the use of stimulants and tranquilizers is far more widely practiced than is usually recognized,[26] and some physicians have been caught up in this undesirable practice. The only drug which has been reliably shown to increase a champion's efficiency is amphetamine sulfate. In a dosage of 14 mg/70 kg body weight this improved the performance of 75 percent of swimmers, runners and weight throwers, in a carefully controlled double-blind study.[27] No harmful effects were observed. However, it is believed that an occasional death has resulted from uncontrolled use of this drug. Moreover, as the AMA states, its use is "inconsistent with the practice and ideals of sportsmanship."[28] Drug usage is strongly condemned by the AMA, the U.S. Olympic Association, the Amateur Athletic Union, the International Amateur Athletic Federation, and recently by the National Collegiate Athletic Association. Although more than a decade has passed since this AMA statement, "none of our pro baseball, basketball, football or hockey leagues has rules banning doping, nor has the National Athletic Trainers Association laid down a policy."[29] Physicians have made extensive studies on all aspects of sports in thousands of published medical papers. These are concerned with "biology, anatomy, anthropology, biomechanics, Kinesiology, physiology, hygiene, medical control, traumatology, rehabilitation, first aid, massage and psychology related to physical education, games, sports, training, and competition of children, adults, and women, and old age."[17] With dentists,[30] engineers and others, they have also proposed and helped to devise safety equipment. They have recommended changes in rules when current procedures have proved too dangerous. With physiologists and physical educators, physicians have effected enormous improvements in physical training techniques, as the continual breaking of world records attests.[31] Between 1900 and 1967, world record performance improved 55 percent for throwing, 23.7 percent for swimming, 13.9 percent for jumping, 11.0 percent for long-distance running, 9.4 percent for middle-distance running and 7.1 percent for sprints. During this time, not a decade went by without an improvement in every one of these groups.[32] In addition to its direct value in recreation, this vast accumulation of knowledge now makes it possible to provide a scientific, practical and enjoyable program of physical fitness from the cradle to the grave. It has also offered amazing new techniques for rehabilitation after cardiac disease, even in the elderly.

However, the views of sports physicians have not always won acceptance. They have run up against traditions and vested interests in trying to reduce accidents, especially among professional athletes. There have often been delays of years between recommendations and their acceptance. There is also the problem of compliance. As in too many other aspects of our national life, it is one thing to have a rule on the books and another to get it regularly enforced. A good example is spearing and but-blocking in football. For about seven years this has been illegal, that is, a player may not strike another with his helmet-covered head. However, the rule has been variably interpreted and deliberate injuries have continued. In November, 1970, the AMA committee on the Medical Aspects of Sports strongly recommended abolition of all varieties of this procedure. It remains to be seen whether the rules committees will accomplish this in all levels of football. It has also long been known that the protective face mask tends to force the head back at a collision or fall and has caused serious damage to the spinal cord, sometimes with sudden death. Teams that have abandoned it have had fewer serious injuries and the players can see and function better. However, unless this practice receives very strong support from many official organizations, the coach or school which removes this protection may be liable to a law suit in the event of injury to a players face. Unfortunately, logical improvements are being hampered by certain lawyers who specialize in advising injured athletes to seek compensation. In 1969 through 1970 two new organizations[33,34] began research to develop better equipment, with the help of Richard C. Schneider, M.D., a neurosurgeon with research experience in head injuries. The initial project is the improvement of football helmets. Incidentally, physicians played a role in making the use of helmets mandatory in amateur hockey in North America. There is a strong feeling that the helmet should also be required equipment for baseball batters and runners. With such active and expanding efforts to increase safety, it is probable that more attention will be paid to the recommendations of sports physicians in the future. This is vitally important, for football today is considerably more dangerous than it was twenty-five years ago.

We must now consider five moral issues which face the physician in any attempt he may make towards increasing the positive health values of sports and reducing their negative effects.

MORAL ISSUES

Commercialism and Win-ism*

The concept of the amateur originally put a premium on wealth. In the ancient Olympic Games, every winner (or his family) had to provide a victory banquet as well as provide his own horse and chariot or other necessary equipment. To this day, lack of money undoubtedly limits participation. Many students find all their energies drained by putting themselves through school or helping to support the family. Thus, they never reach Olympic standards. While the wealthier nations may be able to collect donations for the athletes' travel, and governments may sponsor some, others lack money for dispatching all potential competitors. Thus, pressure has increased for liberalization of the rules. Unless this is wisely done, it could open a Pandora's box. It is hard enough to retain high ideals when fame is the spur. When financial rewards also enter the picture, it is even harder. The course of college sport is a case in point. From its clearly amateur beginnings it has strayed so far that it has even undermined the structure of education in many American universities. Tunis[8] refers to the "submerged professionalism" of basketball, a game in which 950 college teams played before 15 million spectators in 1958. He traces development of "industrialized sport" back to the cost of enormous sports stadia which were required by any colleges which planned to participate in big-time sport. To finance this, the stadium had to be filled and adequate entrance charges made. To fill the stadium there had to be a winning team. This required first rate coaches, who could virtually name their own price, and excellent players. To obtain the latter, the athletic scholarship was invented, and more coaches were hired to act as talent scouts. Add to this the rapidly rising cost of equipment, and one can see how the universities got onto a treadmill. A head coach might be paid as much as the chairman

---

*The author defines "win-ism" as a concept and practice which places more emphasis upon winning than upon sportsmanship. A win-ist may boast, lie, break the rules, berate and even deliberately injure an opponent if he thinks he can get away with such behavior. Typically, he is full of excuses as a loser, blames others, exhibits self-pity and rarely has any genuine good feelings towards the victor.

of an academic department, and then he would calmly break his contract if offered more elsewhere. The tail began to wag the dog with a vengeance! It was costing 3,000 dollars per year to prepare a college athlete for sport. At the same time, the median cost of library services per student was 43 dollars. It transpired that even the college with the winning team could barely break even, and many were far into the red. Becoming desperate, the colleges put more and more emphasis on winning (hereafter called win-ism), thereby compromising their vaunted adherence to the principles of sportsmanship. Coaches were hired who reflected the win-ism philosophy and inevitably persuaded vast numbers of students to their way of thinking.

"How can you be proud of a losing team?" asked Jim Tatum, the football coach. Another coach, Woody Hayes of Ohio State, has said, "Anyone who tells me, 'Don't worry that you lost, you played a good game anyway,' I just hate." A major league manager tells his team, "Cheat a little bit, especially at first and second when you're going to tag up after a fly ball." American sport has nothing comparable to the English maxim, "That's not cricket." Instead, all too many honor Leo Durocher's wisecrack, "Nice guys finish last." This successful manager of the Chicago Cubs baseball team also said, "If it's under W for Won, nobody asks you how."[5]

The college president may have to swallow this sort of philosophy as the price of having a college football team. When next he instructs the graduating class about standing by their principles in a tough world, he must have his tongue in his cheek. "The college itself is involved in such a tangle of evasions, compromises and downright surrenders that it is jeered at by the sporting world at large and its ethical pretensions laughed at by its own undergraduates." (Christian Century.)[8] Here is a sizable credibility gap for the protesting student. The president must also be concerned at the inequality in the distribution of college funds between sport and academic concerns; about the fate of the college if it cannot balance its budget because of the costliness of its sport; about the anger of the alumni and its effect upon his own job if the team hits a losing streak; and about the fact that the Soviet Union has paid for its students to become linguists, administrators, scientists and economists, while he has been paying the way for football halfbacks and basketball forwards. Truly, the colleges have a tiger by the tail. Small wonder that an increasing number of them have dropped athletic scholarships and even followed California Tech and Johns Hopkins and dozens more (NYU, Fordham, St. Johns, for example) in getting right out of competitive football. Not only many college presidents but two-thirds of the high school principals also consider that sport is overemphasized. In October, 1970, the Florida Council of Student Body Presidents asked the state's board of regents to reevaluate the role of intercollegiate athletics.[14] This trend has been accelerated by disaffection amongst the athletes themselves. They object to racism and bossy coaches who have an anti-individualist and anti-intellectual attitude. Recent scandals at the University of Iowa and at Kansas State athletic departments have done nothing to help matters.[35] Dave Meggyesy, a former St. Louis linebacker turned pro with the Cardinals, recently quit to write an exposé of football.[36] This includes illegal payoffs, medical malpractice (drugs to keep an injured man playing in spite of the serious risk of making the injury worse), authoritarianism, hypocrisy and racism. Winning was everything, and it imposed a frightening and deliberate inhumanity upon the players. In the process he turned from an innocent *success-oriented* American youth to a disillusioned radical.[37]

It is not only at the colleges that sport has led to exploitation. Dr. Fred V. Hein, an official of the American Medical Association's Committee on the Medical Aspects of Sports, criticized "highly organized sports for children, such as Little League Baseball. He also opposed night games, events far from home, and commercial promotions that 'seek to exploit youth for selfish purposes'."[8] Professional sport also has its problems. Periodically a scandal occurs, a new commissioner is appointed and steps are taken to prevent a recurrence. On the whole, each professional association runs its own affairs under well-considered rules and with effective supervision from a state commission. The system by which clubs purchase players tends to keep the teams in reasonable balance. Eventually even the New York Mets made it to the top. The individual player's record shows his ability even if he is on a losing team. The pressure to win is of course very great, but excessive violence and fouls can usually be checked by enforcement of the rules. While sportsmanship needs emphasizing here too, frank professionalism is morally superior to pseudo-amateurism. And it certainly provides a splendid spectacle, potentially free of the moral conflict which assails college sport. Professionals must keep to the same standard of sportsmanship as amateurs. They are in the business of mass entertainment, and they are watched by millions who are amateurs. If they use unfair methods they will be copied by amateurs, and this will spoil the sport and mar the character of the fans. Moreover, if they fail to use recommended safety equipment, amateurs will copy them and many will be hurt and some killed. Not until a basic change has been made in motivation in school children can we hope to see much improvement in the attitude of some fans. Excessive partisanship can spoil the game. It should be axiomatic that while the fan primarily roots for his own side, he should always applaud brilliant play by the other side and should never jeer the opponents except perhaps for an obviously deliberate foul. Beisser[10] reports that in Italy "jeers and profane comments so upset foreign players that some refuse to play there." Worse than this, even judging and umpiring have not escaped the tarnish. The astonishing bias shown by some judges, especially those from the Iron Curtain countries, at the 1972 Olympics evoked official protests, and some judges were subsequently suspended. However, the injustice which they had perpetrated was allowed to stand. Millions witnessed this on television, and Mike Mansfield, leader of the Democratic majority in the U.S. Senate, even called for abolition of the Olympics because of this and other politically oriented intrusions.

The combined effects of commercialism and win-ism on sports are to strengthen aggressiveness without encouraging the self-control of the true sportsman. It has tended to produce a person who cares little about the rights of others. He has never learned that it is better to lose with honor than to win unfairly. These same traits are then carried forward into life and "The admiration of society is directed towards those who get, not toward those who give."[38] This is of course in direct contrast to the Christian maxim, "It is happier to give than to receive." The expectation that happiness will come through success produces an interminable rat race "trying to keep up with the Jones" or get a little ahead of them. Also significant is the sense of failure imposed on those who do not come out on top. So little is taught about how to be a good loser that millions of people must be shattered by this frequently repeated experience. These two conflicts may have much to do with the high incidence of mental breakdown in the United States.

Gambling

Many sports are chiefly or notably indulged in for the purposes of gambling. They vary from horse racing, gaming tables, card games, numbers games, bingo and raffles. It is claimed that more millions change hands over basketball than any other game. A strict puritanical attitude regards all gambling as basically immoral, since it encourages people to look to chance as a source of success instead of relying on work. There is also the wastage of money and time on what is a losing proposition for the majority, coupled with the encouragement given to organized crime and police corruption. Even those with more flexible consciences find little to commend in gambling. With highly dubious historical support, the state has at times assumed that its employees are less liable to corruption than other citizens and has taken over a sizable share of this profitable business, with specious arguments about lowering taxes. In a fascinating study of why people gamble, Charlotte Olmsted concludes that gamblers as a class "seem to find the world an appallingly dull place, and their lives intolerably empty."[39]

By way of solution she sees no help in legislation. "In the case of *self*-injury—suicide, drug addiction and the like—ordinary law enforcement techniques become a farce." She sees far more hope through agencies such as Gamblers Anonymous which aim to restore self-respect and justifiable self-confidence. Debunking the pleasures of gambling in a first-rate program like the present anti-smoking publicity might gradually wean the public from its mesmeric attraction. However, for maximum effect, all types of addicts need to gain a whole new idea about the meaning of life

—and about-face towards positive ideals such as a religious experience may offer.[40]

Injuries

The National Safety Council publishes information about prevention of sports injuries, gives statistics on accidents,[41] and has a Public Safety Conference whose membership comprises organizations which maintain continuous safety programs in sports and recreation. However, there is no central source of information about *all* sports from which one can find out their total cost in life and limb. It would probably be very disturbing. We know that skiing accidents exceed 100,000 a year.[42] Spaderman, who personally treated 617 skiing accidents at Squaw Valley, reported that 428 involved the lower extremity. The initiating factor was skiing out of control, due to lack of confidence, training or experience, poor judgment, and sometimes fatigue. Beginners learning the snow plough accounted for 55 percent. The safety bindings commonly failed to release the foot before a fracture occurred. The author discusses the defects of the present release mechanisms.

As a source of injury, football is even more impressive. A former US Air Force physician reports 290 injuries, (111 being major) in twenty games. No less than thirty-eight players were hospitalized, twenty-two had surgery and sixty-five were out for the season. Thus, for every game played there was an average of one operation, 1½ fractures or dislocations, and three men knocked out for months.[43] Obviously this is too rough. Considering the larger number of participants, today's record may not be as bad as in 1905 when eighteen footballers were killed, but it surely needs some drastic action such as Theodore Roosevelt[8] took in 1906. He called a White House conference, which led to new rules, doing away with mass pushing and fighting, banning freshmen from competition, discouraging tramp athletes, and introducing the forward pass. Perhaps a word from some distant observers may help here. At a sports medicine conference in England it was observed, "U.S. football seems to condone tackles designed to rupture the medial ligament of the knee joint."[44] Perhaps we condone a great deal more than this in our variety of the game. But note here that there were twice as many fatalities from baseball as from boxing or football during the period 1918 to 1950.[45] For college and high school males aged fifteen to twenty-two, it has been shown that hours spent motoring are nine times as likely to end fatally as are hours spent on football. The latter was barely 20 percent more lethal than the ordinary risks of daily life.[46]

In the 1968-9 season three Canadian ice hockey players died of head injuries, two of them in spite of wearing helmets. There would doubtless have been more deaths had helmets not been worn. The refusal of the professionals to wear helmets sets a bad example to the amateurs who watch them on television.[47]

Amongst newer sports, snow mobiling is taking its toll. It is estimated that there were 82 deaths in three to four months in the winter of 1969-70 in the USA, along with at least 306 injuries.[48] It is expected that these figures will rise rapidly with the vast increase in popularity of this sport, unless it is better regulated.

The relative risk of some other sports can be judged from the following figures from the 6th British Empire and Commonwealth Games.[49] Most of the injuries were minor. Only 2.5 percent required hospital admission, and there were only five fractures. There were 392 injuries amongst the 1122 athletes. The number of injuries per 100 participants were wrestling 81.3, jumping 50.4, throwing 49.2, boxing 44.9, running 44.8, fencing 35.0, weight lifting 34.4, swimming and diving 24.3, rowing 10.9, cycling 9.7, and bowls 1.2. It is generally considered that the better the training, the fewer the injuries. From his observations, Dr. Kenneth Lloyd suggests that sprains and strains may be related to a failure to develop skill at the same time as strentgh during training.

In spite of the fact that baseball and football are claimed to be more lethal[50] (boxing being 7th[51] on a list of sports fatalities), and wrestling, jumping and throwing cause more injuries, boxing is the sport about which many people have a bad conscience. The criticism is directed more against professional boxing than amateur boxing where skill receives more consideration. However, an unfortunate fatality at the University of Wisconsin in 1960 robbed it of a fine student. The emotional reaction which immediately followed virtually sounded the death kneel of college level boxing throughout the United States,[52] and boxing is officially frowned upon at all school levels.[53] Professional boxing "is the only sport where victory is achieved through the deliberate infliction of bodily injury."[54] At the present time the activities of the American Humane Society have provided more protection to cattle in a rodeo[55] than is often given to a professional boxer in the ring. It is not the frequency of injury which is the problem, but its deliberate nature and its potential severity when it occurs. In a fine paper on 1043 professional boxers it was reported that 1400 electroencephalograms (EEGs) showed a normal brain wave pattern, even immediately after a knockout. Concussion was shown to be reversible and careful medical examination revealed no brain damage.[56] These findings have been supported by many other studies, including one in which there were 132 head injuries in 2400 boxers. Only forty-two had cerebral symptoms, all of which were transient.[57] However, it has also been shown that the brain waves may appear normal even when brain damage has occurred. It is now clear that more detailed studies such as encephalography are needed. In this procedure air is introduced into the ventricles (fluid-filled cavities) of the brain. This test is considerably more reliable. It is a more formidable procedure which would not normally be done unless a serious brain injury were suspected. It was positive in eight out of nine cases of brain injury after boxing.[50] Another paper reported on fifteen exprofessional boxers with an average retirement of twenty-two years, who had persistent symptoms since one specific bout. The author points out that these injuries dated from the 1930s when there was scarcely any medical supervision of boxing.[58] There is still uncertainty as to whether multiple small injuries eventually lead to the serious "punch-drunk" state of irreparable damage. Most of the evidence is against this possibility. It is therefore wrong to base arguments about the morality of boxing upon the assumption that it almost inevitably causes cumulative damage to the brain.

A strong case can be made for preserving boxing and other sports concerned with self-defense. We live in a violent world where we are still liable to be attacked. However,

> As physicians, we surely have a duty to help bring about a revision of this sport . . . by increasing protective measures, by altering the rules and by placing greater emphasis on good

boxing techniques. A fighter should be obliged to abstain from the sport and from training for a specified time after a knock-out . . . under medical surveillance.[54]

Unfounded Expectations

It is a common misconception that sport *of itself* gives one a good start in life. In 1962 this idea appeared to be supported by publication of a report on 1391 Pitt lettermen who had performed between 1900 and 1960. A questionnaire showed that many had achieved preeminence in their fields,* which varied from finance to academic. As many as 37 percent had taken masters degrees or higher.[59] Unfortunately we do not have control figures regarding their nonathletic class mates. Note, however, that at least in the one-third who obtained higher degrees, their success was largely dependent on academic achievement, which may not have been casually related to their sports background. Of the remainder, one wonders how many went through considerable tribulation before they found their niche in life. Hero worship in our culture often places the ex-athlete in a job which is beyond his capabilities. He may become principal of a school, where he adds nothing to its academic standing. His competitiveness, transferred from sport to all that he does, may thus make him a first rate example of the "Peter Principle" by which we tend to attain our "level of incompetence."[60] He may be quickly dropped when the facts emerge. One of Dr. Beisser's[10] patients was a brilliant college athlete whose life had been so built around sports that he underwent mental collapse when faced with the pressures of life. When finally he was restored, he spoke to his old high school football team, "Don't forget, boys, its a great game, but it's only a preparation for living." He had learned his lesson the hard way.

Not only the athlete, but the whole university suffers from this overemphasis on sports with its distorted values and unfounded

*One who answered this questionnaire is my friend and colleague, Herman J. Bearzy, M.D. In a personal communication he says "I would never have had an opportunity without an athletic scholarship." He became Athletic Team Physician at the U. S. Military Academy, West Point, New York, prior to specializing in rehabilitation medicine. In 1969-70 he rose to the top in the USA in his chosen field, becoming President of the American Academy of Physical Medicine and Rehabilitation.

expectations. This is best shown by comparing our present American culture, where paradoxically we put more effort into our sport than into our work, with a previous culture in France.[61] Andre' Maurois suffered from scoliosis as a child and could take little exercise. As soon as he could discard his iron corset he exercised so vigorously that he won a medal as the best gymnast at the Lycee. He did this, not just for the fame, but to prepare his body for the infinitely more important activities which he intended for his mind. By his early teens he had read "All of Taine, Flaubert, Maupassant, Anatole France, Prevost and Michelet." At an age when our present students are yelling support for teams—or maybe having a high on pot—he was "dizzy and intoxicated, blind and drunk with power" as he was "deliciously borne along in the whirlwind of ideas." He revelled in the writings of "Epictetus and Epicurus, Plato and Aristotle, Descartes and Spinoza, Locke and Kant, Hegel and Bergson." With teachers who showed him how to learn, how to think, and the wisdom to apply knowledge to life, his innate talents soared to an amazing pinnacle. He became one of the most readable and prolific biographers of all time, and he never lost his modesty or good humor.

Every true teacher longs for a pupil like Maurois. However, in the sports-oriented American schools, a true scholar must not only have ability but the courage to buck the system. He has to be willing to stick out like a sore thumb and to be considered a square, if he prefers such things as art, music, mathematics or biography to college sport, or even if he prefers to swim, run or cycle alone rather than cheer with the crowd. Our system, with a number of fine exceptions, does not inspire the depth of enquiry needed by the prospective man of letters, the psychologist, the research worker or scientist, nor the firmness of moral purpose needed by the philosopher, sociologist or seminarian. Too much effort is drained off for unproductive sport. It may produce a demon competitor, but not *of itself* a full man.

A second popular but erroneous idea is that sport keeps one physically fit. In fact, sports are more likely to produce injury than fitness. As a prominent English surgeon has said, "We must get fit to play games, not the reverse."[62] As Cooper and others have pointed out, the vitally important cardiovascular aspects of physical fitness are only produced by such rhythmical activities as running, swimming, cycling, and brisk walking. Weight lifting and brief intermittent activities such as most ball games have little effect. For physical fitness training, it is necessary to drive the pulse up to a rate of 150 for a period of over five minutes, or a somewhat slower rate for a longer period. To attain and retain such fitness, one must devote thirteen to forty minutes to such activities, at least three to five times a week.[63] There is strong evidence that this reduces the incidence of heart attacks; lowers high blood pressure, high blood fat, and obesity; lessens the tendency to diabetes, peptic ulcers, emotional imbalance and fatigue; improves sexual function and even mental performance. It makes for a longer, happier and more productive life. None of these things can be counted on by the former all-American who gives up exercise and smokes, eats and drinks too much. When he quits competitive games he must continue in an appropriate activity program and not overindulge. Otherwise his fitness will speedily dwindle. Fortunately, a measure of physical fitness can be regained at almost any age, even after a heart attack, but there are serious risks involved in inactivity, especially after age thirty in men and fifty in women. There is no truth in the fear that the athlete's heart tends to fail prematurely. On the contrary, he has a distinct advantage, *provided he continues appropriate activity all his life.* A follow up of 294 oarsmen[64] who rowed for Harvard more than fifty years ago revealed that at age twenty-two they had a life expectancy of sixty-seven, and the man who stroked the teams had an expectancy of sixty-nine. These men lived six years and eight years respectively longer than their classmates, who were used as controls. The less active coxswain had a considerably shorter life span. Honor graduates also live long, but not as long as the rowers. It was noted that the rowers tended to keep themselves fit throughout life.

There is no more important aspect of health for the physician to stress than lifelong fitness. In doing so, he will go far beyond the customary level of treating diseases and beyond the usual bounds of preventive medicine. He will be in the forefront of advance. Better still, if he sets an example of fitness himself he may challenge his patients more effectively. He will be meeting head-on the causes of degenerative cardiovascular disease which result in 55 percent of all fatalities in the USA. He may save many from a crippling heart attack or stroke. He will often see a remarkable improvement in hypertension and even after a coronary thrombosis. He will be using natural means more than medication and will be teaching people how to live healthily.

Cruelty to Animals

Just over 100 years ago animals were regarded purely as property. They had no rights to protection against all types of cruelty. In 1866 the American Society for the Prevention of Cruelty to Animals (ASPCA) was organized, and later the American Humane Association (AHA). The latter is the national body.[55] The succeeding years of hard effort have seen a phenomenal trend towards really caring for animals. Laws in every state protect them. Experts from the AHA supervise rodeos, films where animals take part, and arrangements for housing, feeding and transporting animals. The greatest battle concerned the slaughter houses. Not until 1958 did humane killing methods become mandatory. The new federal law covered 90 percent of the meat animals. The pattern was set, and further improvement followed.

The AHA is committed to total elimination of animal exploitation, and has long been at odds with the medical profession in the use of animals in research. The present compromise imposes stringent rules to limit animal suffering, but fortunately does not ban their use, as this would be a disaster to the advance of medical science. Animals used in sport are also protected, for example a horse may not be raced to exhaustion. Bullfighting, cockfighting and similar events are banned, and attempts have been made to prevent them being shown on film. This is an unfinished struggle, as film of part of a bullfight has recently been shown on television. Moreover, cockfighting and dogfighting have not been entirely eliminated in the rural areas.

The hunting of deer, foxes, rabbits, birds and other wild animals may be justified by the biological need to keep their numbers down or by man's need for food. Moreover, their suffering is minimized by laws and the ethics of hunting which protect the female and the young, limit the numbers which a hunter may kill, prevent dogs from tearing animals to pieces, and assure a quick death. Nevertheless, the instinct which regards killing as sport is surely cruel. It is more evident when a safari or hunt seeks out wild animals to kill, without any attempt at justification. In rebellion against this residual cruel streak in civilized man, many modern explorers shoot with a camera instead of a gun. This has given us magnificent animal photographs which are increasingly popular on film and television. Hopefully this trend will continue, and one day the sport of hunting will be over. The new emphasis on conservation may help. Man's actions have led to the extinction of an average of one animal species per year since 1900.

SUMMARY

Moral Advantages

Some sports require the type of training which leads to physical fitness, which of itself tends to produce far better functioning of the person as a whole, with less mental and physical disease. Many sports necessitate self-discipline in maximum development of a latent capacity. This prepares for the average life work and also for feats such as exploration—Scott's expedition to the Pole, Hillary's conquest of Mount Everest, and the return of crippled Apollo 13 from space.

Under good leadership, sport provides an opportunity to develop and express true sportsmanship, with a sense of fair play, good will and poise which neither the heat of competition, the elation of victory nor the experience of defeat can upset. Team events teach cooperation, with subordination of the ego for the common good—a valuable, well-known but currently underemphasized lesson.

Immoral Aspects

Commercialism and win-ism have largely undermined sportsmanship, amateur status, and the credibility of those educational institutions which have athletic teams. It has redirected vast amounts of time, energy and money, a great deal of which could have been better spent on solving national and international problems. It has squeezed out most of the average competitors in the schools and colleges, in favor of a handful of experts who are idolized. Gambling is firmly entrenched in many sports and in some is the major attraction. This plays into the hands of organized crime and periodically leads to scandal. It is a sickness indicative of inner emptiness and lack of a goal.

Injuries are an inevitable by-product of activity, but in some instances are deliberate or are needlessly severe because of bad rules or poor enforcement.

Unfounded expectations lead the naive to suppose that sport is *necessarily* a good preparation for life. This idea has been exploded by the observation that the demand for victory further emphasizes the win-ism attitude which is already too strong in the average American. Very few can actually win, thus it can be a cause of the widespread mental illness amongst the vast majority who are failures by these standards. In any event, excessive competitiveness can make a battle out of a game, and lead to fouls, tricks, deceit, boastfulness, self-pity, and a host of other logical but unpleasant results. Many sports are equally inappropriate as a means of keeping fit, since they do not provide enough of the right type of activity.

Cruelty to animals is still exhibited, especially in hunting, and in some films of bullfighting imported from abroad.

RECOMMENDATIONS

With abuses as varied as those which beset sport, it is obvious that the physician can only influence change in the right direction if he works along with community leaders. However, the physician's special knowledge in the field of mental health, physical injury and the value of physical fitness make him an important member of any group which sets out to resolve some of the problems. In the following section no further comments will be made about cruelty to animals, which is being well handled by the appropriate agencies, nor about gambling, which involves law enforecment and crime syndicates to the point that it would require a separate treatise.

Schools and Colleges

All educational institutions should follow the lead of those which have already rid themselves of the stigma and burden of being in the professional entertainment field. They could take the following steps:

Firstly, they could hand over at market value to private enterprise (sports clubs) the training of competitive sports teams, the organization and conduct of interclub competitions and all the finances, buildings, and equipment concerned therewith. No attempt would be made to recruit promising athletes in preference to other pupils of equal scholastic and leadership standing, nor would they be offered any fee reduction or academic advantages. It may well be argued that we need an alternative to the athletic scholarship. Agreed, but others besides athletes also need such help, and scholarships should be made available to all who have the academic ability. A new system which might well replace the athletic scholarship is now developing. Promising athletes are being trained as professionals at the cost of the promoter. During their training they are able to continue academic studies. This frankly professional approach has much to commend it and may provide equal academic opportunity.

Secondly, their future athletic program would provide for frequent participation by *all pupils*. The school coach would be paid a sum appropriate to his training and experience, in line with the rest of the faculty. He would no longer be specializing in producing one first rate team, but scores of teams. All competition would be intramural. The physical education program would major in those activities which are known to be especially beneficial to mental and physical health. Other sports would be optional electives. Coaches and all the faculty would emphasize *lifelong fitness of body, mind and spirit* as the primary goal of civilized man. This logically includes both sportsmanship and maximum achievement.[40] Win-ism would be despised. The idea of the good sport helping others, for example coaching beginners, the handicapped or the underprivileged would be highly commended. (Marilyn Bell, the 16-year-old Canadian who was the first to swim across Lake Ontario, gave time to teaching handicapped children to swim.) A service attitude and sportsmanship could be paired with informed patriotism and internationalism in preparing tomorrow's citizen. He would be taught that only in war is a "win at almost any price" attitude justified. To practice win-ism in ordinary life, let alone in sport, is to live in a jungle. Even in war, hatred should be directed against the enemy's ideals and objectives rather than against the individuals who make up his nation, even though many of them will have to be killed. To do more is to make one's self as hateful as he is and to risk losing the peace even if we win the war. Many experts claim that the peace of Versailles was vengeful and did in fact cost us the peace after World War I. Certainly we did better after World War II with its generous Marshall plan and other measures which made our erstwhile enemies our friends. Ideals like these might well capture the imagination of today's youth which rejects our subservience to pressure groups and the almighty dollar.

Thirdly, extramural competitions would be reserved for sports clubs. Pupils whose academic standing was high enough could receive a certificate from the school, renewable annually, allowing them to join a sports club outside the school. The schools would help to maintain ethical standards of these sports clubs by giving or denying their students the right to belong, based on the reputation of the club for real sportsmanship. The new ethical attitude of the schools would then permeate the sports clubs, so that win-ism would be downgraded there also. These clubs could put on competitions and charge for admission in order to raise enough to cover operating expenses, but would be nonprofit corporations. Having no university funds to fall back on, they would be less ambitious and no doubt operate far more economically than is the case in many college sports programs now. Already there are more than 2½ million undergraduates who belong to sports clubs outside the varsity, "because they want to be real amateurs."[65]

In this reorganization of school sports the author would not favor, as some do, the abolition of competition amongst the younger students, and he does not feel that it need be harmful physically or emotionally. In fact, the lessons of competition, healthful activity and sportsmanship are probably easier to learn in the pre-teens than in the teens. Reasons given for avoidance of pre-teen competition include physical injuries, the greater pressure required to make them go all out, and the excessive involvement of their parents in their own success-by-proxy. Well-run Peewee sports may have to include some *adult* education in sportsmanship. Hateful as win-ism may be, when seen in a 10-year-old who deliberately injures a rival, is it any real solution merely to defer this behavior for a few years? A well-brought-up child should have learned cooperative behavior and a give-and-take attitude by the time he is four. Competitive games thereafter can strengthen rather than weaken his character, provided he has a coach who is interested in the *total* development of his team, not merely in his own reputation for winning games. Such a man can show one child how to teach another. Children are not professionals and should share their knowledge for mutual benefit. They may sometimes need to be reminded "this is only a *game.*" Care must be taken that physical training does not usurp the place of homework or other responsibilities, even if the parents connive at an excessive commitment to sport. Character development in preparation for life must be the central consideration. It is possible to make too big a sacrifice for an Olympic gold medal or even for a Pop Warner football team. If pressure is exerted to enforce a training program which is too intensive, the pupil may come to hate the sport, and it may do him physical and psychological harm.[66]

In two admirable articles, an orthopedic surgeon argues against win-ism[67] and details the excellent recommendations of the American Academy of Pediatrics[68] and adds some of his own, but mentions the "utter disregard of such expert advice" by coaches and others. Nine national educational associations have made policy statements on sport.[53,69,70] However, clear guidelines on pre-teen sports have not solved the problems of coordination and enforcement, and the carefully reasoned proposals of the National Education Association[53] are frequently ignored:

> Interscholastic competition should be permitted only in senior high school. In elementary school and in junior high school there should be no "school team" (in the varsity sense), no leagues, no tournaments, no interschool championships. In

senior high school there should be no postseason championship tournaments or games.

Athletic games, in all cases, should be played with emphasis on fun, physical development, skill and strategy, social experience and good sportsmanship. High-pressure competition, with overemphasis on the importance of winning, should not be sanctioned in any part of the school program.

Amateur Status

To be an amateur is to participate for the thrill of competition,[71] whereas professionals play for a living. To some people the difference has little meaning, and periodically an amateur unwisely accepts money for advertising and loses his status. However, the International Olympic Committee (IOC),[72] the Amateur Athletic Union and many other agencies are deeply committed to retaining the distinction. It gives an opportunity to those who can only spend a limited time in training; it promotes the ideal of sport for sports' sake; it fosters a fine type of patriotism, leads to friendly international rivalry, and aims at giving no advantage to the richer competitors or countries. It has not been easy to retain amateurism, and its survival is largely due to fine leadership in the major amateur organizations. Periodic changes in the Olympics are made, as games gain or lose popularity. For example, football, basketball and ice hockey have become so professionalized at the top that it is questionable as to whether they should remain in the Olympic program, since it is no longer possible to assemble amateur teams of Olympic calibre.[71]

The Olympic rules preclude accepting any prize of over 50 dollars in value or converting prizes into money or its equivalent; capitalizing on athletic fame; acceptance of an athletic scholarship or a paid job with no real work but ample time for sport; payment for playing; teaching athletics or coaching; special training camp for over three weeks; expense accounts which include a manager, coach, relative, friend, or are padded. The rules allow the competitor to receive actual travelling and living expenses for a three weeks training camp, pocket money for petty daily expenses during the games, and clothing and equipment for his sport. Political, nationalistic and commercial use of the games is illegal. Voluntary effort is their mainstay.

Such rules as these can hardly be improved upon, but occasionally they have been unfair. Approved minor adjustments include awarding of a hardship allowance to an athlete's dependents, corresponding to their lack of support during a period up to thirty days; permitting an amateur athlete to teach sports to beginners or school children on a temporary basis without changing his usual occupation; permitting an amateur athlete to be a full-time professional journalist, radio or television reporter, or a full-time manager of or worker in an athletic facility.

In view of the hardship which may result from a serious accident sustained during competition or practice and to counteract the increasing tendency towards law suits in such cases, the author of this chapter recommends that consideration be given to permitting an approved amount of accident insurance coverage to be taken out for competitors by supporters, clubs or other organizations, without loss of amateur status. It would be required that similar insurance coverage be offered to all members of his club, school or other athletic group (including the Olympic Team as a group), so that no favored treatment was given to the more outstanding competitors. Specifically, the insurance may apply to injury sustained during organized training and competition and include medical and hospital care, disability benefits and permanent injury insurance, sufficient to give him a life income not less than the average income in his country at the time the contract is made. If he is married, he may also be given term life insurance sufficient to provide for a spouse for her life expectancy in the event of his being killed. In the event that he has dependent children, additional insurance may be provided to cover their needs through college and advanced degrees. Essentially, all such provisions for the amateur are designed to protect him from loss, but not to give him any financial gain.

Unfortunately there are many who are insistent on much more radical changes.[73] Maurice Martel, French President of the Federation Internationale de Ski (FIS) approves of cash awards for members, and they are permitted to accept money for lending their names to advertisers. The International Olympic Committee (IOC) has therefore cited virtually the entire French, Austrian and Swiss ski teams for breaking the Olympic code. Avery

Brundage, as president of the IOC is dedicated to the principle of amateurism, but Martel feels that his "first responsibility is to assure the present and future financial security of the competitors." It is felt likely that this clash of principle which marred the winter games in 1972 may eventually undermine the Olympic ideal. Such an occurrence would be a serious set back to amateurism. It is uncertain as to how long the IOC will be able to withstand the constant pressure to let in professionals. Brundage retired at 85 after the 1972 Olympics. After him the flood? We hope not.

To Brundage, amateurism goes far beyond sport.[65] He sees it as dedication to the task in hand; as pride of accomplishment; as basic reliability, as producing the man who doesn't have to be watched but will finish any job to the best of his ability, not for the reward but because the job is part of him and it would be beneath his dignity to do a shody job even if he lost money on it. Such a man may dislike his boss, but he will still do his best, because the discipline of sport has got into his bones, and he is determined to do his duty, and more. In war, he shows the same courage as on the football field. Wherever there is a hard job to be done, he will volunteer. Are we loking for such men today? Are there too many professionals to ask, "What's in it for me?" Are we increasingly materialistic? If so, let us guard and strengthen the principle of amateurism. Let us undergird it with religious faith and unselfish ideals, and we shall build better citizens. We shall retard moral decay and shall produce men of whom we can be proud.

Control of Accidents and Heart Attacks

To reinforce and expand the activities of the National Safety Council, a Federal Commission on Safety in Sports could help in developing national standards as to what are acceptable risks and in proposing measures to reduce the dangers in all sports. Sports associations could be encouraged or required to obtain standardized annual reports from each of their members or membership groups regarding deaths and nonfatal accidents sustained, and the number of days of inactivity resulting from injury, together with an estimate of the total number of people-hours spent on the sport during the year. They would also report the steps taken to prevent accidents, to provide first aid, and their plans and proposals for further improvements. In this way each sports association would monitor its own affairs, but would be subject to inspection and review. If it consistently failed to reduce a high accident rate, it could be subject to moral or legal pressure. Figures from all sports could be published in a single national report, giving the incidence of deaths, nonfatal accidents, and recovery days for 1,000 person-hours of participation, so that their relative dangers could be easily assessed.

While vast numbers of papers have been produced by physicians concerned with sport accidents, it is in the last analysis the responsibility of government to take action in the matter. Doctors can rarely do more than advise. If the government does not take action, it is most improbable that the average citizen or even the sports associations will be able to resolve it, any more than the American Automobile Association has resolved the enormous problem of road accidents. Where necessary, radical changes in conduct of games should be initiated. For example, a number of changes are long overdue in the rules governing football.[74] Tradition and less worthy motives have delayed acceptance by coaches who dominate the rules committees. Face masks should be made illegal. A "no blocking below the belt" rule is essential to cut (probably by 75%) the shocking incidence of knee injuries. More important still, these proposed new rules and all existing rules must be enforced. At present, many coaches are actually teaching students how to break the rules, and weak refereeing allows the cheating to succeed. So we have butting, spearing, piling on, hitting late, and tackling out of bounds continuing to mar the game in spite of the belated and hard-won rules.

There is a general feeling that "professional boxing needs a face lifting,"[75] as Dr. Max Novich so aptly puts it. His suggestions include abandonment of gloves. It seems that these have unexpectedly added to the dangers of the sport by allowing a harder blow to be struck without pain to the striker. A small leather mitten over gauze-bandaged hands would be a compromise. It is claimed that there was no death from a head injury from boxing in 100 years, when it was carried out with only a narrow leather band across the knuckles in ancient times.[76] Use of grease

on the face is another safety measure. He also advises better physical training, closer supervision by physicians who have been
given complete authority to stop a bout, more rigid standards of
matching the weight of boxers and excluding those who have
had recent or severe head injuries, regardless of EEG findings.
Perhaps the most important recommendation is that professional
boxing become more scientific and less a matter of brute force.
In this it could follow the lead of fencing.[76] Since dueling, which
was often fatal, has given way to the modern sport of fencing, all
the thrusts are recorded electrically at contact and the protective clothing makes injury a rare event. A similar measure with
boxing would make heavy blows needless, since victory would
depend on points scored by skill and speed. The reduced carnage
would also protect the spectators from feasting their eyes and emotions on violence-for-its-own-sake, better called savagery, barbar-
ism,[77] or sadism. While some claim that violence-by-proxy eases
tensions and reduces the likelihood of the spectator using violence
himself, precisely the opposite usually occurs.[77-79] While the placid
person may receive no emotional damage, the potentially violent
activist may gain incentive and learn techniques for aggression.
Unlike the western movies or the comics, sports seen on the
screen are for real—with the possible exception of some wrestling.
Thus, even if people can avoid contagion from the fantasy violence of the former, they cannot but be brutalized by seeing potentially serious injuries deliberately inflicted.

While professional boxing is currently the whipping boy, the
commission should consider all sports. There should be more
emphasis on what constitutes adequate training for each sport.
With half a million deaths a year in the United States from coronary disease, some of them precipitated by nothing more vigorous
than snow shovelling, it is obviously foolhardy for the overweight,
heavy smoking, sedentary person suddenly to sally forth into such
activities as mountain climbing, water skiing, or even cycling,
without some preliminary training. Even a teenager should never
be pushed hard without training, as this may precipitate a very
rapid or irregular heart, in addition to other strains. A well-
developed system of attaining physical fitness suitable for all
sports on a do-it-yourself-basis is available[63] To this should be

added the specific techniques needed for each sport. For example, in training for skiing, it is important to strengthen the hip and thigh muscles for weeks before participating. There is a need to systematize and publicize suitable systems for all sports, along with simple tests by which the individual can tell when he is ready for the season. Pulse recovery time after a specific activity is a favored one for general fitness.[80] The patient can readily learn to count his pulse. A simple test is to count it for exactly ten seconds, two minutes after the end of exercise. A count of more than twenty indicates that the activity was excessive for his degree of training. Tests of muscle power against a spring scale resistance could serve in many sports. Training exercises under experts and the giving of certificates for various levels of achievement could be used more widely, the more dangerous ski runs, climbs, dives, and so on being reserved for those who have passed the test. Every participant in a potentially dangerous sport should be expected to join the appropriate sports association, really know his sport, and keep up to date in developments. Moral pressure of this sort would be easier to exert if each club had to account for accidents sustained by its members. Supervision and penalties minimize the risks as does the use of reliable equipment and facilities. Finally, the nontherapeutic use of drugs should be made illegal, as it is in horse racing.

A WHITE HOUSE CONFERENCE ON THE PLACE OF SPORT IN AMERICAN LIFE

The implications of sport in American life are so important and the problems so far from solution, it might well be the subject of a White House conference. This could usefully have the widest terms of reference, including all the problems described in this chapter. Subcommittees could consider various groups of sports, sports in the schools and colleges, professional sports, physical fitness, sports medicine, ethics in sports, gambling and sports, amateur status, and sportsmanship. This would serve to publicize and document the many facets of the subject and should reach firm conclusions. It might be held in connection with the President's Council on Physical Fitness and Sports,[81] an organization with which Richard Nixon has close ties, historical and avocational. As Vice President of the USA in 1956 he was chairman of the first conference and of the resulting Council. As President of the USA, on September 24, 1970, he greatly expanded it, adding fifteen nationally recognized fitness and sports figures. With such new life, it may well be the ideal moment to inspire Americans with a new enthusiasm for true sportsmanship. This should be a major goal of the Council. However, victory will not be won by inspiration alone. The follow-up action after White House conferences on most other subjects has been disappointing in the extreme. Entrenched forces must be faced—forces which feed upon the present system with its win-ism and dishonesty. Much moral strength will be required of the leadership, along with tact and wisdom, and unflagging support from the White House.

In theses turbulent days decisions are often made because of threats, violence, emotion or vested interests rather than as a result of wise judgment. There could be adverse public reaction to any significant changes in rules regarding spectator sports, because of their popularity. The public educational value of a top level conference would be considerable in offsetting such emotionalism and would promote national discussion in the news media, making for smoother passage of any new legislation. It would help to keep the balance between those avant-garde educationalists who would like to outlaw all competitiveness, and those who have no patience with sportsmanship and are win-ists. It could also highlight the need to break the influence of organized crime which reaches even into the nation's sport. Finally, it would show that the executive branch is aware that all is not well in that most American of all American traits, its dedication to sport.

SPORTSMANSHIP: A GRASS ROOTS APPROACH

Any ideal which loses popular support is virtually dead. Internationally, de Coubertin's ideal is not dead. Indeed its success is fantastic. The cream of the athletes of some 125 countries renew their dedication to fair play at the modern Olympiads. Those who would spoil this spirit have failed, so far. Thanks to the vision and courage of the International Olympic Committee and its national affiliates, there has been steady support for the

Olympic ideal. Where does America stand in this? Officially we are in the clear. However, there are skeletons in the closet at home. Avery Brundage, an outstanding American upon whom the mantle of de Coubertin has long rested, has harsh words to say about American college sports. In a speech[65] he referred to repeated widespread scandals including bribery and stated that "educational institutions, taking advantage of the loyalty of their students to pile up gate receipts are [still] engaged in a sordid swindle." He pointed out that the situation is no better than that revealed in a 400 page report by the Carnegie Foundation forty years ago. A very recent report shows that things have grown worse rather than better.[82] Ferruccio Antonelli, President of the Second International Congress of Sports Psychology, pleaded with 1400 of his colleagues "to keep alive sport as a school of courage and fair play."[83] Brundage proposed a nine-point program to achieve this and urges us to return to fundamentals—hard work, self-discipline and emphasis on character, rather than money and success.[65]

We are passing through a period of self-denigration, imagining that everything American is bad—the war, the ugly American abroad, the credibility gap, discrimination and the like. May not the time be ripe for us to put our concepts of sports on the line for true evaluation? We sorely need action. We have had plenty of words.

Edmund Burke wrote in 1795, "the only thing necessary for the triumph of evil is for good men to do nothing."[84] Apply this to sport. What is the evil? It is win-ism. Who are the good men? Surely those who believe in good sportsmanship and in a live-and-let live attitude to an opponent. Burke's voice of experience from the past warns us that we must not keep silent. We must reintroduce respect for true sportsmanship as the code of every sports activity throughout the land. We must militantly and publicly decry those strident voices of win-ism that would drag us all down to their own contemptible level of self-interest. In this way we may not only save competitive sports as a great human activity, but all of us may regain real self-respect—based on a good conscience. Such a change might, within a few decades, build an admirable society out of our social jungle. It would increase respect for everyone's rights, including the poor, the minorities, and the police. Sometimes we feel helpless to influence change, but here is something we can all do, *now*, ourselves, and can influence others in our home and community to do likewise.

For decades Drew Pearson, and now his successor, Jack Anderson, and their associates have used their syndicated column to attack wrongdoing by public figures, fearing neither politicians nor organized crime. As a result, many corrupt people are now behind bars, or at least are stripped of their power. In 1966 Ralph Nader, a young American lawyer, shook up the vast automobile industry.[85] We are still benefiting from the impact, and meanwhile he has successfully challenged other entrenched abuses, all in the interest of the public. Such men keep American Democracy alive at a time when you can be attacked in the street, and the chances are that no observer will even phone the police, much less come to your aid. However, citizens who are not afraid to get involved have fed information to the columnists or worked as "Nader's Raiders." Let each person who cares and dares solemnly resolve to work determinedly for reform of American sport—come what may.

> "And the world will be better for this
> That one man, scorned and covered with scars
> Still strove, with his last ounce of courage,
> To reach the unreachable stars."[86]

REFERENCES

1. Webster, F. A. M.: *The Evolution of the Olympic Games 1829 B.C.—1914 A.D.* London, Heath, Cranton and Ouseley, 1914.
2. Kieran, John and Daley, Arthur: *The Story of the Olympic Games, 776 B.C. to 1968.* New York, Lippincott, 1969.
3. Bryan, J. III: *The Colosseum: World's Bloodiest Acre.* New York, Perfect Publishing, 1969.
4. Bryan, J. III: *The Colosseum: World's Bloodiest Acre.* Condensed from *Holiday* (Dec., 1969), *Readers Digest,* June 1970, pp. 234-240.
5. Boyle, Robert H.: *Sport—Mirror of American Life.* Boston, Little, Brown, 1963.
6. Owens, Jesse and Neimark, Paul G.: My life as a black man,

condensed from *Blackthink* (see ref. 7), *Readers Digest,* May 1970, pp. 126-131.

7. Owens, Jesse and Neimark, Paul G.: *Blackthink: My Life as a Black Man and White Man.* New York, W. Morrow, 1970.

8. Tunis, John R.: *The American Way in Sport.* New York, Duell, Sloan and Pearce, 1958.

9. Adams, James T.: *Dictionary of American History.* New York, C. Scribner's Sons, 1940.

10. Beisser, Arnold R.: *The Madness in Sports.* New York, Appleton-Century-Crofts, 1967.

11. Ryan, Francis J.: (a) An investigation of personality differences associated with competitive ability. (b) Further observations on competitive ability in athletics. In Bryant M. Wedge (Ed.): *Psychosocial Problems of College Men.* New Haven, Yale University Press, 1958, pp. 113-139.

12. Stewart, Jackie and Dymock, Eric: *Jackie Stewart: World Champion.* Chicago, Henry Regnery, 1970.

13. Peale, Norman Vincent: *Faith Made Them Champions.* Carmel, Guideposts Assoc., 1954.

14. Are sports good for the soul? In *Newsweek,* January 11, 1971, pp. 51-52.

15. Miles, Surgeon Rear-Admiral Stanley: Medical criteria in the selection of athletes, symposium on sports injuries. *Proc. R. Soc. Med., 62*:921-924, 1969.

16. Ryan, Allan, J.: A medical history of the Olympic Games, symposium on sports contributions: 1968 Olympics. *J.A.M.A., 205*: 715-720, 1968.

17. Smodlaka, Vojin: Sports medicine in the world today, Symposium on sports contributions. 1968 Olympics. *J.A.M., 205*:762-763, 1968.

18. Cureton, Thomas K.: *Physical Fitness of Champion Athletes.* St. Louis, C. V. Mosby, 1947.

19. Stiles, Merritt H.: Medical preparation for the Olympic Games, symposium on sports cotnributions: 1968 Olympics. *J.A.M.A., 205*:771-774, 1968.

20. Dill, David B.: Physiological adjustments to altitude changes, symposium on sports cotnributions: 1968 Olympics. J.A.M.A., *205*:747-753, 1968.

21. Editorial: Survey of status of team physicians in the United States. *J.A.M.A., 184*:981-984, 1963.

22. *A Guide for Medical Evaluation of Candidates for School Sports.* Chicago, AMA, 1966.

23. *Tips on Athletic Training, I-XII the Committee on Medical Aspects of Sports.* Chicago, AMA, 1970.

24. Novich, Max M.: A physician looks at athletics: *J.A.M.A., 161*:573-576, 1956.

25. Reiheld, Robert E.: The high school team physician, pp. 50-51, proceedings of the seventh national conference on the medical aspects of sports, Nov. 28, 1965. Chicago, AMA, 1967.

26. Novich, Max M.: Doping in sport: In *Abbottempo,* vol. 2. North Chicago, Abbott Laboratories, 1964.

27. Smith, Gene M. and Beecher, Henry K.: Amphetamine sulfate and athletic performance, I. Objective effects. *J.A.M.A., 170*:542-557, 1959.

28. *Tips on Athletic Training II.* Chicago, Committee on the Medical Aspects of Sports, AMA 1960.

29. Editorial: Drugs: their use and abuse by athletes. *J. National Athlectic Trainers Assoc., 5* (No. 4):5, Winter 1970.

30. *Mouth Protectors for use in Contact Sports: A Responsibility of All Dentists.* Chicago, American Dental Association, Bureau of Dental Health Education, 1970.

31. Faulkner, John A.: New perspectives in training for maximum performance, symposium on sports contributions: 1968 Olympics. *J.A.M.A., 205*:741-746, 1968.

32. Craig, Calvert B., Jr.: Limitations of the human organism, symposium on sports contributions: 1968 Olympics. *J.A.M.A., 205*:734-740, 1968.

33. F-8 Committee on Protective Equipment for Sports. American Society for Testing and Materials, Washington.

34. National Operating Committee on Standards for Athletic Equipment. National Federation of State High School Associations Office, 7 South Dearborn Street, Chicago, Illinois.

35. Padwe, Sandy: Big-time college football is on the skids. *Look Magazine,* Sept. 22, 1970, p. 66.

36. Meggysey, Dave: *Out of Their League.* Ramparts Press, 1970.

37. Rebel with a cause. In *Newsweek,* Nov. 16, 1970, p. 68.

38. Tawney, R. H.: *The Acquisitive Society.* New York, Harcourt, Brace and World, 1948.

39. Olmstead, Charlotte: *Heads I Win, Tails You Lose.* New York, Macmillan, 1962.

40. Kanaar, Adrian C.: Lifelong fitness: A positive approach. *J. Assoc. Phys. Ment. Rehabilitation,* Nov.-Dec. 1962. (Reprints available from the author.)

41. Accident Facts, Annual Report, Public Safety Conference, National Safety Council, 425 North Michigan Avenue, Chicago, Illinois.

42. Spaderman, Richard: Lower extremity injuries as related to the use of ski safety bindings. *J.A.M.A., 203*:445-450, 1968.

43. Allen, Maurey L.: Air Force football injuries, a clinical and statistical study. *J.A.M.A., 206*:1053-1058, 1968.
44. Smillie, I. S.: Knee injuries in athletes, symposium on sports injuries. *Proc. R. Soc. Med., 62*:937-939, 1969.
45. Gonzales, Thomas A.: Fatal injuries in competitive sports. *J.A.M.A. 146*:1506-1511, 1951.
46. Clarke, Kenneth S.: Calculated risk of sports fatalities. *J.A.M.A., 197*:894-896, 1966.
47. Editorial: Ice hockey can be safer. *J.A.M.A., 207*:1706, 1969.
48. Snowmobile Accident Summary, 1969-70, Winter Season, Public Safety Department, National Safety Council, 425 N. Michigan Avenue, Chicago, Illinois, 1970.
49. Lloyd, Kenneth: Some hazards of athletic exercise. *Proc. R. Soc. Med., 52*:151-158, 1959.
50. Mawdsley, C. and Ferguson, F. R.: Neurological disease in boxers. *Lancet, 2*:795, 1963.
51. Editorial: Statement on boxing: *J.A.M.A., 181*:242, 1962.
52. Flinn, John H.: *The Wisconsin Boxing Story.* Madison, University of Wisconsin, 1960.
53. School Athletics: Problems and Policies, (p. 82) Educational policies Commission of the National Education Association of the United States, and the American Association of School Administrators, 1201 16th Street, N.W., Washington, 1954.
54. Frey, U.: The relationship between anatomical site of injury and particular sports, symposium on sports injuries. *Proc. R. Soc. Med., 62*:917-919, 1969.
55. *To Protect Rodeo Livestock: Uniform Supervision Standards.* The American Humane Association, Denver, Colorado.
56. Kaplan, Harry A. and Browder, Jefferson: Observations on the clinical and brain wave patterns of professional boxers. *J.A.M.A., 156*:1138-1144, 1954.
57. Blonstein, J. L.: Boxing injuries. *J. R. Coll. Gen. Prac., 18*:100-103, 1969.
58. Johnson, F.: Organic psychosyndromes due to boxing. *Br. J. Psychiatry, 115*:45-53, 1969.
59. Litchfield, Edward H.: Saturday's hero is doing fine. In *Sports Illustrated,* Oct. 8, 1962, pp. 68-80.
60. Peter, Lawrence: *The Peter Principle.* New York, W. Morrow, 1969.
61. Grebanier, Bernard: *Memoirs 1885-1967 by Andre Maurois.* Translated from French by Denver Lindley. New York, Harper and Row. pp. 439, 1970.
62. Capener, Norman: Introduction and appraisal, symposium on sports injuries, *Proc. R. Soc. Med., 62*:915-917, 1969.

63. Cooper, Kenneth, H.: *The New Aerobics.* New York, Bantam Books, 1970.
64. Prout, Curtis: Life expectancy of crew members. A paper presented at the Twelfth National Conference on the Medical Aspects of Sports, Nov. 29, 1970.
65. Brundage, Avery: The fumbled ball: Some constructive suggestions. A speech delivered at California State College, Hayward, California, Dec. 1, 1966. In *Vital Speeches of the Day, 33*(No. 13):411-416, 1967.
66. Van Huss, W. D., Heasner, W. W., and Michkelsen, O.: Effects of prepubertal exercise on body composition. In *Exercise and Fitness.* Chicago, The Athletic Institute, pp. 201-214, 1969.
67. Giannestras, Nicholas, J.: *To Win or to Play? that is the Problem.* Bulletin, American College of Surgeons, July-Aug., 1967.
68. Giannestras, Nicholas J.: *Pee Wee Baseball and Football—Good or Evil?* Bulletin, American College of Surgeons, June 1970.
69. Recommended Standards and Practice of a College Health Program, American College Health Association, Evanston, Illinois, 1969.
70. Policy Statement: Desirable Athletic Competition for Children of Elementary School Age. American Association for Health, Physical Education and Recreation, Washington, 1968.
71. Brundage, Avery: Personal communication from president, IOC. Chicago, Illinois, Oct. 22, 1970.
72. Eligibility Rules of the International Olympic Committee, Chicago, Illinois, 1962.
73. Amateurs on the skids? In *Newsweek,* Jan. 11, 1971, p. 55.
74. Nelson, David M.: Forum on football rules and injuries: in the college contest. Paper presented at the twelfth National Conference on the Medical Aspects of Sports, Nov. 29, 1970.
75. Novich, Max M.: Professional boxing needs a face lifting. *J. Sports Med. Phys. Fitness, 5*:82-87, 1965.
76. Official publication: *How to Understand and Enjoy the Sport of Fencing.* Amateur Fencers League of America, West New York, New Jersey.
77. Lukacs, John A.: America's malady is not violence but savagery. In Thomas Rose (Ed.): *Violence in America.* New York, Random House, 1969.
78. Marmor, Judd: Some psychosocial aspects of contemporary urban violence. In Thomas Rose (Ed.): *Violence in America.* New York, Random House, pp. 338-348, 1969.
79. Scott, John P.: A symposium on aggression and sport. In Gerald S. Kenyon (Ed.): *Contemporary Psychology of Sport.* Proceedings

of the 2nd International Congress of Sports Psychology. Chicago, The Athletic Institute, 1970.

80. Kasch, Fred W. and Boyer, John L.: *Adult Fitness: Principles and Practices.* All-American Productions and Publications, Greeley, Colorado, 1968.

81. A Brief History. The President's Council on Physical Fitness and Sports, Washington, 1970.

82. DuPree, David: Playing the game: subtitles: sports-crazy colleges continue to lure stars with improper offers—cash, cars, girls proffered; some coaches get fed up, but few tattle on peers; a stingray and a sure degree. In *The Wall Street Journal,* vol. 176, No. 71, Oct. 8, 1970.

83. Antonelli, Ferruccio: Presidential address, In Gerald S. Kenyon (Ed.): *Contemporary Psychology of Sports.* Proceedings of the Second International Congress of Sports Psychology (1968 meeting). Chicago, The Athletic Institute, 1970.

84. Burke, Edmund, from a letter to William Smith, Jan. 9, 1795.

85. Nader, Ralph: *Unsafe at Any Speed: The Designed-in Dangers of the American Automobile.* New York, Pocket Books, 1966.

86. "The Impossible Dream" from the musical play "Man of La Mancha," based on Don Quixote by Miguel de Cervantes y Saavedra.

INDEX

Abortions,
  birth control method, 58-59
  illegal, maternal deaths, 74
  Lusitanus' oath, 9
  Oath of Hippocrates, 9
  population control method, 54
  sterilization as preventive measure,
    73-74
  United States, 73-74
Acceptable sports, foul play's effect, 271
  see also Sports
Accident injury, child, 251
Accident-prone persons, unconscious
  death wish, 117
"Accidental deaths," many suicides, 103,
  111
Actions, thought controlled?, 133
Adolescents, girls, suicide attempts, 120
Africa,
  low suicide rate, 114
  population growth, 50
Age, dread of as suicide cause, 107
Age of Chivalry, sportsmanship, 272
Aged persons,
  ill, right to die, 126
  life prolongation problems, xii
  suicide approved among Eskimos, 113
  suicides, 104
AHA,
  action on animals used in sports,
    294-295
  sports injuries action, 290
Alcohol, dependency on, 144
Alcoholics, suicide risk, 119, 144
Alcoholism,
  clue to suicide tendency, 121
  suicide relationship, 104, 137
All Union Thoracic Surgery Congress,
  lung transplant report, 189
AMA, see American Medical Association
American Athletic Union,

drug use condemned, 281
  sports status interest, 300
America,
  sports' importance, 277, 292, 307
  suicide categories and rates, 135
American Academy of Pediatrics, sports
  recommendations, 299
American College of Sports Medicine,
  reports on research, 280
American Humane Society, see AHA
American Indians,
  alcholishm and suicides, 105
  Cheyenne, suicide rate high, 115
American Medical Association,
  amphetamine sulphate use in sports
    condemned, 280-281
  Committee on Medical Aspects of
    Sports, 280
  Criticism of junior sports, 285
  deliberate sports injuries condemned,
    282
  drug use in sports condemned, 281
  experiments, ethical considerations,
    13
  Judicial Council, experiment regu-
    lations, 13
  medical ethics, 5, 9, 11, 12
  National Congress on Medical Ethics,
    3
  sports guidance, 280
  sterilization stand, 69
American Society for the Prevention of
  Cruelty to Animals, see ASPCA
Americans,
  birth control, abortion views, 59
  deaths, suicide rate, 129
Amphetamine sulphate, sports use and
  dangers, 280-281
Anabolic effect, HGH, 258
Ancient philosophers, "natural metaphysic," moral law, 8

315

Killers of the Seas

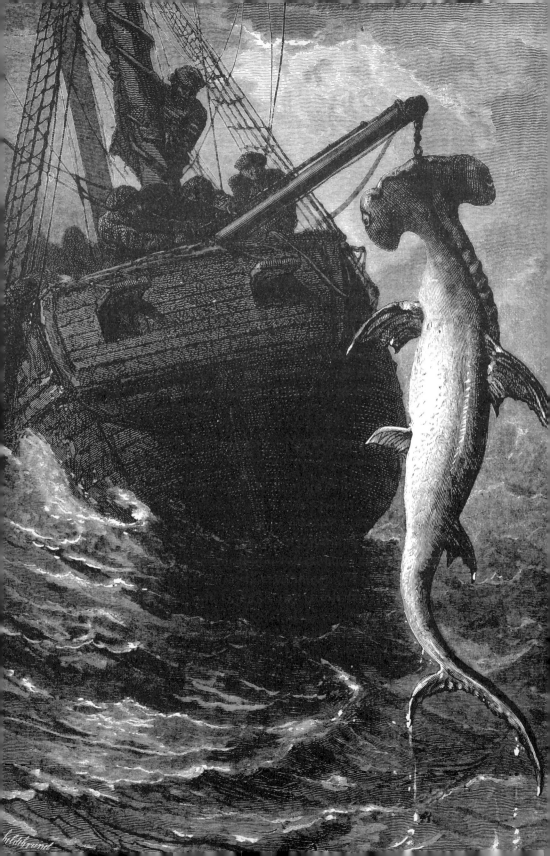

Killers of the Seas

Edward R. Ricciuti

 WALKER AND COMPANY · New York

First published in the United States of America
in 1973 by the Walker Publishing Company, Inc.
Published simultaneously in Canada
by Fitzhenry & Whiteside, Limited, Toronto

ISBN: 0-8027-0415-8

Library of Congress Catalog Card Number: 72-95785

Printed in the United States of America.

10   9   8   7   6   5   4   3   2   1

To Dominic Napolitano
who has many sons

CONTENTS

PREFACE

Perhaps there was a time when I was not fascinated by the water world and its creatures, but I cannot remember it. One of my clearest memories of my very early years, on the other hand, is of my father showing me a horseshoe crab on a sandy beach in Milford, Connecticut. By the time I was age six, I had an aquarium with multihued little fish swimming in it, and had begun to peer under rocks in streams to see what kind of creatures hid there.

The years have done nothing to diminish the sense of mystery and beauty that for me makes the water world so compelling. Until about a decade ago, however, my involvement with creatures of stream, lake, and sea was that of a fisherman, aquarium hobbyist, and amateur naturalist. But then, as a science journalist, opportunities opened to go to sea aboard research vessels and military craft, and to interview scientists engaged in the various disciplines that constitute the science of the sea.

In 1967, I joined the curatorial staff of the New York Zoological Society, which in addition to the Bronx Zoo operates the New York Aquarium and the Osborn Laboratories of Marine Sciences, near the Coney Island boardwalk in Brooklyn. As curator administering the society's popular and scientific publications, film-making, and public relations, I worked closely with the staff of the aquarium and laboratories, which were named in honor of Fairfield Osborn, long-time president of the society and one of the leading conservationists of the century. During my five years with the society and in the years since I have been able to write extensively on the natural history of the water world.

It was only a matter of time after joining the society that I learned to dive with scuba and began to take advantage of every opportunity to work with water life. Even more exciting were the associations and friendships with the members of the staffs of the New York Aquarium and the Osborn Laboratories and of similar institutions around the world, who have always been generous with their knowledge.

For my years with the society, and thereafter, I have been the beneficiary of the tutorial abilities of a man with almost unequaled grasp of the intricate web of aquatic life, Dr. Ross F. Nigrelli, for many years head of the New York Aquarium and founding director of the Osborn Laboratories. Sometimes with chalk and blackboard, sometimes over a dish of *squid marinara* at Gargiulo's, a restaurant in Coney Island near the aquarium, Ross Nigrelli has shared some of his knowledge and insights with me. And so, with utmost patience, has Dr. George Ruggieri, S.J., now director of the Osborn Laboratories. In conversations with both of these dedicated scientists, I formed the germ of an idea, which led to the development of this book. I am deeply grateful.

I also owe special thanks to Dr. James Atz of the American Museum of Natural History, and to his wife, Ethel. Not only did they welcome me into their home so I could use their unique library, but they provided food, drink, and warm hospitality.

The author of a book that covers such a wide range of material as this one must depend on many people for assistance and must draw on many sources of information. I owe a debt to many people and institutions, most of which are mentioned in this book, and all of which, I sincerely hope, I have credited. In addition to those mentioned above, I am especially grateful to the following: D.W. Bennett and Virginia Steiner of the American Littoral Society, Sandy Hook, N.J.; Edward Dols and Peter Fennimore of the New York Aquarium; Perry W. Gilbert, director of the Mote Marine Laboratory, Sarasota, Florida; Nixon Griffis, president of the American Littoral Society; David Hancock of Hancock House, Saanichton, B.C., Canada; Robert Morris of Cornell University, former curator, New York Aquarium; James A. Oliver, former director, American Museum of Natural History, director, New York Aquarium; John Prescott, director, New England Aquarium; Dorothy Reville, New York Zoological Society; William Walker, curator, Marineland of the Pacific, California; Robert Wicklund, project manager, Hydro-Lab, Freeport, Grand Bahama Island; and finally, Gary Nault, who helped with research, and Don and Carol Sanders, for their editing abilities.

The following institutions were especially helpful: the library of the New York Zoological Society, the library of the London Zoological Society, the library of the British Museum of Natural History, the United States Navy Office of Information, the library of the University of Bridgeport, and the Killingworth (Conn.) Public Library.

E. R. R.
Roast Meat Hill
Killingworth, Connecticut
June 20, 1973

Life and Death in an Alien World

Beneath the beryl-blue ocean that washes the beach at Freeport, Grand Bahama Island, a bottom of white sand slopes gently seaward. About a mile from the shore the sandy bottom is strewn with boulder-size chunks of coral (called heads) which are fringed with gorgonians—sea whips and sea fans whose delicate branches belie their membership in the animal kingdom. The scattering of heads continues seaward for about 200 feet and then gives way to a series of parallel coral ridges which extend, fingerlike, away from the shore. The ridges are separated by channels and alleyways 6 to 10 feet wide and as deep as a man is tall. As the distance from the shore increases, the ridge complex grows in mass until it builds into the great outer reef that edges this part of Grand Bahama's southern shore.

The reef teems with life, much of it beautiful, some of it dangerous, and very often possessed of both qualities. Clouds of midnight parrotfish school over the coral, their blue-black forms etched against the lighter blue of the water. Permits, coveted as gamefish for their craft and fight, flash like winged moons through the passages between the ridges; and here and there prowls a great barracuda, snaggletoothed, jut-jawed but incredibly sleek and graceful.

One sunny spring morning I looked out over the inner margin of the reef from inside a yellow steel chamber, resting

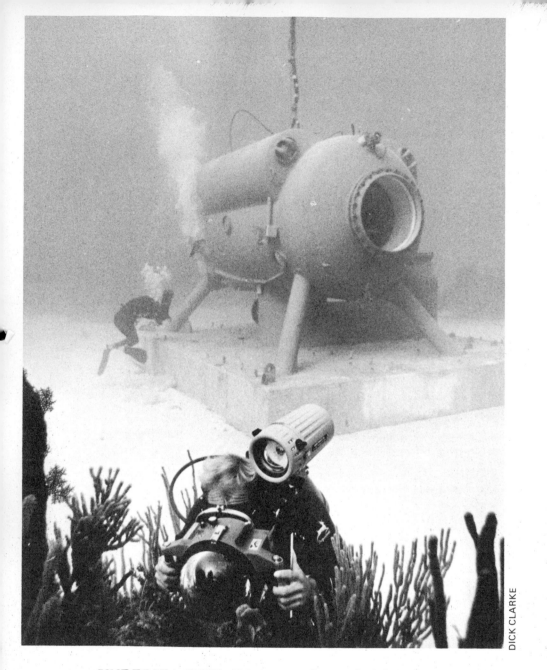

UNDERSEA BASE: Divers use the Hydro-Lab manned habitat as an undersea station for scientific study and photography of marine life off Freeport, Grand Bahama Island.

4

on the bottom among the coral heads. Built by the Perry Oceanographic Corporation and dubbed Hydro-Lab, the chamber is made available to a wide variety of people, from sports divers to scientists, who want to observe the rich and varied life of the reef, as if watching from a living-room window, for hours or even days at a stretch. Accessible to divers with scuba equipment, Hydro-Lab receives air, electricity, and other essentials through a life-support system from a buoy floating on the surface 50 feet above the chamber. With its life-support equipment operating, Hydro-Lab is an island of survival for humans in the hostile environment of the sea.

As I stood within the chamber, watching a steel-gray Bermuda chub meander past the 4-foot viewing port, I felt an ironic kinship with the small fish that swam in my living room aquarium at home. They too were alive by virtue of an encapsulated simulation of their natural environment, maintained by machines in surroundings vastly different from those in which their kind had evolved. The room outside the glass panes of their aquarium was as alien to those small fish as the water on the other side of Hydro-Lab's viewing port was to me. The water was their home, not mine, and millions of years of evolution had molded their bodies and behavior for life in an environment where, without artificial aids, I would perish.

To humans, many of the ways in which fish and other aquatic animals have evolved for survival seem strange and sometimes frightening, but that is because we view them from a human perspective, in our own terms. Yet the deadly stinging batteries of the sea wasp jellyfish, or the tentacles of a giant squid writhing 30 feet from its boneless body are as natural for these creatures in the context of their way of life as a hand with five fingers is in ours. This does not diminish the fact, however, that many such characteristics of aquatic animals make them dangerous to humans who confront them in the water.

5

The assorted stings, teeth, and other unpleasant attributes of dangerous aquatic creatures certainly did not evolve for the purpose of harming humans, but rather as the result of vastly complex processes, working over millennia, that have given these creatures a means for survival in their watery home. Only when we trigger these instincts, these automatic mechanisms for survival, do they endanger us. It is the nature of these potentially dangerous characteristics of aquatic animals, and their relationship to humans in the water, that is the subject of this book.

Knowing One's Enemy

Most, if not all, of the major groups of animals in the sea include members that can endanger humans. They range from tiny blobs of protoplasm to some of the largest and most intelligent animals on earth. Some of them can poison entire human populations; some can swallow a man whole; some kill in seconds with a deadly dart hardly felt by the victim; some are so monstrous they have dragged entire ships down into the depths.

Stories about the terrors of the deep are as ancient as man's ability to tell them. Certainly the hazards of encountering various forms of aquatic life have concerned people ever since they first began to live near large bodies of water. Only comparatively recently, however, has there been organized investigation of the dangers, alleged and actual, that the animal inhabitants of the water present to man.

Much of the interest in dangerous aquatic animals arose as a matter of military necessity during World War II. For the first time in history, millions of men from nations with high technological development traversed regions, particularly in the tropics, where dangerous aquatic animals abound. Moreover, many of these men were put in survival situations due to the downing of aircraft or to maritime disasters, in which they were much more likely to encounter dangerous aquatic creatures.

Many wartime accounts of such incidents seemed contradictory. Unquestionably, large numbers of men lost at sea were indeed victims of sharks—yet by the war's end it remained arguable whether the shark was, as some experts insisted, "a sissy" or whether it was indeed a savage killer. Conflicting stories were told by survivors of disasters at sea. Many told of shark attacks, or at least of seeing the killer fish circling their rafts. Yet one airman spent 12 days aboard a life raft without seeing a single shark. A U.S. Navy pilot who with his gunner was downed at sea, drove away a shark by hitting it on the snout. But sharks pulled down the gunner only a few feet away. Another downed flier, stranded on a raft, saw no sharks but was menaced by a huge sea turtle that batted his raft about for 20 minutes.

The chances of contact between humans and potentially dangerous aquatic animals are increasing in proportion to the number of people who take to the water as divers, surfers, swimmers, yachtsmen, and sports fishermen. As their ranks widen so does their jet-age mobility. Never before, for example, have boatloads of tourists wandered along the Antarctic ice fronts where leopard seals prowl the water's edge hoping to make a bloody meal of a penguin. The availability of scuba, and too often the lack of control over its distribution and use, has enabled almost anyone with even slight athletic ability to venture into depths that only a few years ago the most experienced divers seldom visited. The water world holds far more grace, wonder, and beauty than terror, but it would be unrealistic to dismiss the danger that does exist, particularly for the unwary.

It is most perilous to venture into the water without an

awareness of the characteristics that make some aquatic creatures dangerous to man, and how one's own actions in relation
to these animals can increase the danger. Aquatic animals that
menace humans do so because of adaptations in their behavior
and physical makeup that result from evolutionary processes.
In most cases the adaptations have enabled them to continue
as a species while countless other species have failed. Whether
these adaptations be in the shape of an animal, or in the way it
senses prey, or in its ability to move rapidly, they contribute to
the animal's success in coping with the world of water.

The Water World

The world under water—the hydrosphere—has often been
considered analogous to outer space, the region beyond the
earth's atmosphere. But there are great differences between
the two worlds. Simply by dipping your toe into the water of a
pond you can enter the hydrosphere; space, on the other hand,
has been reached only by a very few humans, and then only
with the resources of entire nations behind them. Space is a
cold, black void, while the hydrosphere teems with life in
varied and wondrous forms.

As terrestrial creatures, humans often fail to appreciate the
immensity of the hydrosphere, which contains considerably
more living space than the part of the earth above the water.
Not counting water locked in glaciers, in ice and snow, in the
crust of the earth, and in the atmosphere, the hydrosphere comprises about 329,055,000 cubic miles, all of which is ocean except for some 55,000 cubic miles in lakes and rivers. The
ocean, which covers almost 71 percent of the earth's surface,
has 3,000 times more living space than does the land. Its deepest parts are more than 36,000 feet in depth, while the continents have an average height of less than 3,000 feet. Even Mt.

Everest, with an altitude of slightly more than 29,000 feet, is not as high as some ocean trenches are deep. Most of the animals that inhabit the land live on or under the surface, or in trees within 50 feet of it. Birds, while they may fly to great heights, carry on most of their vital functions on or near the surface. In the ocean, however, life in a multitude of forms exists everywhere from the froth that tips the waves to the abyssal muck.

Until recently, scientists believed that marine life petered out at depths greater than a few thousand feet. But during the past few decades, deep-sea explorers have found evidence that life thrives even on the floors of the deepest trenches. In 1960, the Swiss oceanographer Jacques Piccard and Lieutenant Don Walsh of the United States Navy peered through the porthole of the bathyscaphe *Trieste* 35,800 feet down in the Pacific Ocean's Challenger Deep and saw a flatfish the size of a frying pan. Two years later, Commander Georges Houot and engineer Pierre Henri Willm descended in the 70-foot-long bathyscaphe *Archimede* to a depth of 31,300 feet in the Kuril-Kamchatka Trench north of Japan. On the oozy bottom of that ocean deep they found several small animals. In 1964, members of a bathyscaphe crew in the Puerto Rican Trench spotted small fish swimming in the gloom at 17,700 feet and again at 27,150 feet.

Oceanographers have divided the ocean into various living zones, some of which are classified according to the ecology of the habitats they provide and others according to depth or distance from shore. Some of the zones overlap and thus tend to confuse, but their existence is logical because of the three-dimensional aspect of the ocean's living space. Perhaps the best way to consider them is to begin at the shore, where the salt spray rains on organisms of the land that have ventured to the edge of the sea, and on those of the sea that have gained a foothold upon the land.

The Many Faces of the Shore

Many types of shore lie at the water's edge, some rocky, some muddy, some battered by surf, and some washed by gently lapping wavelets. They are alike, however, in a very important way—the shore changes continuously and animals that inhabit it are under great pressure to adjust to the ever-present change. The shore has a *splash zone*, land above high water that regularly is moistened by sea spray but never covered by waves, except when the storm surge booms up the beach. Below the splash zone, between high and low water, is the *littoral zone*, true meeting ground of land and sea, where the tides hold sway.

Even in the *tidal zone*, at the very edge of the water, one may come in contact with sea creatures that can cause a variety of harm, from death to but a few moments of unpleasantness. The mishaps involving dangerous life forms that occur in the shallows greatly outnumber those that take place in deep water, largely, of course, because greater numbers of people congregate near the beach. Sharks, for instance, commonly cruise into water that is only knee-deep on a man, and even killer whales roam just beyond the breaker line. Danger from the sea even can lurk high up on the beach, sometimes in the form of jellyfish, stranded but still capable of delivering painful stings.

The Richest Region

Beyond the tidal zone, to a depth of 600 feet, lies the region of the sea most important to humankind. This region comprises the continental shelf, which juts seaward like a pouting lower lip from the world's great land masses. Exposed during geologic periods when the sea level is low and submerged when the sea level rises, the continental shelf—if all the various shelves are considered as one—covers 10 million square miles, an area equivalent to 20 percent of the planet's dry land.

The waters of the shelf surpass any other region on earth in richness of life. Some scientists estimate that four-fifths of the organisms that inhabit our planet live in the waters over the continental shelf. These coastal waters teem with the billions upon billions of tiny floating plants and animals that constitute the base of the sea's food pyramid. The abundance of light in the relatively shallow shelf waters makes possible lush plant growth on a microscopic scale. The key members of the microscopic plant assemblage are diatoms, brown or yellow specks of protoplasm, each composed of a single cell encased in a silica box, an external skeleton. Viewed under a miscroscope, these skeletons have beautiful and fantastic shapes.

The microscopic plants, which together are called phytoplankton, provide the food for hordes of tiny animals that float with them at the whim of wind and wave. Some of these minute creatures are preyed upon by other living motes, and these in turn are eaten by larger creatures as the food pyramid builds. The largest concentrations of fish in the sea occur in these rich coastal waters, where food is abundant. In contrast, the waters of the open ocean seem a desert.

Little of the nutrient material washed into coastal seas from the shore ever reaches the open ocean, nor does the fertile mix of dead organisms from the coastal waters enrich the open ocean to a significant degree. This is not to say that the open ocean lacks life, for many fast-swimming fish—tuna, billfish, and some sharks—rove the waters far from shore.

Below the surface waters, light gradually fades into a zone of twilight, and then disappears in a realm of enternal blackness. During the night when the surface waters dim, some of the creatures of the nether zones rise from the depths, like banshees slipping out of the darkness, to feed at the lower margins of the zone of light. Some of the creatures of the depths are fantastic in appearance, carrying coldly glowing lights, and having expandable stomachs that enable them to swallow creatures as large as they. Fortunately, most of these monsters are small, measuring a foot, perhaps two or three in length. But giants prowl the depths too, huge squid scores of feet long that are hunted by great sperm whales, and sharks, weirdly shaped and of mysterious nature. Perhaps other monstrous creatures, yet beyond human ken, also hide in the ocean deeps, a subject that will be considered later in this book.

Coral Constructions–Reefs

Within the various zones of the sea are a multitude of habitats, of which one, the coral reef, supports the greatest variety of life, including many of the creatures most dangerous to humans in the sea. Coral reefs thrive in a band that girdles the globe between 30 degrees north and 30 degrees south latitude, beyond which, to north or south, the water is too cold to support the growth of the fragile polyps that build them.

As a habitat, the coral reef has been likened to the tropical rain forest on land. Like the rain forest the reef supports life in extravagant diversity. The analogy is especially apt for the fishes of the reef rival the birds of the forest in their dazzling color and form. The forest's splendid blooms are mirrored by the flower animals of the reef, creatures resembling colorful plants more than animals. Like the rain forest, the reef can be a deadly place, too, where savage predators search for prey and where hidden crannies conceal creatures whose touch means quick, agonizing death.

Although the surface of the reef teems with living creatures, the greater proportion of its animals live and die within   ·

its recesses, honeycombed with caves and crevices. Moray eels, aggressive and powerful, wind sinuously through the pathways in the coral. Lobsters wedge themselves into crannies, and worms of many types make their homes in holes and burrows. The honeycombed nature of a reef seldom is apparent from above. Underwater you can explore a cave deep within a reef, and after emerging and flippering back over the surface of the coral you can see bubbles from your own scuba still filtering through what appears to be a solid mound of coral.

Adaptations for Aquatic Survival

Animals have adapted, in the evolutionary sense, to every sort of niche in the water world. The various species adapt, i.e. change over the eons, not only physically but in the manner by which they reproduce, seek food, or protect themselves. Individual adaptations may result in unusual size, shape, or color, or in the way each creature responds to what it senses in the surrounding water.

One of the most obvious adaptations for an aquatic life is the torpedo-like form of the fish. This form endures even in the pancake body of the flounder, except here the torpedo has been flattened. The shape of a fish's body helps the creature push through the resistance offered by water, which is 800 times more dense than air. Aquatic mammals such as whales and penguins have developed similarly streamlined bodies, showing that a particular type of adaptation is not limited to any one class of animals.

The schooling of some species of fish is a behavioral adaptation that long has interested scientists. One reason why fish school is that many small fish, by schooling, take on the form of a large animal, thus discouraging predators. Konrad Lorenz, in his classic book, *On Aggression,* described how he was

13

fooled in this way by a school of fish while skin diving in the Florida Keys. Lorenz was approaching a pier when a huge form, many yards deep and wide, slid out from under the structure. Lorenz described himself as terrified by the approach of this great shape—until it broke up into a crowd of little grunts and snappers.

The adaptations of some aquatic animals that make them dangerous to humans do not fit any single classification. Stinging spines, sharp teeth, ravenous feeding behavior, large size, poisonous flesh have evolved for various reasons and under vastly different conditions. The venom glands of venomous fish, for instance, evolved from the cells that produce the slime which coats the skin of most fish. The slime is mildly antibiotic; that is, it kills certain disease organisms that might infect the fish. The glands that manufacture such slime in venomous fish have been modified by the processes of evolution so that their secretions are vastly more toxic. Similarly, some of the spines that deliver the venom are merely modified arrangements of fins. The spine at the end of the stingray's tail, however, probably evolved from one of the denticles, which in sharks and rays cover the body as scales do in most other fish. Coupled with the instinctive manner in which the ray lashes about with its tail when molested, its spine becomes, to man, a highly dangerous adaptation.

Killer whales, as has been their fashion for countless generations, sometimes feed by bumping seals or penguins off of ice floes. Such behavior makes them dangerous to any humans who happen to be strolling about on the ice. Generally, to be injured or killed by an animal, a human must place himself, intentionally or not, in a position where he can be attacked. To imply that animals of any type want to attack humans because of a reasoned enmity for people is utter nonsense. There is no malice aforethought, or afterthought, in the animal kingdom. A shark that savages a swimmer is merely acting out an instinctive pattern of behavior triggered by a combination of circumstances, including the fact that the swimmer happened to be in the wrong place (for him) at the wrong time. A venomous fish whose spines penetrate the foot of a beachcomber did not lie there waiting for a careless human to tread upon it. The shark and the venomous fish virtually have no choice but to react as behavior and physiology instructed.

Robert Morris, former curator of the New York Aquarium and a veteran diver, told me of an experience he had a few years ago with sharks that illustrates how an understanding of the nature of a creature can eliminate the hazards of encountering it. He was diving with a group of graduate students from the University of Hawaii, collecting fish off Palmyra Island, a dot of land in the tropical Pacific. Each day when they descended into the water, five to ten sharks gathered nearby. "We respected them and watched them carefully," Morris says, "but did not note any aggressive behavior. One day, however, Morris and two diving companions noticed that one shark had been observing them closely for an hour, and appeared ready to attack. Deciding to return to their boat, they grouped for protection. "No sooner had we grouped together than the grey [shark] came for us," Morris relates. "It swam straight at the three of us. We swam back to back extending our spear guns towards the shark and made it to the boat after several charges by the shark. I am sure that we avoided severe injury by understanding the behavior of the shark and knowing that it was time to exit." Had the shark caught Morris or any of his party alone and unaware, the results might have been tragic.

Animals that most of the time are quite harmless may, under certain conditions, be terribly dangerous. A swordfish or a whale that has been harpooned may ram a boat which otherwise it would have ignored. A bull sea elephant, which ordinarily would scarcely notice a man's approach, becomes a horrendous antagonist if his territorial boundaries are breached during the mating season. The mating season, in fact, makes the males of many species especially alert and bold; at that time they should be avoided. Animals in captivity may act in a fashion entirely out of tune with the way they behave in the wild, and certainly the females of many species will stand and fight when with their young; if alone they would flee.

All of these theoretical considerations make no difference, however, to the person who is being devoured by a shark or is writhing in pain from the stings of a man-of-war. Whatever the reasons for the disaster, the damage has been done. The first line of defense in such situations is of course to avoid them or at least to keep in mind that in the water a human is operating in an essentially alien environment, although if approached intelligently it need not be particularly hazardous. But foolhardiness and carelessness compound the risk, and it usually is the person who grabs the shark by the tail who is bitten.

CHAPTER 1

The Shark: An Ancient Horror

A spectral shark lurks in the backwaters of my consciousness. It is an image that is ill-defined but always there, like a phantom half-hidden in a forgotten corner, ready to reveal itself when the time is appropriate. I do my best to avoid this shadowy creature, for confronting it unnerves me—although I never have been rattled by watching live sharks glide sinuously through the water or by wrestling one of these primitive killers onto the deck as occasionally it has been my job to do. This does not mean that if a real shark attempted to use me as sustenance I would not prefer the imaginary one, but I sincerely wish I could be rid of the phantasmal creature. It seems to intrude upon my thoughts without warning, and if it does so while I am in the water it will drive me ashore, although I seldom admit this to myself.

I know divers and diving biologists who seem to lack any special concern for sharks, even while swimming with them. Wish as I might that I could be like them, I now accept the fact that, with so many of my fellow humans, I have a deeply rooted fear of, and fascination for, sharks. Possibly that fear is rooted in some primal memory of a time when our ancestors shared the water with sharks; we have changed considerably since then, but not the sharks. Sharks survive today by reason of adaptations that serve as well now as they did almost 400 million years ago. Ironically, sharks are quite primitive biologically; yet they are among the world's most efficient, and dangerous, predators—savage, powerful, and sometimes nearly invincible.

The terror inspired by sharks doubtless relates to the fear of being eaten alive, which often happens in shark attacks. From Asia to the Americas, human fear and fascination regarding sharks has engendered a vast body of legend and lore, much of it fanciful but much also true. Various accounts by voyagers of a few centuries ago describe alleged food preferences of sharks for either Caucasians or blacks, Frenchmen or Englishmen, with the sharks' choice generally being a race or nationality other than that of the teller. The shark, it seems, always favors the other fellow as a meal.

Probably the part of the world richest in shark lore is Polynesia. The late Charles Haskins Townsend, who headed the New York Aquarium early in this century, noted that the Polynesians of his day had the same regard for the shark as some of the African tribes had for the lion. Polynesian legends often describe the activities of shark gods, and it is said that the ancient Hawaiians staged gladiatorial bouts between men and sharks penned in shallow water. The Hawaiians made practical use of the shark, too: women wore gloves studded with the razor-sharp teeth of sharks to discourage would-be rapists.

Among the South Seas legends of sharks are those linked to the widespread belief that some people are reincarnated as sharks after death. One story tells of an islander who was attacked by a shark while out in his canoe. The shark jumped into the canoe and the man reached for an axe to attack the fish. Before he could dispatch the shark, however, the man noticed that the fish was regarding him with a highly human gleam in its eye. Fearing that he might be about to axe someone he might have known, the canoest sank his boat and swam for shore while the shark headed in the other direction.

Medieval European accounts tell of sharks whose bellies held men in full armor, a situation whose truth is debatable. A truly odd assortment of junk, however, has turned up inside sharks. The list includes a roll of roofing paper 30 feet long, telephone books, pots and pans, a potable bottle of Madeira, sail canvas, a keg of nails, and a ship's papers.

The discovery of the latter item in a shark sent the captain of an American privateer to the gallows in the 18th century. The American vessel, the brig *Nancy*, was cornered by a British man-of-war in the Caribbean Sea; but before the British caught up with him, the Yankee captain, Thomas Burggs, tossed his ship's papers into the sea. The *Nancy*, with her captain and crew, was taken to Port Royal, Jamaica, where Burggs was placed on trial for his life. The authorities had no hard evidence to convict Burggs of privateering, however, so they prepared to release him. Meanwhile a second British vessel had sailed into port, bringing with it the ship's papers of the *Nancy*. The papers were introduced as evidence, and Burggs was convicted and sentenced to hang. The captain of the second vessel explained that crewmen on his ship had caught a shark off Haiti, opened it up, and found the *Nancy*'s papers in its stomach. The papers were placed in a museum in Kingston, Jamaica.

Legend and lore aside, biologically the shark compels admiration and attention. The living sharks belong to a class of fishes known as Chondrichthyes, the cartilaginous fishes. Taxonomists, who make their living arguing about such things, classify the various sharks, and their pancake relatives the rays, in a variety of subcategories. Some taxonomists put sharks in the subclass Elasmobranchii and the order Selachii, and others describe the subclass as Selachii and the order as Pleurotremata. All this name-changing makes no real difference to anyone but the taxonomists who would be out of work if they had no new

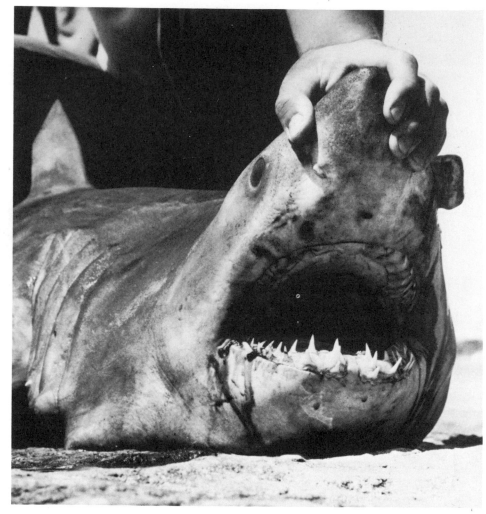

NATIONAL MARINE FISHERIES SERVICE

MAN-KILLER: The jaws of even a young great white shark can easily dispatch a man. Its teeth are triangular—and razor-sharp.

animals to classify or old ones to reclassify. The chief characteristic that sets the sharks and rays aside from the higher fishes is that their skeleton consists of cartilage, without a single true bone. Cartilage allegedly is more primitive than bone, but the cartilaginous skeleton of a shark weighs less than one of bone would and thus is more bouyant, an advantage in the water.

Sharks first arrived on the scene during the Devonian Period, almost 400 million years ago, when fishes were the dominant forms of life on the earth. Vast, shallow seas covered much of the earth, including a great portion of what today are the continents. On the land, primitive plant life was establishing a foothold; during this period, too, the first vertebrates emerged from the water to begin life on land.

No one knows how sharks originated but by 300 million years ago several shark-like fishes sought their prey in the sea. Many of these were encased in complex armor, and most passed from existence before the sharks reached their zenith. Cartilage is a poor raw material for fossils, so ancient sharks generally are represented in fossil deposits only by their teeth or spines. Such relics have been discovered in various parts of the world, with the oldest dated at about 300 million years. From them paleontologists have pieced together a sketchy picture of how some early sharks must have appeared. Some were remarkably like the sharks of today, except for the fact that the mouth opened at the fore part of the snout and was not underslung as in modern sharks. By the time the dinosaurs kicked their last on the land, about 60 million years ago, sharks like those of today prowled the seas.

Among the best fossils of an early shark is one discovered by W.D. White of Omaha, Nebraska, and described by Gerald R. Case, an amateur paleontologist who ranks with the professionals in his expertise on fossil sharks, in the Fall-Winter 1970 issue of the *Underwater Naturalist,* a publication of the American Littoral Society. The fossil, a 22-inch-long specimen, estimated to be 300 million to 325 million years old, was dug from a limestone quarry south of Omaha. It is unusual because it faithfully depicts the outline of the shark's body, which had a prominent dorsal fin of the same triangular shape as that of most sharks today. Another fossil, taken from much younger beds at Calvert Cliffs on the western shore of the Chesapeake Bay, has teeth 5 inches long. Based on the size of the teeth, the jaws must have gaped so wide that a tall man could have stood upright between them. Several indications exist that near the beginning of the age of mammals, some 60 million years ago, huge sharks ranged the sea. Fossil shark teeth half a foot long have been discovered. The size of their owner can be imagined when they are compared with the 3-inch-long teeth of a contemporary 36-foot great white shark whose jaws are on display in the British Museum of Natural History.

Giants and Dwarfs

Generally sharks are large animals, and the whale shark (family Rhinocodontidae), with a length of 60 feet and a weight of 10 tons, is the largest living fish. At the other end of the scale, the midwater shark (*Squaliolus laticaudus*) of the Gulf of Mexico is only 6 inches long when mature.

Sharks inhabit a surprisingly wide variety of aquatic environments, even freshwater lakes and rivers. They cruise the cold, dim abyss more than 12,000 feet deep and range the sun-washed surface waters as well. They penetrate several hundred miles up some of the world's major rivers, and they rove the ocean far from land. Some sharks seek their prey on reefs, others forage on the bottom, and still others pursue fast-swimming schooling fish, such as tuna and bluefish. World citizens, sharks range from the Arctic to the northern margin of the Antarctic. The presence of such a murderous predator on a global scale means that sharks will at times encounter and attack humans. Although only a score or so species of shark have been implicated in direct attacks on man, any large shark is best considered dangerous because of its size if not its predatory nature. That certainly was the attitude taken by the authorities charged with protecting President Richard M. Nixon when fish described as "sand sharks" slipped inside the protective net surrounding the swimming beach at his home in Key Biscayne, Florida. Divers were dispatched into the water to kill the sharks with explosive-tipped harpoons. According to newspaper reports, the construction of a swimming pool at the President's residence may have been linked to a reluctance to bathe in waters containing sharks.

Various groups have at times kept records of shark attacks, although there is no central shark-attack file. The U.S. Navy's Office of Information reported that, according to its data, shark attacks on a global basis had averaged 40 to 50 a year in the five years preceding 1973. "The trend," a Navy spokesman said, "was an average of about one or two attacks more per year during this period," then during the half-decade before.

The nearest approach to a central shark-attack information file was made by the Shark Research Panel of the American Institute of Biological Sciences. The panel expired in 1970 when it was no longer funded by the Office of Naval Research. Formed in 1958, the Shark Research Panel brought together the world's leading authorities on sharks in an attempt to coordinate various shark research programs. The panel conducted a lengthy analysis of shark attacks on a world-wide basis and enabled experts in the field to pool their information, and in some cases their resources. By the time its funding was cut off, the panel appeared to be making major contributions to its field of endeavor.

The panel was only three years old when, in the journal *Science*, a team of panel members published a significant analysis of 790 shark attacks from the year 1580 to December 31, 1960. The researchers concluded that of the total, 599 attacks

25

were unprovoked, 42 were provoked, and 30 followed air or sea disasters. Fifty-three of the attacks may not have involved sharks, and 76 involved assaults on boats rather than on persons.

Varieties of Attack

Most shark attacks on boats involve a creature which, without exaggeration, merits being called a monster of the sea. It is the great white shark (*Carcharodon charcharias*), of all sharks the only species known universally by the name man-eater. This it undeniably deserves. Some of the most harrowing encounters between the great white shark and men in boats have occured in Canadian waters and have been described in the journal *Copeia*. Among the worst was an attack on a 14-foot dory carrying two men in the waters off Cape Breton Island, Nova Scotia, on July 9, 1953. A large fish smashed into the dory, punching a hole 8 inches in diameter in the bottom of the boat. Both occupants were dumped into the water, and one drowned. On the basis of a tooth imbedded in the wood of the boat's hull, William C. Schroeder, of the Museum of Comparative Zoology at Harvard University and the Woods Hole Oceanographic Institution, identified the fish as a great white shark. Based on the size of the tooth, the shark must have been about a dozen feet long.

The chances of being attacked and killed by a shark approximate those of being struck and killed by lightning. Just as one would not go about in a thunderstorm holding a lightning rod, it is unwise to act in a fashion that attracts sharks when in waters where they may be lurking. Sharks attack a human when he triggers the appropriate patterns of feeding behavior in the fish. Of course, someone who has been dumped into a sea full of sharks may have little control over whether or not he elicits a predatory response from the hungry beasts, but many people invite shark attack when there is no need to—by trailing a string of speared fish while skin diving, for example.

Too often over-confident divers minimize the hazards from smaller sharks. Even a shark 3 or 4 feet long is tremendously powerful and potentially dangerous. I have had occasion to hold living sharks of this size while a researcher took blood samples from them. Even though I had a firm grip on the shark's gill openings—I wore gloves—it was difficult to prevent even a 3-footer from breaking loose and using its gaping jaws.

Shark attacks can occur almost any place where men and sharks share the water. Although incidents seem more prevalent in the seas of the tropics, they are not restricted to regions of warmer water, or even to the ocean. In 1936 a shark capsized a sailboat in Carradale Bay, Scotland, causing the boat's three occupants to drown. Seventeen passengers and crew members of the vessel *Durao* were attacked by sharks when the boat sank in Africa's Zambesi River on July 30, 1910.

Generally, however, most shark attacks occur within a broad belt between latitudes 30 degrees north and 30 degrees south. During the warmest months of the year the attack zone edges slightly beyond its usual boundaries, to southern Canada in the northern hemisphere and into New Zealand waters in the Southern Hemisphere. Within this belt, South Africa and Australia seem to have the most serious shark problem. The head of the New York Aquarium early in this century, Charles Haskins Townsend, writing on sharks in *Animal Kingdom*, magazine of the New York Zoological Society, noted a 1929 report by an Australian zoologist that hardly a summer passed without fatal shark attacks in that nation's waters. Despite continuing efforts to shark-proof the beaches, Australian swimmers still face a relatively high risk of shark attack.

Sharks have been known to upset canoes of the type used

27

by South Sea islanders by grabbing the outriggers in their jaws. Once, a party of 40 islanders in several canoes were overtaken by a squall which capsized one of the craft, pitching its occupants into the sea. Sharks immediately attacked the people in the water and then began to ram the canoes, upsetting every canoe and killing all but two of the party.

Sharks also claimed countless victims during the days of the African slave trade when slavers approached by British naval vessels would rid themselves of evidence by tossing their human cargo overboard. Due to the slavers' practice of jettisoning slaves who died in the stinking holds of their vessels, slave ships were frequently followed by large numbers of sharks.

Man-sized animals constitute a regular part of the diet of many sharks. Ravenous feeders, sharks have even been known to bite hooks baited with their own entrails after they have been gutted and thrown back into the sea. Although many shark attacks involve but one animal, large numbers of sharks sometimes swarm about a source of food, igniting a feeding frenzy which observers say is perhaps the most bloodcurdling sight on earth. Gangs of sharks mob their victim or victims in a literal frenzy of destruction, tearing huge chunks of flesh from prey and even from each other. A shark bitten by another in the midst of a frenzy stands little chance of survival for it will probably be ripped to pieces by its fellows. During a frenzy, sharks churn the water to a bloody froth, leaping high in the air and swirling around and around as they complete the slaughter. Scientists do not understand all the elements that create the feeding frenzy, but undoubtedly reciprocal stimulation among the sharks plays a significant role. When a ship or aircraft goes down at sea, and large numbers of people, some injured, are flailing about in the water, there is real danger that a feeding frenzy will happen.

Even in the absence of a frenzy, attacks by sharks on sur-

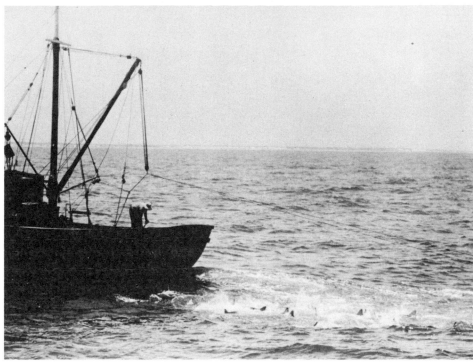

FRENZIED FEEDERS: Blacktip sharks, some 7 feet long, feed on trash dumped from a shrimp boat in waters off Georgia.

vivors of marine disasters are horrible to contemplate. A grisly tale is recounted about a shipwreck in November, 1819, in the Caribbean Sea when sharks picked off survivors one by one as they clung to wreckage in the water. The ship *Una* had struck a rock 60 miles from land, smashing its bow and forcing the crew and 65 black laborers who were on board to abandon ship. The crew took over the lifeboats leaving the blacks to climb on hatches and other pieces of wreckage that floated on the water. The sea, which was quite calm, rapidly filled with sharks, reportedly 8 to 16 feet long. Many of the laborers hanging on to the wreckage fell into the water and into the jaws of the sharks. Little by little, apparently emboldened by the easy pickings, the sharks began to pay more attention to the larger pieces of wreckage which still held men. Before long the men were screaming in terror as the sharks thrust their snouts out of

29

the water and plucked their horrified victims off their make-shift life rafts. The unfortunate laborers tried desperately to hold on as the sharks submarined and rammed the wreckage on which they had taken refuge, but one by one the men slid or tumbled into the water, and perished.

Wartime Tragedies

Disasters at sea, horrifying in themselves, become far more ghastly when sharks enter the picture. The fear of shark attack and especially of the feeding frenzy had a serious effect on morale during World War II, to the extent that the United States Navy published a manual downgrading the shark as a menace to life. The apparent unpredictability of shark attacks, or more properly the lack of understanding as to why they occur, fueled increasing debate as the war progressed.

Often it seemed that sharks possessed an uncanny sense that led them to be seen almost immediately after downed fliers had launched life rafts. Some of the more perceptive airmen noticed, however, that perhaps the sharks were after not the rafts but the schools of little fish that took shelter under them. As the sharks went after the fish, they bumped and joggled the rafts and sometimes leapt into them. During one such incident, a 4-foot shark in pursuit of fish inadvertently hurtled into a raft full of survivors and, as it flailed about, bit one of them. The victim was gashed so severely that he died in a few hours.

A Navy flier downed in the South Pacific fought a three-day battle with sharks that originally had approached his raft to get at the small fish that accompanied it. The sharks did not appear until three days after the flier had ditched his aircraft. Shortly after they closed with the raft, however, the sharks began to bump it with their heads and snouts as they swam below. The flier shot one at point-blank range with his .45 caliber pistol, and the sharks vanished. By nightfall, however, sharks again appeared around the raft and began butting it. The flier shot at more of them but this time they stayed with the raft. The pilot's ordeal climaxed the sixth night after he had left his aircraft, when one shark, 7 feet long, assaulted the raft viciously. As the shark slammed the raft, spinning it about and lifting it from the water, the flier found that his pistol had rusted and would no longer fire. Screaming, the flier hammered the shark with the butt of the pistol, but the fish continued the attack until, in desperation, the pilot dumped the contents of a dye marker on the shark's head. At this, the shark departed.

The unpredictability of sharks was demonstrated when two other Navy airmen were forced into shark waters after their aircraft went down taking their life raft with it. One, a radioman, managed to inflate his life vest and that worn by his companion, the aircraft's pilot, who had been knocked unconscious. For an hour the pair floated in the sea, drifting away from the dye markers they had dumped to show their position to rescuers. Hearing the drone of an aircraft engine, the downed flyers began to kick, yell, and splash to draw attention. The commotion failed to attract the aircraft but instead summoned a pack of sharks, one of which immediately slashed at the radioman's foot. The pilot swam to his comrade to help him stay afloat but even as the two men clung together the shark—or sharks—struck the radioman again, twice jerking both men underwater. The force of the attack wrenched the radioman from the pilot's grasp and the pilot, whose face had been battered by a shark's tail, drifted away from his dying companion. The horrified pilot watched as sharks surged through the water, passing him by to maul the radioman. Time and time again the body of the radioman was jerked about as the fish tore away mouthfuls of flesh. Still the pilot was ignored, except for an occasional bump as a shark passed by his legs, which dangled in the water. The sharks stayed with him for several hours, until he was pulled from the water by the crew of a patrol boat.

More recently, other people have narrowly escaped being eaten by sharks. An amateur scuba diver, exploring off California's Farallon Islands in January 1962, was grabbed by a 14-foot shark as he surfaced. The shark held the right side of the diver in its jaws and shook him like a dog shaking an old towel. The diver smacked the shark on the snout with his spear, and, surprisingly, the shark released him. In August 1962, a 24-year-old man was attacked by a shark as he swam 30 yards off the beach at Manasquan, New Jersey. Pulled from the water by a lifeguard, the victim had 20 toothmarks in one leg. In October of that same year a 35-year-old woman fell from the family cabin cruiser while she and her husband were fishing in Catalina Channel off southern California. She was not as lucky as the swimmers described above. Her husband in the stern of the boat reversed course on finding that his wife was missing—but by then she had vanished. Two hours later, two miles from where she fell overboard, her body was found by the Coast Guard. It had been mutilated by sharks.

Super-Predator

What is the physical nature of the creature responsible for such tragedies? Basically, much of the efficiency of the shark as a predator stems from its primitive simplicity. Its intestine, while short compared with that of many plant-eating fish, has superb digestive powers. The length of an intestine generally determines the amount of surface over which food can be absorbed, with longer intestines absorbing more food. Within the intestine of the shark, however, there is a corkscrew-shaped valve which, because of its spiral design, slows the passage of food and exposes it to many times the absorptive surface that such a short intestine otherwise would provide.

Sharks lack the swim-bladder of most higher fishes. The swim-bladder, a gas bag that has evolved from a portion of the alimentary canal, serves as a hydrostatic organ. When a fish with a swim-bladder descends in the water, the volume of the bladder decreases, increasing the overall density of the fish and decreasing its buoyancy. Conversely, when the fish travels upward, the gas within the bladder expands and gives the fish greater buoyancy. The swim-bladder, therefore, enables a fish to ascend and descend or remain at a given depth while expending less energy that would be required of a fish that lacks this organ.

Although the swim-bladder represents an advantage for the fish that has it, it also causes a problem in that it adjusts only slowly to changes in depth, and therefore prohibits rapid ascent. If a fish with a swim-bladder is caught by net or hook and brought up rapidly from a substantial depth, its swim-bladder may rupture. A fish with a swim-bladder can be likened to a balloon, whose altitude is controlled by the expansion or contraction of gases within it. The shark, on the other hand, is like an airplane; it ascends or descends by its own motive power. Most sharks must swim ceaselessly to stay off the bottom. But the shark has great mobility since it can change its depth quickly without swim-bladder rupture.

The shark swims with powerful sideways sweeps of its tail fin, a motion that tends to thrust the head of the shark downward. This downward tendency is offset by the lift provided by the rigid pectoral fins which also help steer the shark. Some sharks, particularly those that range the open sea in search of fast-moving fish schools are spectacular swimmers. It has been calculated that the mako shark must reach a speed of 22 knots to launch itself from the water in its breathtaking leaps, which it often makes when it takes an angler's hook. For this reason, the mako is increasingly popular as a game fish.

Sharks reproduce by internal fertilization. Males carry a double sexual organ in the form of elongate tubes, or claspers, of considerable size. These penetrate corresponding openings in the cloaca of the female and introduce sperm through a groove in each clasper. The females of many species give birth to live young. Others produce eggs but retain them within the oviduct until they hatch. Some sharks—a minority of species—reproduce by laying eggs which, in most species, are in a tough, membranous egg case.

When a female shark is ready to give birth she moves to a nursery area—usually a region where the water is warm, shallow, and not frequented by other adult sharks. It is believed that females that are giving birth do not feed, an adaptation that prevents them from preying on their own young. After giving birth, the female leaves the nursery for feeding grounds, but the young remain where they first came into the world until they grow to a moderately large size.

The young of at least one species of shark begin their struggle for survival even before they leave the body of their mother. The sand tiger shark (*Odontaspis taurus*), of the Atlantic coast of the United States, begins its life in a pea-size egg, one of about 15 within each of the two uterae of the female. One of the 15 embryos in each uterus develops more rapidly than the others, and shortly eats its siblings and any other eggs that are produced by the female. For almost a year the embryonic sand tiger shark exists on the eggs that the female produces with regularity; if perchance the uterus contains another embryo of approximately the same state of development, the two lilliputian cannibals battle for survival within their mother until one is killed and eaten. Eventually, one young shark emerges from each uterus.

People who literally have had brushes with sharks usually

come away with scrapes and cuts resulting from contact with the shark's rough skin. No wonder, for the skin of the shark is covered not with scales, as in most higher fishes, but with structures called denticles that biologically are akin to teeth.

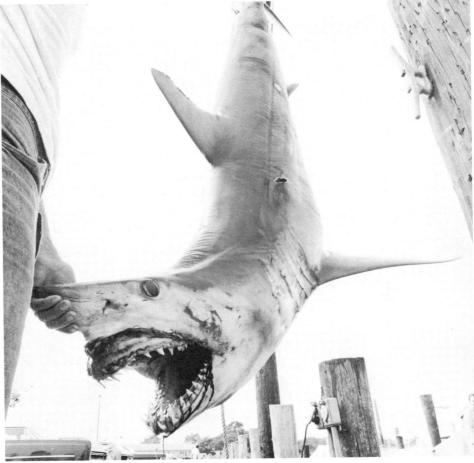

THE TOOTH MACHINE: The cutaway jaws of a mako shark, caught off Montauk Point, New York, reveal several ranks of teeth behind the first set. As the front teeth are lost, those in the rear move forward to replace them.

35

The teeth of the shark, in fact, probably evolved from the denticles, which have a bone-like base and a core of pulp surrounded by dentine, and are coated with enamel.

The shark's teeth, of course, are the part of its anatomy that concern most people. Shark teeth are razor-sharp in most species, and since they are set in jaws that can exert a pressure of several tons per square inch they easily shear through flesh and bone. The shape of a shark's tooth depends on the nature of its owner's diet. Sharks that feed on mollusks have teeth with flat surfaces that are adapted for crushing and grinding shells. Sharks that prey on lobsters and fish of moderate size generally have spike-like teeth that transfix and hold their squirmy prey. Sharks that hunt large animals such as tuna and seals have blade-like teeth, with serrated edges that shear off huge chunks of flesh, much like a carving knife.

The supply of teeth in a shark is almost inexhaustible, and indeed sharks can be described as living tooth factories. Lacking sockets, the teeth fall out easily—but no matter, for they are replaced almost immediately. In the jaws behind the first line of teeth wait row on row of others in various stages of development. Like soldiers replacing the fallen in the front rank lines, teeth from the rear of the jaw move up to fill the position of those that have been lost.

Taxonomical authorities, as so often is the case, differ on how many main groups of sharks exist. They generally recognize four to seven main groups, and, within this context, they debate whether the different groups represent families or suborders. For reasons of simplicity, the categories described here are those used by Paul Budker, the French marine biologist in his 1971 book *The Life of Sharks*.

The so-called typical sharks belong to the suborder Galeiformes, the largest by far of the four major groupings. The other suborders are the Hexanchiformes and Heterodontiformes, extremely primitive and relatively rare creatures, and the Squaliformes, some of which resemble creations out of a bad dream.

Man-Eater: The Great White Shark

The Galeiformes, however, include the true living nightmare, the great white shark. This species caused the worst shark scare in the history of the United States when a series of five attacks terrified the New Jersey shore in 1916. The first victim, a 24-year-old man, was fatally injured off the community of Beach Haven on July 2. Another man died four days later at Spring Lake, 20 miles north of the scene of the first attack. And 20 miles north of Spring Lake, on July 12, a 10-year-old boy was killed by a shark at Matawan Creek, and a man who tried to save him was bitten so badly on the thigh that he also died. Farther down the creek, on the same day, a 12-year-old boy was bitten by a shark on his foot, which had to be amputated. It appeared as if the attacks were the work of a single shark, which was moving slowly north up the New Jersey coast. Entire seaside communities were in a state of near panic, and the authorities launched a massive hunt which resulted in a huge catch of sharks. One, an 8-foot-long great white shark caught off South Amboy two days after the last attack, had human bones and flesh in its stomach. No more attacks occurred after it was caught, and it is believed to have been the shark responsible for the New Jersey scare, which authorities on shark behavior call one of the most remarkable series of attacks ever recorded.

Unquestionably, the great white shark attacks more humans than any other species of shark and is by far the most dangerous of its tribe. Not only is it a bold predator but it grows to huge size, often longer than 20 feet. A great white shark caught in Australian waters measured more than 36 feet in length. Great white sharks also have considerable heft for their length. One specimen which was 16¾ feet long, hooked by a fisherman off Australia in 1959, weighed 2,664 pounds. And a 21-footer caught off Cuba is reported to have weighed more than 7,000 pounds.

Great white sharks are so big that they regularly prey on animals as large as sea otters, tuna, and seals. One 30-foot-long great white shark taken off California had a 100-pound sea lion in its stomach. The larger great white sharks often swallow their prey whole, but with their triangular, saw-edged teeth they can easily bite huge pieces of flesh out of a victim too large to swallow at one gulp.

Inshore visits by the great white shark are not at all unusual, and sometimes this great brute voyages quite far up estuaries. In 1966, a great white shark turned up in Cobequid Bay, an almost landlocked body of water in Nova Scotia. The incident was reported in 1968 by Gerald Case in the magazine *Underwater Naturalist*. The shark, 11 feet 10 inches long, apparently entered the bay through the Bay of Fundy and the Minas Basin, which extends far inland from Fundy itself. Fisherman Aubrey Scott and his cousin, Gerald Scott, discovered the shark entangled in their salmon nets. Lodged in the jaws of the shark was a three-pronged fishing hook manufactured in Oslo, Norway. The shark still lived when it was found by the Scotts, who towed it behind their 22-foot skiff for seven hours until they reached their home port where other fishermen helped them beach it and hang it from a pole.

"Savage" and "aggressive" are the words used by the United States Navy Diving Manual to describe the great white shark. The words fit even immature individuals less than 6 feet long, which have menaced divers.

As with other sharks, however, the great white sometimes shows its back. Donald R. Nelson, a diving biologist from California State College at Long Beach, reported such an encounter in 1969. Dr. Nelson was diving in 40 feet of water off Grassy Key, Florida, when a great white shark, 12 feet long, began to circle him. After swimming around Dr. Nelson the shark headed directly for him, but turned aside about five feet away when the diver shouted and brandished his spear gun. The shark circled and approached again, and once more Dr. Nelson's aggressive moves turned back the beast. The harrowing sequence of events was repeated several more times before the shark turned and swam away.

Besides the great white shark, the Galeiformes include the porbeagle, mako, basking, thresher, nurse, sand tiger, great blue, whale, and hammerhead sharks, as well as about a hundred other species. The oddest of the assortment is the goblin shark (*Mitsukurina owstoni*), which grows up to 14 feet long and bears a long, horn-like projection which extends from its forehead over its snout. Scientists believed the goblin shark long extinct until, in 1898, a specimen was discovered in deep water off Japan. Later, under somewhat unusual circumstances, the range of the goblin shark was found to extend to the Indian Ocean. A telegraph cable strung across the bottom at a depth of 4,500 feet had failed and was hauled to the surface, where it was found that the damage had been caused by thin, spike-like teeth embedded in the coils of wire that sheathed the cable. The teeth were identified as those of the goblin shark.

Sand Tigers, Brown Sharks, and Makos

The Galeiform shark encountered most frequently on the Atlantic coast of the United States is the sand tiger, which seems the very picture of the man-eating shark. It is up to 9 feet long, with awl-shaped teeth and a pointed snout. Nevertheless, the sand tiger has not been found guilty of attacks on man, although close cousins elsewhere in the world have many human lives to their credit. I believe that given the opportunity, however, the sand tiger well might try to sample human flesh, along with the flatfish, bluefish, squid, lobsters, and other wriggly creatures it regularly consumes. The Navy Diving Manual, in fact, rates the sand tiger as dangerous as the feared tiger shark, a proven man-eater.

Sand tigers often are displayed at public aquariums, for they seem relatively adaptable to captivity. Generally they prowl the bottom at a moderate depth in search of food, but occasionally vast packs of sand tigers, sometimes numbering hundreds of animals, have been seen operating in organized fashion as they drive bluefish, corral them, then chop them to shreds.

When not devouring prey, sand tigers seem to be sluggish beasts, but they are extremely powerful. Helping to collect and tag sand tigers during my years with the New York Zoological Society, I found that while they do not fight the line in the tackle-busting manner of the mako, big specimens nevertheless resist relentlessly. The easiest way to collect live sharks—or to catch, tag, and release them—is to fish for them with hook and line. Before the hooks, baited with slabs of fish, are dropped into the sea, perforated plastic bags of chum, chiefly chopped fish intestines, are swished through the water, leaking juices that trail off into the depths. Usually this action brings sharks in minutes although they often remain out of sight, circling around below the boat. This is not the time to fall overboard.

The largest sand tiger I have caught weighed more than 200 pounds and was 8 feet long. Hooked in the murky waters of Delaware Bay, the shark fought with such tenacity that it gave me a lasting impression of the brute strength of its species. The shark first indicated its presence by a slight tug on the line, at which I started to slowly crank at the reel, waiting for a chance to set the hook. The opportunity came as the

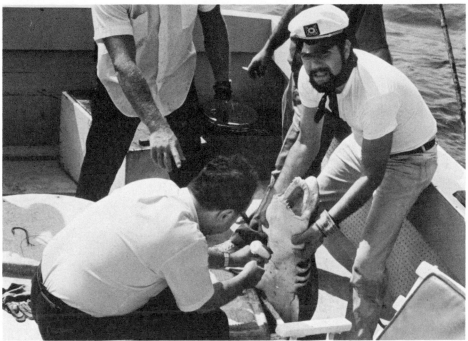

SHARK'S BLOOD: The author holds a live sand tiger shark while a biomedical researcher takes a blood sample for comparative blood studies. The shark was caught in Delaware Bay.

shark tugged again, with a bit more force, and I yanked back hard on the heavy fishing rod, jamming its butt into the socket of the harness that I wore around my back and waist.

Now, in the hot midsummer sun, I engaged in a wearying contest of endurance with the shark, which lay on the bottom and fought my efforts to bring it in with unyielding power. The next day I wrote words in my journal to describe my impressions of the contest: "I had the sensation of brutal, primeval strength, that was somehow insensitive to my efforts. There was little sport, just exhausting work that wrenched and strained almost every muscle in my back and arms." As I set the drag tighter on the line and continued to crank, the shark exerted more pressure against me. After a quarter of an hour of what appeared to be a standoff, suddenly the shark's resistance eased, and soon it was hauled alongside so that a marker tag could be placed behind its dorsal fin with a small harpoon. The tags that are used to trace the movements of fish—much as bands are used to mark and track birds—are contained in small plastic tubes the size of a cigarette. The tube is attached to a pointed pin, which is held in a socket at the end of a hand-held harpoon and slips free of the harpoon when it is inserted into the fish.

Fishermen looking for sand tigers often catch brown sharks (*Carcharhinus milberti*), which are somewhat larger than the sand tiger. Brown sharks cruise Atlantic coastal waters and inhabit the Pacific Ocean and Mediterranean Sea as well. Many East Coast fishermen and divers dismiss the brown shark as harmless, but a tragic incident that occurred off Cuba in 1932 militates against this belief. In January of that year a fishermen reeled in a 12-foot-long brown shark whose stomach contained a fresh human arm and right hand, a patch of blue cloth from a man's coat, and other grisly items which showed that the shark recently had consumed a human meal. The identity of the victim remains speculative, but quite probably an incident that occurred a few days before the shark was caught reveals what actually happened.

Edwin F. Atkins, a wealthy planter, had left Key West for Havana aboard the twin-engine seaplane *Columbus*. With Atkins were his wife and two sons, a nurse, a governess, and Otto Abrahams, a New York banker, along with the aircraft's pilot and mechanic. Twenty miles from Havana, over the ocean, the aircraft developed engine trouble and was ditched at sea near a passing ferryboat. The youngsters were lost in the ditching, but Atkins and the governess, Grace McDonald, scrambled atop one of the aircraft's wings. Meanwhile the ferry, the *H.M. Flagler*, had launched a lifeboat which picked up Mrs. Atkins, the nurse, Abrahams, and the aircraft's crew. As the waves swept over the wing of the aircraft, Atkins and Miss McDonald fought to keep their hold but were swept into the sea and vanished. They were never seen again. Atkins, friends said, had been wearing a coat of blue cloth, similar to the cloth found in the shark. The question was not so much whether the shark had eaten Atkins, but whether he was eaten while still alive. In addition to being highly predacious, sharks are scavengers as well.

The mako shark (*Isurus oxyrinchus*), of nearly world-wide distribution, is highly specialized for a life of active predation. It even chases down small swordfish. It is considered a man-eater and seems prone to attack boats. When hooked it can leap 20 feet into the air, and it tailwalks in the manner of a billfish. Deep blue on its back and white below, the mako is a slim, sharp-snouted creature. It is the basis of a growing sport fishing industry in Rhode Island and on New York State's Montauk Point.

The Montauk shark fishery was featured by the American Broadcasting Company on Dick Cavett's television program in 1971, when I took Cavett, his wife Carrie Nye Cavett, and Percy Heath of the Modern Jazz Quartet on a New York Aquarium shark-tagging expedition. Forty miles east of Montauk, in waters south of Block Island, we hooked three makos, all of which fought viciously, even as they were brought alongside our chartered fishing vessel. The qualities that make a mako a prince of the sea are evident when it is hauled alongside after being caught. The mako lashes its tail, thrashes about powerfully, and, jaws agape, lunges at anyone within reach. In contrast, the sand tiger lies passively in the water, almost as inanimate as a log.

Graceful Killer: The Blue Shark

On that same tagging voyage, Carrie Nye Cavett tagged her first shark, a blue shark, (*Prionace glauca*), 10 feet long, which offered surprisingly little resistance as it was brought alongside. If any shark can be described as beautiful, it is the blue, or great blue as it often is called. Its back is an incredibly deep shade of blue and its belly is snow white. The pectoral fins curve from the slender body like long, graceful sickles; their exceptional length gives the blue shark exceptional mobility and grace in the water. Like the mako, it is a creature of the open sea.

As the blue shark neared our boat, Mrs. Cavett grasped the tagging harpoon, leaned over the port gunwale, and prepared to thrust home the pin attached to the tag. A cameraman stood in the bow, recording the moment. As Mrs. Cavett leaned precariously over the side, I began to fear that the pitching of the boat might send her into the water, and, keeping on my hands and knees to avoid entering the picture, I scuttled across the deck and held her ankles.

My action was filmed, however, and subsequently broadcast, causing a number of associates to inquire about my apparent proclivity for grabbing women by the ankles. I explained that sailors long have feared the blue shark, which, some believe, trails ships in hopes of being on the scene if someone should fall overboard. Although it is debatable whether the blue shark actually can be credited with killing people, the animal certainly is not a desirable companion in the water. It grows to a length of 20 feet and has been involved in several incidents in which boatmen have had to discourage its attention by wielding their oars. One researcher from the Scripps Institution of Oceanography was taking a sample of blood from a blue shark on the deck of a boat when the creature snapped at him, missing his leg but taking a piece of his trousers.

Because of their pelagic habits, blue sharks generally fare poorly in aquariums—but small ones survive if they are given sufficient room, as in so-called shark channels, which are circular canals that enable sharks to swim around and around with-

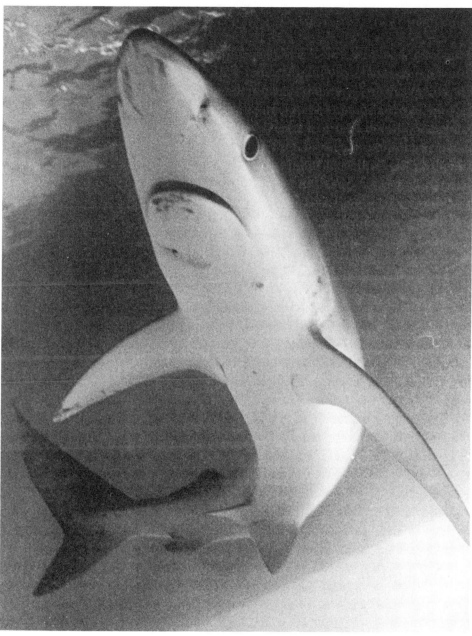

GRACEFUL KILLER: A blue shark over 6 feet long maneuvers with the aid of its long pectoral fins.

out meeting a barrier. A few years ago I accompanied a team of biologists from Marineland of the Pacific as they captured a small blue shark in the water between the California coast and Santa Catalina Island. We boarded the 20-foot collecting boat shortly before noon, when a heavy fog that had hung thickly over the sea cliffs began to dissipate, and motored westward across the channel. As the fog dispersed, we could see a group of pilot whales converging in a small area on the horizon. Two or three at a time, flukes lifted momentarily before they submerged. The whales dove, then reappeared again, apparently feeding on squid somewhere below the surface.

Suddenly, a few hundred feet from the boat, a triangular fin broke the surface of the water. William Walker, then one of curator John Prescott's assistants at Marineland and now curator there, lowered a bag of chum into the waves. As the juices from the bag snaked through the water, the shark—a 6-foot blue—changed course and flashed by the boat. Then, unexplainably, it disappeared. We saw no more sharks until a half hour later, when a second blue shark, about the same size as the first, was sighted cruising on the surface. Again the chum was lowered, and the shark veered toward the baited hooks set out on handlines. Twice the shark flashed under the boat, regarding the bait. The third time, it seized one of the hooks and ran with it. Prescott set the hook and hauled in the hand line, and finally the shark rested in the water alongside the boat. We lowered a canvas stretcher into the water and worked it under the shark, then raised the animal and heaved it into a holding crate on deck. Water, with its life-giving oxygen, was sluiced into the shark's mouth and over its gills through a hose with a fan-shaped nozzle. Less than an hour later, the shark was cruising in the water of Marineland's shark exhibit.

Blue sharks have been studied extensively by scientists of the Narragansett (Rhode Island) Sports Fisheries Marine Laboratory, a federal institution that carries on a long-range pro-

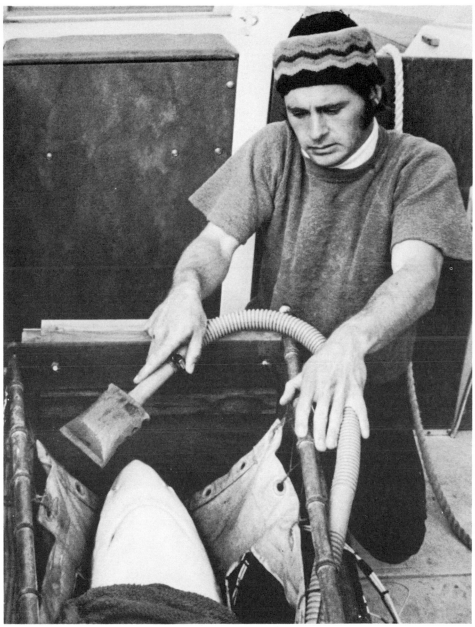

CAPTIVE SHARK: *Robert Poorman of Marineland of the Pacific prepares to insert a nozzle into the jaws of a blue shark we captured in waters south of Los Angeles. The nozzle pumps water over the shark's gills to keep it alive until it arrives at the aquarium's shark pool.*

gram of tagging research. Tags returned to the laboratory indicate that the blue shark is indeed a wanderer. One blue that had been tagged off the Canary Islands was recovered off South America, the first known example of a shark that voyaged across the Atlantic Ocean. Blue sharks tagged in New England waters have been caught 1800 miles to the north, off Labrador, and 2200 miles to the south, off British Guiana.

According to data compiled by the Narragansett laboratory, the age and sex of a blue shark may determine the pattern of its travel. Juveniles and some adult males from New England waters winter in and around the Gulf Stream, while other mature males travel the 2000 miles to wintering grounds off northeastern South America. The females appear to winter at least 700 miles south of their summer range off the New England coast.

The Tiger and Other Requiem Sharks

Blue sharks belong to a family of Galeiformes known as the Requiem sharks. The origin of the name is obscure, but, recalling the name of the religious service for the dead, it tells much about the reputation of the family. Among the Requiem sharks, the most dangerous are the tiger shark (*Galeocerdo cuvieri*), the Galapagos shark (*Carcharhinus galapagensis*), and the bull shark (*Carcharhinus leucas*).

The tiger shark, primarily a warm-water species, grows to a size almost equal to that of the great white shark. Chunky, with a monstrous maw and a blunt snout, the tiger goes after almost any kind of food that comes its way. To appease its hunger it gulps down garbage, dolphins, sea turtles, sea birds, crabs, and even other tiger sharks.

Eugenie Clark of the Cape Haze Marine Laboratory in Placida, Florida, has written in the journal *Copeia* about an 8½-

48

year-old boy who was the victim of a tiger shark in the Gulf of Mexico. He and his 12-year-old brother were swimming less than 10 feet from the shore of Longboat Key, near Sarasota, Florida, while their parents and uncle watched. Suddenly the youngster screamed and went under while the water around him reddened with blood. The adults ran into the water as the boy's brother reached for him and held his head above the surface. The shark, about 5 feet long, had a grip on the boy's left thigh. A desperate struggle began for the boy's life as his uncle held him tightly by the shoulders, trying to drag him from the water, while his father grabbed the shark's tail and tried to wrench it away from the boy. Finally they were successful, and the shark swam off toward deeper water while the rescuers carried the victim to the beach. The shark had bitten his leg three times, shearing off flesh and damaging blood vessels so severely that the leg had to be amputated.

Tiger sharks have been caught off Florida on at least two occasions with human remains in their stomachs, and in Australia they have killed several people. An 18-foot specimen attacked a 28-foot skiff off Palm Beach, Florida, and sent it to the bottom after the shark was struck by an oar; and off Miami, a 14-foot tiger shark punched a foot-wide hole in a small boat.

The Galapagos shark, which congregates in great numbers around certain Pacific islands, acts quite aggressively toward divers. The species was unknown in the Atlantic until April 21, 1963—but then it made its presence known in gory fashion. John Gibson, a U.S. Navy lieutenant, was visiting a beach on St. Thomas in the Virgin Islands with a friend, Donna Waugh. Gibson decided to swim the seven-tenths of a mile across a bay while Miss Waugh walked along the shore. Gibson seemed to be doing well, but suddenly Miss Waugh noticed him thrashing wildly in the water. As he flung his arms about, she saw to her horror that one of his hands was missing. Bravely she plunged into the water and swam to help Gibson who even as he was being attacked urged her to return to shore. She refused and, with the help of other people who ran into the water, dragged Gibson to the beach. Her heroism was in vain, however. Gibson was dead. His right hand and much of his left shoulder had been bitten off, and one leg was so badly gashed that the femoral artery was severed. A hunt was begun, and the next day a 10-foot Galapagos shark was caught in the bay. Its jaws are now on display at La Parguera, Puerto Rico, in the University of Puerto Rico's marine laboratory.

Several species of dangerous Requiem sharks resemble one another so closely that they may be merely geographical variations of a single species, the bull shark. This rugged, pugnacious shark is particularly interesting because it includes true freshwater sharks, some of which inhabit lakes and rivers a considerable distance from the sea. A chunky, slow-moving creature, the bull shark reaches a length of at least 10 feet and a weight of about 500 pounds. It regularly charges divers who come too close to the reefs on which it dwells, and in aquariums it has been known to snap at keepers. It is extremely common in the West Indies and often enters the estuaries of rivers. Included in its diet are other sharks and, at times, humans. However, Stewart Springer, who has conducted shark research for the United States Fish and Wildlife Service and the Mote Marine Laboratory in Sarasota, Florida, notes that he has often waded waist deep in water surrounded by bull sharks without being bothered. Writing in the book *Sharks and Survival*, a collection of papers published under the auspices of the Shark Research Panel, Springer says he even shoved some of the sharks from his path and that they meekly moved away. The sharks he encountered, however, may have been females in a breeding condition, when their feeding behavior is supressed.

Freshwater Sharks

The majority of human deaths from bull sharks have not occurred in the sea but in fresh water. Bull sharks inhabit Lake Nicaragua, for example. When the Spanish first arrived in Nicaragua they discovered that small sharks about 6 feet long lived in the lake, which lies about halfway between the country's Caribbean and Pacific coasts. Since then, the sharks of Lake Nicaragua have gained a reputation as being highly dangerous because of their frequent attacks on people. The prospect of bathing in a lake or river far from the ocean and seeing a shark knifing towards me strikes me as especially harrowing.

Lake Nicaragua and the Caribbean are linked by the San Juan River, which has bull sharks in its estuary. Apparently, however, the lake and river sharks do not mix, although it seems reasonable that the sharks in the lake are descended from individuals who found their way upstream from the sea.

The Zambezi River of Africa also supports a shark population as do certain rivers in Gambia. The Zambezi empties into the Indian Ocean, and Gambia is on Africa's Atlantic coast. In both regions sharks live hundreds of miles upstream. The sharks of Africa's rivers probably are but another race of bull shark. So, too, most likely, are the Ganges sharks of India, which, while small, have killed countless people. Sharks similar to these riverine races have been caught in streams elsewhere in Asia. Oceanic sharks, as well, have been seen in rivers—far up the Amazon, for example; in the Tigris and Euphrates rivers, and in streams of Southeast Asia and Australia. Some scientists suggest that the ability of certain sharks to adapt to either freshwater or marine environments may mean that the ancestry of sharks is rooted in freshwater stock, but this remains only a theory.

51

The Requiem sharks are closely related to the hammerheads, which have a literally expanded head that probably

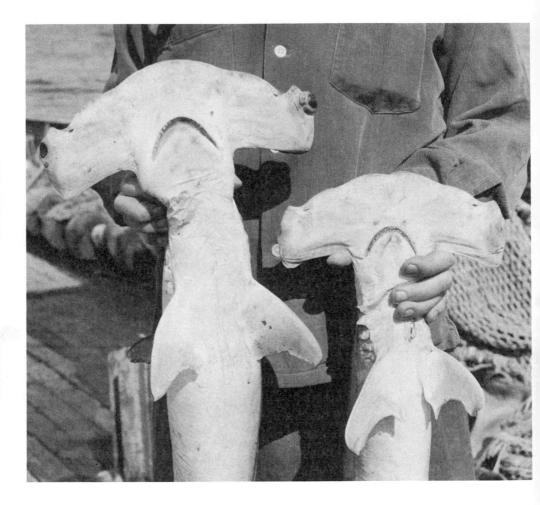

HAMMERHEADS: The hammerhead's eyes are at the end of projections on each side of the head. The evolutionary significance of this is uncertain. These sharks were caught off the North Carolina coast.

52

gives them a more fearful reputation than they deserve. The larger species of hammerheads, more than 14 feet long, have been known to attack people, but only rarely.

Some Galeiformes, on the other hand have such mild reputations they have been treated as pushovers by divers and others who encounter them. Divers often play a game of pull-the-tail with nurse sharks (*Ginglymostoma cirratum*), which long have been regarded as totally harmless—a belief that is dangerously fallacious. The nurse shark is rather flat-bodied and grows to a length of about 12 feet. It feeds on sea urchins, crabs, squid, spiny lobsters, and small fish. Groups of dozens of nurse sharks sometimes concentrate under ledges and in caves, and divers sometimes wander through such assemblages with little more concern than they would in passing through a flock of sheep. However, nurse sharks are not always the placid beasts they appear, and more than once they have mangled people who have bothered them. Theodore Roosevelt III wrote in the March-April, 1973 issue of *Sea Secrets* that he was grabbed on the shoulder by a nurse shark, a foot long, that his wife had picked up and tossed away. As the shark flipped in the air, it fastened its jaws in his flesh, holding on for 20 minutes until it was killed and its jaw ligaments severed.

The Giant Sharks

Ironically, the largest of all sharks, and indeed of all fishes, are inoffensive giants which eat nothing much larger than plankton and even suffer people to clamber over them in the water—although a man could disappear within their huge jaws. The whale shark (*Rhincodon typus*) and the basking shark (*Cetorhinus maximus*), both Galeiformes, have teeth of almost microscopic size, even though the whale shark reaches

60 feet in length and the basking shark is almost as large. On many occasions, divers have climbed aboard these great fish as they basked on the surface of the sea.

The docility of these giant sharks has long been accepted by both seamen and scientists. Icthyologist E.W. Gudger, one of the most prolific writers on fish in the first third of this century, published a lengthy treatise of the whale shark in the March 1915 issue of *Zoologica,* the journal of the New York Zoological Society. The whale shark, he asserted, "has absolutely no offensive habits," and its defensive behavior was "entirely lacking." Gudger declared the animal to be "the mildest mannered shark that swims in the seas."

Gudger had plenty of evidence to support his claims. He knew of several occasions when seamen had routinely harpooned whale sharks and riddled them with bullets, while the sharks had made only a pathetic attempt to escape. Some decades later, the naturalist and explorer William Beebe in *Animal Kingdom* described how his crew aboard the research vessel *Zacca* had attempted to kill a whale shark in the Gulf of California. A harpoon was plunged into the hapless fish, and the explorer then fired two shots from his revolver over the rail of the ship, point-blank into the shark's head. Even though wounded so grievously, the big animal managed to tear loose from the harpoon and escape, leaving Beebe to ponder its strength and tenacity. But no time did the shark attempt to defend itself against its tormentors.

More recent events on the other hand indicate that at least some whale sharks fight back when molested. The late J.L.B. Smith, the South African icthyologist, reported on three sport-fishing boats from Mauritius that had been battered by whale sharks. One shark rammed a 50-foot cabin cruiser in the stern, spinning it completely around. The boat's skipper declined to give battle and sped away.

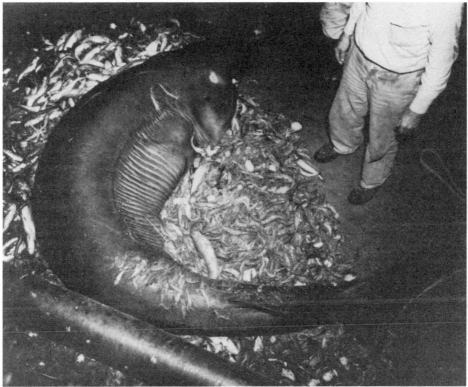

NATIONAL MARINE FISHERIES SERVICE

ANCIENT CREATURE: The cow shark, above, is a primitive Hexanchiforme that reaches 15 feet in length. This 13-foot specimen was caught in the Gulf of Mexico.

The Weird Ones

Few of the non-Galeiform sharks have been thought of as particularly dangerous, although this may be because so many of them are uncommon, or because they live at considerable depths away from humans. Hexanchiformes, for example, are among the most primitive of fishes with a jaw that is attached to the skull more rigidly than in other sharks. An odd-ball member of this group is the weird frilled shark (*Chlamydosela-chus anguineus*), a rare, deep-water creature known to science for only a century. Serpentine in form, about 6 feet long, the

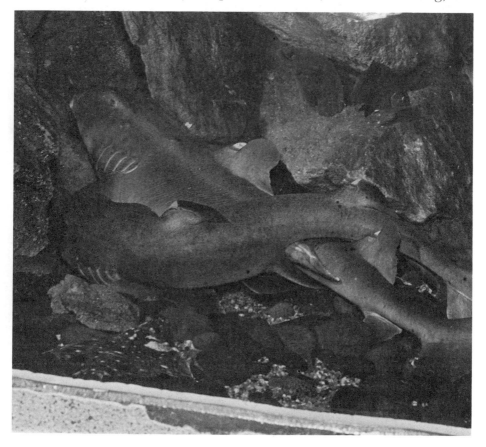

PROPAGATION OF THE SPECIES: Horn sharks mating. Small and not aggressive, horn sharks, nevertheless, should be left alone by divers and swimmers.

frilled shark gets its name from the odd collar formed by its six gill openings. It feeds on octopus and squid, as far as is known.

The suborder Heterodontiform has but one family, the horn or bullhead sharks, so named because of the blunt, heavy head that is characteristic of the group. Small—generally under 5 feet long—these sharks are almost identical to fossils 250 million years old. Their teeth are blunt, but strong enough to crush the shells of the small mollusks and crustaceans which the sharks capture on the sea bottom.

Horn sharks generally are considered harmless but Marineland curator William Walker told me of being attacked by one of them. Walker, at the time 18 years of age, was diving in California waters when he spied a small horn shark, about 2 feet long, swimming along the bottom. Deciding to play with the shark, Walker prodded it with the blunt end of the spear he was carrying to catch halibut. After a few pokes the shark apparently had enough of the game and the little creature turned, swam directly at Walker and attempted to bite the face plate of his diving mask before swimming away.

The Squaliformes include the common dogfish (*Squalus acanthias*), the large and potentially dangerous Greenland shark (*Somniosus microcephalus*), as well as a number of other species that qualify as biological curiosities. A relative of the spiny dogfish known by the scientific name *Centroscymnus coelolepis*, was caught almost 9,000 feet down in the Atlantic, setting a depth record for sharks. The Squaliformes also include the smallest known shark, the midwater shark (*Squalilous laticaudus*), and the odd little saw sharks of the family Pristiophoridae, yard-long creatures whose flat snouts are edged with teeth like those of a comb. The largest of the Squaliformes is the Greenland shark, native to both the Atlantic and Pacific Oceans. It is a 20-foot-long fish which slowly prowls the bottom, eating carrion as well as living prey in large

57

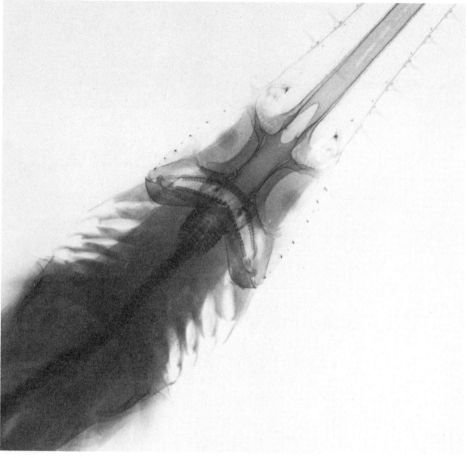

NATIONAL MARINE FISHERIES SERVICE

RARE PHOTO: This unusual X-ray of the head of a saw shark shows how the skull of this strange fish projects forward to give it a beaked appearance.

quantities. Thus far the Greenland shark has not been implicated in attacks on people, but authorities believe that given the chance it might well sample a human meal. Shark attacks seem to be increasing, although slowly, no doubt because more people are venturing into shark waters. If this trend continues, additional species may well be added to the list of sharks known to attack humans.

Solving the Mystery of Shark Attack

Between 50 and 80 percent of shark-attack victims die, according to J.W. Lermond in the U.S. Navy publication, *Science in the Sea*. If he is not consumed alive, the victim usually expires from shock and loss of blood. Scientific investigation of the causes of shark attack may have been hampered by the demise of the Shark Research Panel, but the search for a better way of coping with the problem continues. Marine laboratories and other institutions are conducting studies relating to shark attacks, and the Navy is continuing to support shark-attack research projects.

The core of the problem is to resolve the complex association of factors that produce shark attacks. Certain patterns are evident. The frequency of attacks seems to be greater in waters that are warmer than 65 degrees F. but this may be merely a reflection of the fact that more dangerous sharks inhabit the tropics, and of the disinclination of people to swim in cold water. If more people in northern regions begin taking to the water, the statistics on shark attacks and water temperatures may change.

From the results of a study reported in the journal *Science* it appears that hugging the shore does not protect a person from death at the jaws of a shark. Of 217 shark attacks in which a distance from shore was known, more than half occurred within 200 feet of the beach. In cases where distance from shore was not always known, 75 of 302 attack victims were standing in water no deeper than their shoulders, and 212 victims were struck by sharks in water no more than 5 feet deep.

A person becomes a victim of a shark when he provokes one or when he triggers mechanisms that make the shark go after prey. Built into the shark's being are automatic responses to certain stimuli such as the thrashing about of a wounded or sick fish. Like other animals, sharks make a living in the easiest way possible: if prey can be obtained with little energy expenditure, so much the better for the shark in terms of survival. An injured fish is easy prey, and a human who splashes about erratically may trigger the same response in the shark that a struggling fish does.

Scientists believe that the low-frequency, erratic pulses of sound produced by that sort of movement in the water attracts sharks, which seem able to pick up such vibrations at a range of 600 yards. As vibrations from a struggling fish travel through the water, they can be sensed by the shark through an organ system called the lateral line which the shark has in common with most other fishes. The lateral line consists of a series of mucus-filled canals under the skin along the side of the fish. The canals are open to the water through tiny pores. Vibrations of low frequency, such as those produced by a struggling fish, are transmitted to the canals through the pores. Traveling through the mucus, the vibrations contact tiny hairs which project into the fluid from groups of sensory cells called neuromasts. The vibrations cause the hairs to oscillate, the oscillations trigger a signal from the neuromasts to the brain via the nervous system, and the shark swims off in search of the source of the vibrations. Tests have shown that when one fish approaches another, even while swimming in normal fashion, the nerve cells in the lateral line send a flood of messages through the nervous system.

Another sensory organ in the skin may help the shark find its prey. Pore-like openings on the snout, called the ampullae of Lorenzini, are connected to sacs of mucus and to sensory cells. These openings may help sharks sense the electrical impulses produced by the muscle action of other creatures. The ampullae probably also sense changes in pressure at different depths, and possible temperature changes as well.

Scent plays an important role, too, in helping the shark find its prey. Often called the swimming nose, the shark can sense the barest trace of blood in millions of gallons of water—and no wonder, for two-thirds of its brain consists of cells involved in olfaction. In experiments, sharks with their nostrils plugged have indicated little interest in food; but that may not mean that the shark uses scent to track down its prey. Rather, scent may be merely a signal that sends the shark on its way.

An experiment at the Lerner Marine Laboratory, operated by the American Museum of Natural History on Bimini, in the Bahamas, hints at the role scent plays in shark predation. Homogenized tuna flesh was placed in a corner of a pen housing a lemon shark (*Negaprion brevirostris*). The shark promptly acted as if it sensed a potential meal, but instead of heading for the source of the scent, it swam to another corner of the pen, where the current was strongest, and began to circle. This behavior is not as perplexing as it sounds. Under natural conditions the scent would have drifted with the current, away from its source. By swimming upcurrent, the shark could have come within reach of whatever was producing the scent. Once in the general vicinity of the origin of the scent, the shark might circle until within sight of its prey. Sharks have excellent vision, and the sight of prey might release the final phase of the shark's attack behavior.

The eye of a shark is suited particularly well to the water, for it easily perceives contrast and movement. Because of the high proportion of rods to cones in the retina of its eye, the shark has trouble discriminating between colors and resolving shapes, but that matters little because underwater colors fade and shapes are blurred. The same situation applies to land animals that are active by night, for color means little in the darkness. But an animal's survival may depend on its ability to detect the faint change or the slight movement that may indicate the presence of either prey or predator. Like so many nocturnal animals, the shark has a mirror in the rear of its eye, a layer of cells called the tapetum which reflects light that escapes the retina. In most animals the retina picks up only a portion of the light that strikes it; but if a tapetum is present, light that has escaped bounces back giving the retina a second chance to absorb it. Creatures that possess a tapetum can make the most out of very little light.

Certain actions by people in the water unquestionably increase the chance of attack by sharks. Obviously, the more one acts like an injured fish, the more one invites sharks. Erratic swimming may broadcast vibrations that indicate to the appropriate receptors in a shark that easy pickings await nearby. Juices from a speared fish, or even the flashing of the flanks of fish as they are towed through the water on a string, can draw a shark. In an article in *Underwater Naturalist* of Summer-Fall, 1969, researcher Donald Nelson cautions divers against using shiny air tanks which contrast with the black hue of their wetsuits. The combination may call attention to the diver.

Nelson also reminds divers that the natural response of a shark's legitimate prey is to flee, and if a diver follows this example he further encourages the shark's attack behavior. Nelson writes that he often has discouraged overly inquisitive sharks by waiting until they were about 10 feet away, then shouting and waving his arms. A diver with scuba, fins, and a bubble train may present a somewhat formidable image to a shark. At least one diver in an effort to discourage sharks has carried with him a black umbrella which, when opened, reveals a painted face complete with gaping maw and huge teeth.

The patent absurdity of brandishing an umbrella at a 15-foot man-eater lessens somewhat in the face of the miserable record of most conventional anti-shark devices and procedures. United States Navy life rafts in 1973 still carried World War II "Shark Chaser" as their chief shark deterrent. A brew of copper acetate and black dye, Shark Chaser resulted from experiments carried out by the Navy at the Woods Hole Oceanographic Institution. Faced with a serious morale problem on the part of airmen and sailors because of their fear of shark attacks, the Navy tried various combinations of chemicals to discourage sharks from eating. Some sharks, it was found, seemed to lose their appetite when maleic acid, copper sulfate, and decomposing shark flesh were dumped in the water. Dubbed "Shark Chaser," the concoction was molded into cakes the size of an English muffin and distributed in survival kits. The black dye allegedly hides the potential victim from the shark, and possibly it accomplishes its goal, although it may be more important as a morale booster than a form of concealment. The problem with repellents such as Shark Chaser is that they work only as long as they last in the water in sufficient concentration. A cake of Shark Chaser lasts for less than four hours.

Considerable research on shark repellents has been carried out by H. David Baldridge, Jr., a retired Navy officer now associated with the Mote Marine Laboratory. Writing in the journal *Military Medicine*, in 1969 Dr. Baldridge reviewed attempts to develop a drug that would kill or incapacitate a shark in the water. The problem, he noted, is that such a drug would have to have an immediate effect, especially since a shark moving in for the kill probably would pass quickly through the patch of water containing the drug. The ideal anti-shark drug, Dr. Baldridge noted, would have to act quickly at low concentrations to change the shark's attack pattern before the creature fully committed itself to the pursuit of its prey. Thus far, no drug or other chemical works with complete effectiveness against sharks in the open sea. One of the problems hampering the development of anti-shark chemicals is the lack of facilities for extensive and prolonged experimentation. Because sharks are so difficult to maintain in captivity, few laboratories have the resources to conduct such studies, particularly on the large species that threaten humans.

Promising Prevention

Although the outlook for chemical shark deterrents is bleak, researchers working with the Navy have developed a plastic device that promises to be an effective means of protecting people against sharks. Promoted by the Navy as "a new idea in shark deterrents," it is a man-sized plastic bag that floats in the water by means of an inflatable collar. Called Shark Screen, it is 5 feet long and a yard wide when expanded, but it easily folds into a package small enough to be carried on a life jacket. The collar can be inflated orally in moments. Once the bag is afloat, a person can climb inside and, by pushing the rim of the bag under the surface, fill it with water so that it expands to its full size. The occupant is concealed within the bag, blood from any wounds does not escape into the water, and no arms or legs are left dangling to tempt a hungry shark. From without, the bag floating in the water appears as a solid, bulky, dark-colored object that is calculated not to trigger a shark's predatory behavior.

Shark Screen was developed during the late 1960s under the supervision of Dr. Perry Gilbert, who then was president of the Shark Research Panel, and Dr. A.L. Tester, a panel member. It was subjected to severe testing at the Hawaii Institute of Marine Biology and at various Navy research centers. The sharks used in the tests were starved for several months and kept in an experimental channel. When scientists considered the sharks sufficiently hungry, two prototype Shark

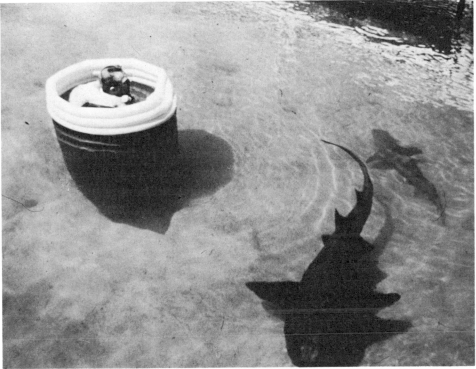

OFFICIAL U.S. NAVY PHOTOGRAPH

SHARK SCREEN: Dr. C. Scott Johnson crouches within the Shark Screen, a plasticized floating bag which he designed to shield its occupant from sharks. In this test, two medium-sized sharks ignore both bag and scientist.

Screens, filled with water, were placed in the middle of the channel. One of the bags, made of fabric, was silvery gray and opaque; the other, made of plastic, was pink and translucent. The sharks, which had been swimming in the middle of the channel, veered away from the bags, avoiding them even when fish and chum dumped into the water triggered a feeding frenzy. Indeed, the sharks often ignored pieces of fish that

65

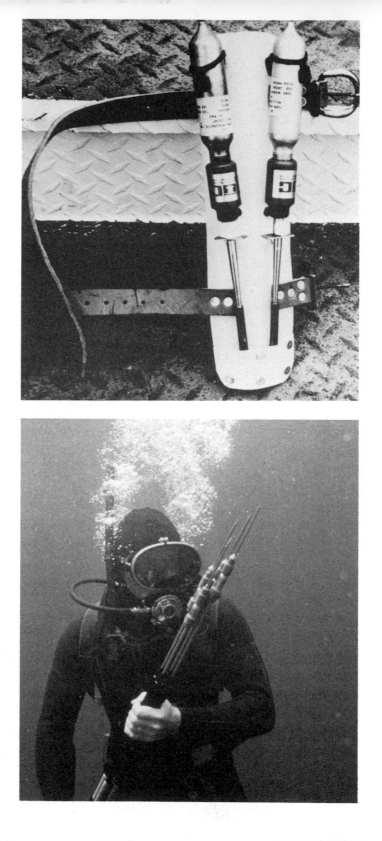

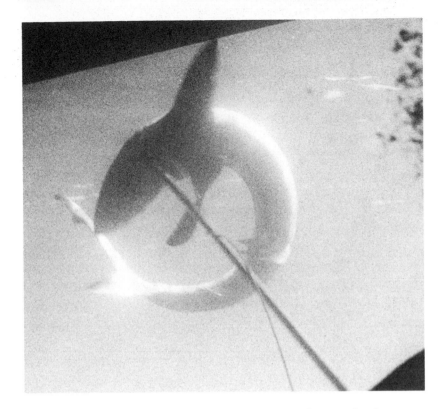

SHARK DART: *Two Shark Darts, personal anti-shark weapons, are shown at the upper left in their sheath. Armed with the darts, a diver sets out after sharks. As a shark comes near, upper right, the diver jabs it with the dart, filling it with compressed gas so that the shark's stomach balloons out, lower right, and it floats to the surface, dying.*

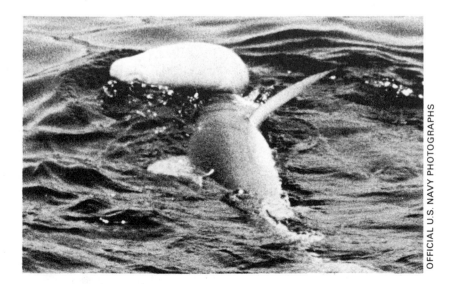

were within a foot of the bags, although one shark rammed a bag once with its snout, and several accidentally rubbed against them.

Later tests in the ocean proved even more promising when several species of dangerous sharks, lured to the vicinity of bags with bait, left the Shark Screens alone. A few sharks inquisitively bumped the bags and bit them on a bottom corner, but did little damage. Eventually, researchers climbed into the bags amidst feeding sharks and were not molested, indicating that Shark Screen works much better than any chemical now in use. In addition, according to the Navy, Shark Screen can serve on land as a pup tent, sleeping bag, lean-to, stretcher, or solar still for making drinking water.

A number of murderous anti-shark weapons for divers are either on the market or in varying stages of development. For a number of years, researchers have been weighing the advantages of hypodermic spears that inject huge doses of poisons such as strychnine into sharks. The most widely used weapon is the powerhead, or "bang stick," a long pole with a chamber at the end that fires a high-caliber bullet or shotgun shell when jammed against a shark. Contact with the shark shoves the cartridge backward against a firing pin. A bang stick can blow a large hole in a shark's body, but to immobilize large sharks it must be applied to the head. It has killed sharks as large as a 14-foot-long, 1,600-pound great white shark. Once the cartridge is expended, however, the diver is weaponless.

Probably the best anti-shark weapon developed thus far is the Navy's "Shark Dart" which has been carried by frogmen since 1971 at the site of Apollo spacecraft splashdowns. The Shark Dart is a hollow steel dart that carries a cartridge of highly compressed carbon dioxide. When the dart, usually mounted on the end of a lance or spear, is plunged into the body of a shark, the cartridge explodes and releases carbon dioxide into the shark's body cavity. The gas balloons the shark toward the surface, leaving the creature floating helplessly with its insides ruptured.

The Navy also has worked on an electric dart in the form of a 10-inch battery-powered spearhead that detaches from the spear shaft after penetrating the flesh and sends a 30-volt current through the shark. The Navy developed the electric dart after preliminary experiments at the Mote Marine Laboratory showed that sharks could be stunned by electric currents. Depending on the size of the shark, the dart either kills the animal or paralyzes it for several minutes. In one test, the dart immobilized a 12-foot-long, 450-pound tiger shark. Unfortunately, the paralysis ceases after the dart's battery-operated power supply expires.

Dolphin vs. Shark

Probably the most imaginative research on shark deterrents has been carried on at the Mote laboratory, where scientists have turned to the dolphin as an ally against the ancient killer. Under contract with the Office of Naval Research, scientists at Mote taught a bottle-nosed dolphin (*Tursiops truncatus*) to attack sharks on command. The dolphin, a 7-foot-long, 450-pound male named Simo, had its pointed snout protected by a rubber cup. At first, when a brown shark of about the same size was put in the tank with Simo, neither creature demonstrated hostility toward the other. But soon Simo was taught to ram a dead 3-foot shark at the command of an electric signal, and he received a reward of fish when he complied. Next, Simo learned to strike a dead 7-foot brown shark that was being towed through the water. Eventually, the dolphin was able to drive a live brown shark, 6 feet long, from the pool. The project raises the possibility that dolphins might be trained as bodyguards for divers and other personnel who work in the water, and they might even be used to guard bathing beaches. It is comforting to think of schools of dolphins, each dolphin with its rubber noseguard, crusing back and forth on patrol along a beach while people swim and surf under their care without fear of sharks. Swimming with dolphins is a marvelous experience at any rate, for these likeable sea mammals will cavort within a few feet of a human swimmer, often

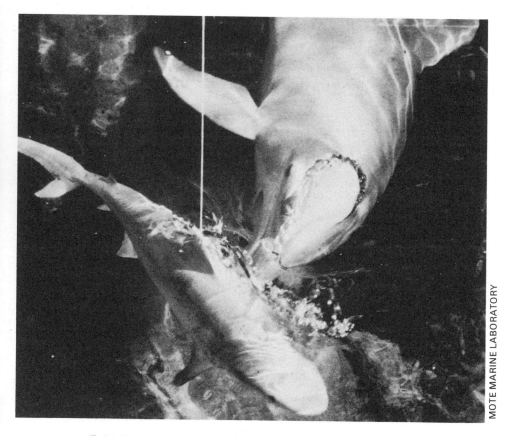

MOTE MARINE LABORATORY

DOLPHIN VS. SHARK: A dolphin trained to attack sharks rams a dead shark towed through a training tank at Mote Marine Laboratory, Sarasota, Florida.

70

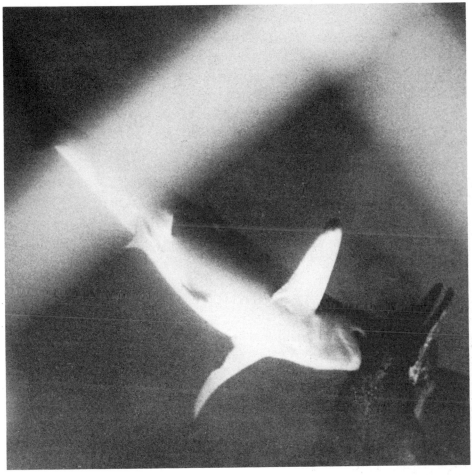

NATIONAL MARINE FISHERIES SERVICE

SHARK VS. DOLPHIN: Contrary to popular belief, sharks will attack dolphins, although the dolphins often fight back successfully. Here a shark rips into a dead porpoise in tests at San Diego Biological Laboratory.

streaking past in the water or surfacing to breathe, but generally staying just out of reach.

Protecting swimmers from sharks remains one of the most serious water-safety problems at beaches where shark attacks are common. At many beaches some years ago, experiments were conducted with curtains of bubbles formed by sending compressed air through a perforated hose lying on the sea bottom. The bubbles were believed capable of discouraging the approach of sharks. However, when Perry Gilbert, now director of the Mote laboratory, exposed tiger sharks to a bubble curtain, the brutes swam back and forth through the bubbles with no concern.

The most effective method of beach protection seems to be meshing, a technique whereby gill nets are arranged in a staggered pattern beyond the breaker line. The purpose is not so much to prevent sharks from approaching the shore as to trap them. Many of the sharks caught in these nets are snagged not when swimming toward the beach, but away from it. Meshing was first used in Sydney, Australia, in 1937, and since then it has proved successful in Australia and South Africa. During 1968, 1,377 sharks were caught off 39 Australian beaches. The first year meshing was attempted, however, 1,500 sharks were netted at one site alone. The reason for the decline may be that large sharks are being fished out of the meshed areas.

Swimmers, divers, and even victims of disasters at sea can reduce the chance of becoming a shark's meal by keeping in mind the adaptations that make the shark such a superb predator. Since the eyes of the shark are adapted for seeing contrast, it does not make sense to wear a black-and-white swim suit or shiny jewelry in waters inhabited by sharks. Since the shark has receptors that pick up vibrations caused by movement in the water, it is foolish to make erratic movements when sharks may be present. And if you are cut and bleeding, and you can get out of the water, there is little percentage in remaining there and inviting a shark to make you its dinner.

CHAPTER 2

A Mixed Bag

When the British troopship *Birkenhead* sank off Africa's Cape of Good Hope February 26, 1852, 480 men lost their lives in the sea. Not all of them died from drowning—many were devoured alive by the killer sharks that homed in on the disaster from every direction. But sharks were not the only fish to feast on human flesh that day. Amidst the shark packs swam a creature resembling a gigantic porgy with a Roman nose, and it, too, participated in the carnage. This fish was the red steenbras (*Petrus rupestris*), which indeed is a cousin of the common porgy although much removed from it in temperament and size.

The red steenbras averages about 25 pounds in weight, but 100-pounders often are landed by South African anglers who bottom-fish for them in deep holes around rocks and reefs. Specimens weighing several hundred pounds have been reported and some have even attacked fishing boats. While the red steenbras cannot be thought of as a habitual man-eater, it must at least be considered potentially very dangerous, as in fact must any large, rapacious predator. Like the red steenbras, there are many inhabitants of the hydrosphere that do not go about seeking human beings to dispatch but nevertheless present a substantial hazard to human life and limb. And, of course, there are aquatic creatures not generally recognized as dangerous, but that quite possibly are so; and there are others that have unsavory reputations, but whose menace is highly debatable.

Is the Bluefish a Man-Killer?

Included among the latter is the bluefish (*Pomatomus salatrix*), whose nickname "chopper" best describes the way this voracious living torpedo chews its way through schools of alewives, mackerel, herring, and menhaden. Bluefish also school and when they feed at the surface, the water seems to boil with their shining form. They careen through the water, slashing and chopping their victims literally to pieces, leaving the froth abob with bits and chunks of fish. Feeding bluefish were the cause of mangled menhaden which floated ashore on New York City beaches one summer and led city officials to speculate that a Soviet trawler somehow was chopping up fish offshore. What really is the normal feeding behavior of bluefish appears to the human eye like a wasteful orgy of destruction. Bluefish pursue their prey even onto the beach, lunging out of the surf after victims that have stranded themselves ashore.

Often after seeing a school of ravenous blues feeding in this manner, fishermen begin the old debate about what would happen to a man who fell overboard into a horde of them. Commonly it is asserted that a person in the water amidst feeding blues would be severely mutilated, if not eaten alive a piece at a time. So reputable a source as *Man and Nature*, a journal published by the Massachusetts Audubon Society, printed an article in December 1972 describing bluefish as "vicious" and noting, without comment, that "It has been suggested that a school of hungry bluefish would skeletonize a swimmer."

No one knows for sure what would happen if a man were engulfed by feeding bluefish, but an examination of the creature and its way of feeding permits a reasonable guess. The bluefish is a moderate-sized fish, averaging about 10 pounds, although the record is more than 30 pounds. It is sleek and swift, with jaws lined with sharp, conical teeth, and it fights powerfully and runs with the line when hooked. Steel leaders often are used in fishing for bluefish of even moderate size. The bluefish has an extensive range, from Australia to Europe and North America, where it lives in vast numbers along the East Coast.

Bluefish travel in tremendous schools, often numbering in the thousands. A school that passed through Narragansett Bay, Rhode Island, in 1901 reportedly extended for four or five miles. When large schools of bluefish feed, they naturally destroy multitudes of other fish, and very often as the blues streak through schools of prey they take only a chunk or two out of each fish. Sometimes blues merely decapitate or remove the tails of prey, and every so often this behavior prompts newspaper accounts of the mysterious beaching of headless or tailless fish. This behavior has encouraged speculation that blues would tear a man to shreds.

The idea that bluefish are highly destructive of other fish has been encouraged by scientific literature. The ichthyological classic, *Fishes of the Gulf of Maine*, by Henry B. Bigelow and William C. Schroeder, describes the bluefish as "perhaps the most ferocious and bloodthirsty fish in the sea, leaving in its wake a trail of dead and mangled mackerel, menhadden, herring, alewives and other species on which it preys." The authors quote reports, which they admit are "wildly exaggerated," that during the 1870s, when bluefish were extremely abundant, "they annually destroyed at least twelve hundred million millions of fish during the summer months off southern New England." In addition, the book perpetuates the belief

77

that bluefish are deliberately wasteful by quoting a 19th-century source that may have done more to spread the notion than any other. That source was George Brown Goode, who, in the final decades of the last century, produced voluminous scientific papers on fish. Most of his work was of signal quality. However, Goode attributed to bluefish an almost purposeful greed, noting that "not content with what they eat, which is of itself enormous quantity, [bluefish] rush ravenously through the closely crowded schools [of prey], cutting and tearing the living fish as they go, and leaving in their wake mangled fragments." This type of language makes the bluefish seem more terrifying than it is in actuality.

Certainly the bluefish attacks its prey voraciously, but so do other predatory fishes. Is it the sheer violence and ferocity of the bluefish's attack that prompts otherwise detached researchers to ascribe a certain ruthlessness and even malice to a creature quite incapable of having such qualities? Perhaps partially—but it should be pointed out, too, that the bluefish was vilified by New England mackerel fishermen whose catches lessened considerably when bluefish were exceptionally abundant during the 1860s and 1870s.

Among the chief detractors was Nathaniel E. Atwood, a Massachusetts mackerel fisherman who had gained recognition as an authority on fishes native to the northeast coast of the United States. As a mackerel fisherman, Atwood certainly had no love for the bluefish—his animosity toward them supposedly surfaced when he was questioned on the habits of the bluefish by a researcher who was preparing a report for the United States Commission on Fish and Fisheries. Atwood is said to have asserted that the bluefish was so gluttonous that once full, it regurgitated like a diner at a Roman orgy, and resumed its bloody repast. The story stuck, but its truth never has been demonstrated scientifically, although the feeding behavior of the bluefish has been studied quite thoroughly.

Perhaps the most significant research on bluefish feeding behavior has been carried on at the Sandy Hook Marine Laboratory of the National Marine Fisheries Service. The Laboratory is located on the great arm of sand that curves north from the New Jersey coast into the waters of the New York Bight. Sandy Hook researchers captured bluefish, released them in an experimental tank at the laboratory, and observed what happened when live killifish were placed in the water with them. The scientists discovered that bluefish capture and consume live prey so rapidly that the manner in which they strike is blurred. To study the furious action of the feeding blues, the researchers were forced to take pictures of them at a speed of 32 frames per second, then analyze the film frame by frame.

The film revealed that the feeding behavior of bluefish consists of several distinct stages. The blues were schooling normally when the killifish were dropped into the tank, but as the smaller fish splashed into the water the school scattered, and the individual bluefish, which had not yet seen the prey, increased their swimming speed. The blues began to sight their prey as they fanned out through the water. Once a blue perceived a killifish, it fixed its eyes upon its intended victim and gave chase, swimming faster and faster until the killifish was about a foot away. With the prey at that distance, the bluefish dropped its lower jaw, arched its head, and with gill covers flaring out to each side snapped up the prey. In that furious instant, even as the killifish disappeared down its maw, the blue veered sharply aside and resumed its original course.

After the bluefish had swept the water clean of killifish, they gathered about the place where they first had sighted the prey. If the researchers did not introduce new killifish, the bluefish moved off, swimming randomly about the tank as if looking for more victims.

The experiments at Sandy Hook also revealed a direct relationship between hunger and the attitude of bluefish toward prey of greater size. Bluefish that had appeared satiated after a half hour of gobbling up small killifish resumed feeding vigorously when larger killifish were dumped into the tank. These experiments indicate that bluefish have excellent vision and can discriminate readily the size of potential prey. Dr. Bori L. Olla, of the Sandy Hook laboratory staff, notes that bluefish, unlike many other fishes, seldom err about what they swallow. Sharks and cod often swallow inedible objects, such as rocks and chunks of wood. Bluefish feed on small fish and squid. Nothing in the repertoire of bluefish feeding behavior includes a predatory response to a creature as large as a man, and in fact the presence of a man in the water might send blues fleeing, for the sand tiger shark, which preys the bluefish, is about the size of a man. Despite these reassurances, a person who trails his hand in the water near feeding blues, risks having it mangled. As experienced chopper fishermen know, the jaws of a boated blue are to be avoided at all costs.

Barracuda: Deadly Results of Mistaken Identity

Like the bluefish, the barracuda depends largely on vision to find its prey. However, the barracuda sometimes errs with respect to the nature of its prey, and such cases of mistaken identity have, on occasion, been fatal to people. Of some three dozen known attacks on people by barracudas, most of them appear to have happened because the fish mistook some object worn by the victim, or a part of the victim, for smaller prey.

When speaking of attacks on humans by barracudas, one is talking about the great barracuda (*Sphyraena barracuda*), the largest of 20 species which inhabit tropical and subtropical waters around the globe. The great barracuda, at maximum size 6 feet long and weighing about 100 pounds, looks much like a huge pike, with long, jutting jaws armed with thin,

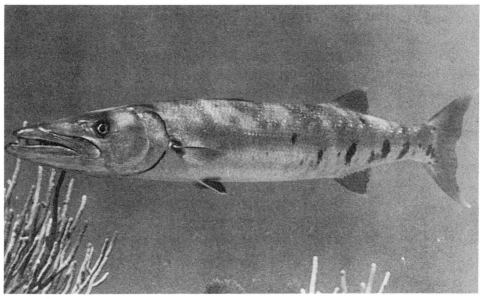

NATIONAL MARINE FISHERIES SERVICE, DR. WILLIAM H. LONGLEY

SLEEK HUNTER: The great barracuda hunts largely by sight, rocketing after its prey in a single swift charge. The great barracuda is blamed for several human fatalities.

double-edged teeth. So slim that it is almost impossible to see head-on, the barracuda has the nerve-racking habit of disappearing, appearing once again, then disappearing in a brief flash of silver.

The barracuda has a particularly villainous reputation. Lermond, in *Science in the Sea,* a U.S. Navy Publication, refers to it as "extremely pugnacious and dangerous," and L.L. Mowbray, a respected authority on fish, wrote in the November 1922 *Bulletin of the New York Zoological Society* that the barracuda is "without question the most aggressive and voracious of marine fishes." Dr. Mowbray also reported that hundreds of barracuda often swarm to attack large, compact schools of smaller fish.

81

Barracudas swallow smaller prey whole and slash larger victims to pieces, then pick up the pieces one at a time. The terrible wound left by the slashing attack of a barracuda leaves two straight rows of toothmarks, nearly parallel, rather than the U-shaped mark caused by the bite of a shark. Young barracuda often swim in schools, but larger specimens hunt alone unless their prey are massed in unusually large numbers.

The barracuda's bad name goes back to the early exploration of the New World. In 1665 Lord de Rochefort, in his *Natural History of the Antilles*, wrote that "Among the monsters greedy and desirious of human flesh found on the coasts of these islands, the Becune (West Indian name for the barracuda) is one of the most formidable. . . . When it has seen its prey it launches itself in fury, like a bloodthirsty dog, at the men it has seen in the water."

Like sharks, barracudas have been endowed in legends with a preference for the flesh of certain races and nationalities. Englishmen in the West Indies during the 1700s reported that the barracuda preferred blacks, horses, and dogs to Caucasians, while Frenchmen asserted that if the barracuda could find no black, it would consume a Briton, and only in extreme hunger would take a native of France. One story of uncertain origin declared that if a Frenchman and an Englishman were in the water together, a barracuda would sample the Englishman first because his beefy diet produced an emanation pleasing to the carnivorous beast.

J.R. Norman and F.C. Fraser of the British Museum of Natural History in the book *Giant Fishes, Whales and Dolphins*, wrote that the "barracuda will not hesitate to attack bathers" and that it is "among the most formidable of the bony fishes in the sea." Norman's classic book *A History of Fishes*, written in 1931 and revised by P.H. Greenwood in 1963, describes the barracuda as "not only extremely ferocious, but also utterly fearless."

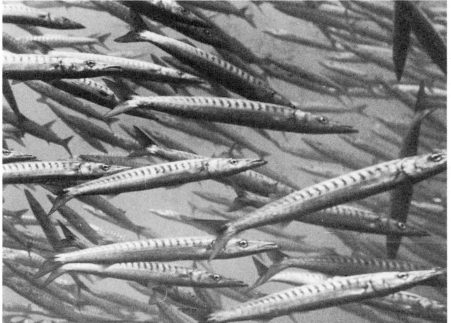

RCN CHURCH, PHOTO RESEARCHERS, INC.

NOT SO DANGEROUS: A large school of smaller barracuda swim in the Pacific Ocean. When in schools, barracuda of small size tend to stay away from humans.

The first officially recorded attack by a barracuda on a human occurred in 1873, off the Indian Ocean island Mauritius, home of the extinct dodo. Another attack, particularly well-publicized, took place in 1922 when a young woman, swimming in Florida waters, was slashed by a barracuda and bled to death. Fatalities also resulted from barracuda assaults in 1947 off St. Augustine, Florida, and in 1952 and 1958 off Key West. The *Miami Herald* reported in July 1956 that a 38-year-old woman was bitten on both legs by a barracuda in the surf along Miami Beach.

Most barracuda attacks on humans seem to occur when the fish's vision is impaired by murky water. Unlike sharks,

83

which often hit a victim again and again, the barracuda seldom makes more than one pass—for that is the way it kills and eats fish: in a single pass, requiring but a few moments of concentrated savagery. In clear water, people usually arouse little more than the barracuda's curiosity. That fact, together with the fact that barracudas strike a person the same way they strike small fish, suggests strongly that the barracuda does not really prey upon man. The real danger of a barracuda's attack is not that the human victim will be eaten alive, but that he will bleed to death or drown in the aftermath of the assault.

Because they hunt by sight, barracudas tend to make passes at flashing objects such as chrome or steel wrist watches or bracelets. The vibrations caused by a fish writhing on a spear also seems to attract them. In 1963 Donald P. DeSylva, of the University of Miami Institute of Marine Sciences, published a careful analysis of barracuda attacks. He reported that he triggered attack behavior in barracudas by spearing small fish and allowing them to wriggle after they were impaled. Yet, DeSylva reported, he often encountered barracuda up to 5 feet long while diving in the Bahamas and the Florida Keys and never was attacked.

Nixon Griffis, the accomplished diver who has served as president of the American Littoral Society, says that solitary sleeping barracudas tend to be nasty when awakened, but that he never has been troubled by barracudas in schools. Barracudas that I have encountered while diving in the Bahamas and Puerto Rico, always in clear water, acted in no way threatening. Countless tourists have bathed in the waters fronting some of San Juan's posh resort hotels while small baracudas swam unseen among them. When approached by a diver, barracudas only 2 or 3 feet long seem fearless, holding their ground, but they seldom act aggressively. I often allow my daughters, both less than 10 years old, to swim among barracudas of 2-foot length.

During my dive to the Hydro-Lab underseas habitat off Freeport, Grand Bahama, a large barracuda, approximately 5 feet long, for a time took up a station over the chamber. Barracudas often lie about the shelter offered by reefs, buoys and rocks, and this particular fish apparently found the vicinity of Hydro-Lab to its liking. While diving to Hydro-Lab, I kept an eye on the resident barracuda, but it hardly seemed to notice me. Robert Wicklund, Hydro-Lab project manager, told me that the creature had displayed no inclination to bother anyone. It should be remembered, however, that the water around Hydro-Lab is extremely clear, often having 100-foot visibility.

All factors considered, barracudas pose little danger when they can distinguish humans from their regular prey. But in murky water the spangle of a bracelet or the sudden movement of a hand or foot, particularly of a light-skinned person, can send a barracuda hurtling toward the object on what could be a deadly errand.

Man and Moray

The moray eel inflicts a wound similar to that of the barracuda, but instead of streaking away after its attack, the moray holds on like a bulldog. Moray eels are the subjects of colorful horror stories—Julius Caesar allegedly tossed recalcitrant slaves into a watery pit full of morays—but generally they do not bite humans unless provoked. I have flippered through the water side by side with morays 6 feet long and as thick as a man's leg, and they paid me no attention. Once while diving in Puerto Rico I aroused a small spotted moray (*Gymnothroax moringa*) from its haven beneath a rock pile. The creature made a slight pass at my hand. Instead of retreating, as I should have, I hacked at it with the knife I had been

85

using to turn over small rocks. I need not have injured the eel, for I could have backed away without danger. There was no reason for my behavior—it was one of those mean little acts against animals that most people perform at one time or another. Although there is little in a moray eel to evoke human compassion, I always have been ashamed of my treatment of that particular creature.

About 20 species of moray eels exist, most of them in tropical and subtropical seas, although a few range north into European waters. Undeniably savage, morays of some species are 8 feet or more long and weigh 100 pounds. During the day, they lurk in crevices in rocks or coral, typically with their blunt heads poking out and turning this way and that. By night the morays squirm out of their hiding places to hunt for fish and an occasional octopus, which they rip to pieces with their long teeth. There is nothing pleasant about the way the moray seizes its prey. Two morays in a Bermuda public aquarium once lunged for the same piece of fish. One of the eels missed its target and instead crushed the head of the other.

Researchers at the Bermuda Biological Station have subjected morays to extensive testing to learn the roles of their various senses in feeding. The results of the study, published in 1959 in the journal *Copeia*, indicate that the moray smells its prey some distance away. Even in daylight, when they seldom venture forth from their crevices, morays have been drawn into the open by the smell of rotten fish. As part of the experiment, the scientists blinded a number of morays and placed them in tanks provided with rockpiles that offered shelter. When the scientists crushed anchovies and allowed their juices to drift through the water, the blinded eels cruised about, searching for the source of the odors.

A telling test of the role of the moray's sense of smell came when two batches of anchovy bits, one batch coated with

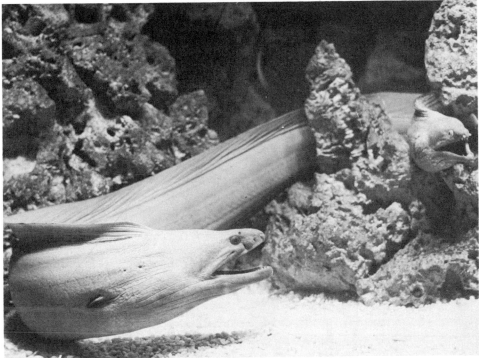

MIAMI SEAQUARIUM

TWO-HEADED MONSTER: Two moray eels, both snaking out of the same crevice, give the appearance of a two-headed beast in the Miami Seaquarium.

paraffin and the other untreated, were dropped into the tank with the eels. Emerging from their hiding places, the morays prowled about the tank until they came upon the pieces of fish. On finding a piece, an eel would nose it with its snout in exploratory fashion. Uncoated pieces were eaten after being touched, but the eels rejected coated pieces even after mouthing them—with one exception, when the sharp teeth of one eel peeled back the coating and exposed the fish. The experiment indicates that once the moray's predatory behavior is triggered by smell, the eel searches until it touches food with its snout,

87

then tastes it briefly before deciding whether it is a suitable meal.

Morays snap up tidbits of carrion and whole small fish in a very neat fashion, but the manner in which they dispatch an octopus—a favorite prey—is horrendously untidy. If it can, an octopus in danger of becoming a moray's next meal will hide in any handy crevice. But often the octopus's haven becomes its coffin, for the moray can insinuate its head into most niches large enough to shelter an octopus. Then all the eel needs to do is seize an arm or any other piece of the octopus in its jaws and spin around forcefully until the hunk of meat is detached. Thus, a piece at a time, the moray eats the octopus.

Small octopuses sometimes try to avoid being consumed by grasping the body of the moray with their arms. The moray sheds the octopus by tying its tail into a knot and slipping its muscular body headfirst through the loop of the knot, dislodging the octopus in the process. Early in this century Walter H. Chute of the Boston Aquarium observed a moray performing a similar contortion as it consumed small bluefish. "Snapper" blues, a few inches long, had been placed in water with a 3-foot-long moray. The eel quickly seized one of the fish by the head, then knotted its own tail into a loop and passed the loop over its head and down the body of the fish, flattening the spines on the fish's dorsal fins. In another example of the eel's ability to tie itself into knots, a moray that had been landed on the deck of a ship supposedly knotted its tail, squeezed its body through the knot, and forced up its last meal—presumably so it could move with enough agility to escape.

An attack by a moray on a person almost always is preceded by the poking of a hand, foot, or other part of the anatomy into a moray's refuge, or by an assault on the moray itself. John E. Randall, a marine biologist at the University of Hawaii and the Bishop Museum in Honolulu, recounted in *Australian Natural History* of June, 1969, several instances in which morays bit people, including four times that he was the victim. Once, as Dr. Randall grasped a reef flat to keep from being tumbled by a wave off the Hawaiian Island of Kauai, he was bitten on the tip of a finger he had thrust into a small hole. Another time, when he placed his hand over the mouth of a cannon in a wreck off northwestern Puerto Rico, a purple moray (*Gymnothorax vicinus*) residing within slashed his index finger. Once again, an eel nipped his heel as he walked on a reef flat, and yet another time a moray that Dr. Randall had just speared bit his knuckle. The eels that attacked Dr. Randall were relatively small and his wounds were not severe, but large morays can seriously mutilate the people they hit.

An especially ugly attack on a diver by a moray eel in 1948 has been recounted so many times that it has become a classic of marine biology. The victim was Vernon E. Brock, who later became director of the Hawaii Institute of Marine Biology of the University of Hawaii. While diving in about 20 feet of water at Johnston Island in the Pacific, Dr. Brock spotted a large moray, which he thought had been killed by rotenone, which had been dumped into the water as part of the study in which Dr. Brock was engaged. He speared the moray, which was about 8 feet long, and the eel, not dead but very much alive, slithered down the spear toward Dr. Brock. The diver quickly dropped the spear and fled, with the monstrous eel pursuing him. The eel soon closed with Dr. Brock and attacked his head. Dr. Brock warded off the attack with his arm, but was bitten badly on the elbow before he escaped to a nearby boat. A surgeon later worked for more than two hours to repair the damage.

Piranha Facts and Fiction

Among fish that men fear, none—with the exception of

the shark—is so vilified as a small resident of South American rivers that is a close cousin of the neon tetra, the silver dollar, and several other small home-aquarium favorites. This fish is the piranha, so often depicted as skeletonizing hapless victims, not uncommonly at the bidding of some arch-fiend or mob chieftain. Mention of the piranha brings to mind stories of jungle tribesmen tying victims to stakes waist-deep in the water, whereupon the killer fish gather and strip them of flesh from the hips down; and of unfortunates who fall overboard from canoes and almost instantly disappear in a welter of foam and blood, the water aboil with crimsoned fish.

Not all such highly colorful accounts originate with creators of horror tales. In November 1916, G. Inness Hartley of the New York Zoological Society's Tropical Research Station wrote in the society's bulletin that "Once blood begins to stain the water [piranhas] become a hoard of blood-crazy demons." Hartley wrote of the piranha when few scientists had penetrated the jungle rivers that the fish inhabits, and probably he relied considerably on second-hand information when he reported that in some rivers swarms of piranhas destroy every living thing they encounter. Hartlet also cites descriptions by "Col. Roosevelt" of how members of the party with which he explored the Amazon were bitten by piranhas. Indeed, Theodore Roosevelt apparently did little to discourage wild tales about the creatures.

Piranhas inhabit rivers in an area that encompasses about 4 million square miles of South America, from the eastern border of the Andes to the Atlantic coast, and south to the northern portions of Argentina, Paraguay and Uruguay. Within this vast area, much of it still relatively unexplored, live more than 20 species of piranha. Most of them are harmless, and they range in length from a few inches to a foot and a half. The black piranha (*Serrasalmus rhombeus*), the largest of the tribe, and three other members of its genus are the only species

90

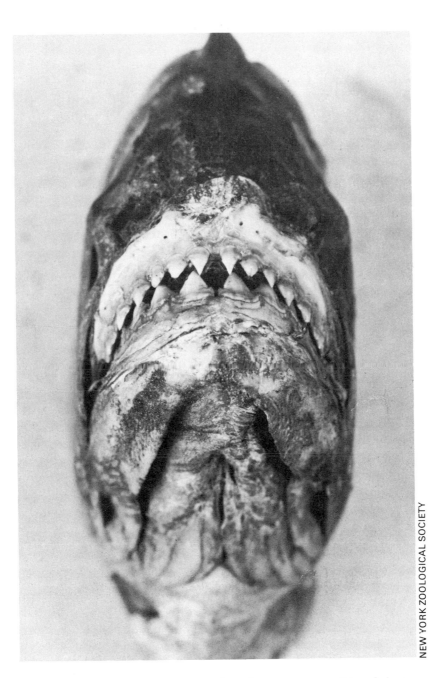

TERROR OF THE RIVER: *With its lips cut away, this adult piranha exhibits the wicked teeth it uses to slice chunks of flesh out of its victims. The piranha lives in the fresh waters of South America.*

that truly threaten man. Unquestionably if enough of these fish converge on a man-sized animal they can skeletonize it; but, although there are plenty of authenticated instances of piranhas biting people, no verified fatalities have been attributed to them.

The very name *piranha*, however, has a menacing connotation. Taken from one of the South American Indian dialects, it means "tooth fish." The name suits the fish, for the most apparent thing about a piranha is its wicked mouthful of teeth, which are readily visible because of the creature's underslung jaw. Driven by powerful jaw muscles, the teeth of a piranha can remove a dollop of flesh with a slice as clean as that of a scalpel. Piranhas do not seize and tear flesh when they bite but rather remove it with surgical neatness. Even creatures with relatively thick hides are vulnerable to the razor-like teeth. Christopher W. Coates, for many years director of the New York Aquarium, reported that piranhas once bit steel tweezers so hard that the steel bore the nicks of their toothmarks.

Normally, adult piranhas do not concentrate in large schools in their native waters. Researchers have swept nets through streams inhabited by piranhas and have caught very few fish, even though the creatures were common there. This may be because when they are not feeding piranhas maintain a rigid system of spacing between individuals. When piranhas were bred at the New York Aquarium, hundreds of inch-long young were packed into holding tanks, and each fish maintained a distance of 4 to 6 inches from its nearest neighbor. At feeding time they converged like pint-sized demons on pieces of shrimp and fish, tolerating the closeness of their fellows—but at any other time, a youngster that violated the personal space of another would be attacked and chased. And when a tank became over-crowded, the young piranhas would turn on one another.

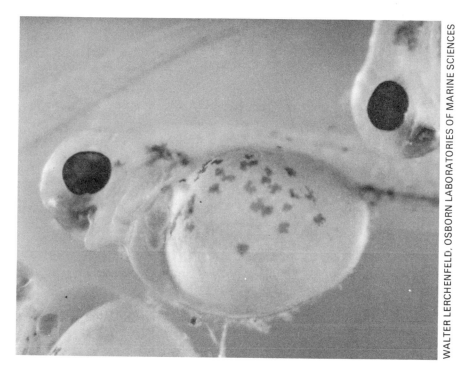

YOUNG CANNIBAL: *This highly magnified photograph of a larval piranha, shows the tiny creature shortly after hatching. A swollen yolk sac still is attached to the larva, which bears little resemblance to the fish in its adult form.*

Piranhas are highly cannibalistic. They will even eat a member of their own school that has been caught on a hook. I have watched young piranhas slice away bits of one another's fins as they crowded about pieces of fish or shrimp. Piranhas belong to the family of characins, and with others of the family —even many of the small species kept in home aquariums— they share the inclination to nibble at objects in the water. Often when I have been tending my home aquarium, the characins among its inhabitants have nipped innocuously at my hand while it was in the water. This tendency reaches its highest pitch among the piranhas, and very probably their furious feeding merely is an exaggerated form of such nibbling behavior.

An assault by a school of piranhas is a gruesome sight. As the water boils with movement, the piranhas' prey disappears among the thrashing fish. Hartley tells of birds falling into the water after being shot by hunters, and being devoured on the spot by piranhas. A motion-picture crew once filmed a school of piranhas as they cleaned the flesh from a 400-pound hog, which had been shot and lowered bleeding into the water. Within minutes it was a skeleton. Paul A. Zahl, senior natural scientist of the National Geographic Society, describes in the November, 1970, *National Geographic* how a dead monkey was lowered into a school of piranhas on a rope. After five mintes, the rope was pulled from the water with only bones attached at its end. Dr. Zahl also describes how piranhas devoured the carcass of a young caiman by eating through its soft underbelly, flopping about within the reptile, and then chewing their way out. Yet, Dr. Zahl declares, people often swim and bathe in water inhabited by piranhas without attracting the little killer fish.

Scientists are unsure what stimuli signal to piranhas that prey is available. Possibly the presence of blood in the water activates their mass feeding behavior, or possibly a specific type of motion on the part of the prey provides the impetus. It also has been suggested that a change in water level or temperature, or some sort of internal clock, determines whether a swarm of piranhas will start to feed.

Although there is not a single documented human fatality caused by piranhas, many people have felt the bite of the razor-sharp teeth of these fish. In May 1920, explorer A. Ha-

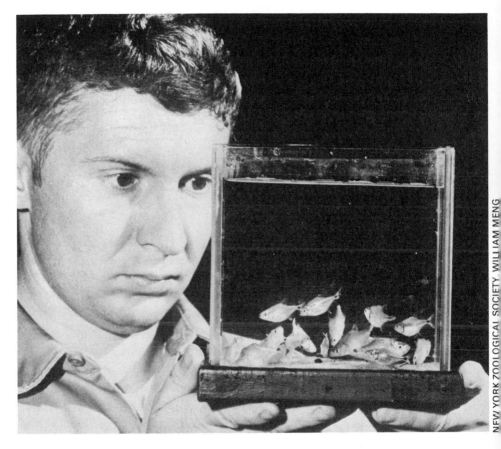

YOUNG ADULTS: Werner Schreiner of New York Aquarium checks on infant piranhas he raised there. They have assumed adult form, but are still small.

milton Rice of New York City reported that a 10-year-old boy, who had been standing knee-deep in a stream, had his penis amputated at the base by a piranha that jumped from the water and in a single slash removed the member. A 16-year-old youth was badly bitten on the thigh by a piranha in the Riacho

95

dos Cavalos Dam of Brazil's Paraiba State.

The Brazilian government waged a campaign of extermination against the piranha in the 1960s because of their supposed damage to livestock. Vast stretches of piranha waters were poisoned. The United States has placed tight controls on the importation of piranhas, which for several decades were a fad of sorts among certain home aquarium buffs. More than one tavern owner has catered to the more perverse appetites of his customers by keeping piranhas in an aquarium near his bar, and occasionally tossing mice or goldfish to them. During the 1930s a club was organized by aquarists who kept piranhas. There was only one membership requirement, and that was to have been bitten by a pet piranha. The first member of this oddly select group was Richard Buettner of the Empire Tropical Fish Company in New York City, who was bitten in 1933. Piranhas are just as hazardous to pet shop employees today. Not long ago Miss Pauline Wilson, a pretty clerk in a British pet shop, was nipped on the little finger of her right hand, an event that was widely covered by British newspapers—although possibly more because of Miss Wilson's pulchritude than the damage done to her pinky.

The laws in the United States controlling the importation and keeping of piranhas have been instituted out of fear that the fish might become introduced into streams and lakes in places of mild climate such as southern Florida and southern California. A variety of South American characins loosed by aquarium owners seem to be thriving in certain streams in Florida, which is approximately as far north of the equator—25 degrees latitude—as the piranha country of Paraguay is south of it. The air temperature near Paraguayan streams that harbor piranhas averages 74 degrees F., only a degree or so lower than that in the vicinity of Miami. And in December 1970, Florida wildlife officials reported an ominous catch in a south Florida canal: the fish was a piranha.

Vampire Catfish: The Candiru

It is not piranhas, however, that are the most feared of the fishes that inhabit river systems in tropical South America. Even more dreaded are tiny catfishes called candirus, which have the unique distinction of being the only vertebrates that parasitize humans. Candirus are bloodsuckers that for the most part belong to the genus *Vandellia*. They are eel-like in appearance and about the size of a thin lead pencil. They have the peculiar habit of entering the human genital opening, of either male or female, and worming their way up into the urethra where they erect prickly spines on their gill covers thus embedding themselves within the body of their human host. Candirus can draw a surprising amount of blood from a victim. Several of these catfish once entered the body of a cow that was being driven across a river on the way to market. Within two hours the cow was so weak that it barely could keep its feet, and when its throat was slashed at the slaughterhouse, hardly a dribble of blood remained in its veins.

The chief danger to humans, however, is that the candiru will reach the bladder and lodge there while its victim dies in agony. Once a candiru has wriggled up into the urethra, the situation becomes so critical that many a male victim has slashed off his penis, preferring life with impaired sexual ability to a painful death.

The candiru and its grisly parasitism first attracted the attention of zoologists in the 19th century, when explorers began to study the life of the Amazon in more detail than they had before. Ethnologist K. von Den Steinen, working in the Mato Grosso, reported that Indians there entered the water to bathe with extreme caution because of their fear of the bloodsucking catfish. Dr. G.A. Boulenger, curator of fish at the British Museum, in 1897 exhibited a candiru that had been collect-

97

ed in a tributary of the Amazon. A physician in La Plata, who evidentally had treated candiru victims, provided Boulenger with a description of the fish's habits. Instant amputation of the penis was the only way to prevent the candiru from gaining access to the bladder once it entered a male, the physician said. The good doctor apparently had administered this severe form of treatment to three boys and a man.

So difficult was it to accept the existence of a fish that could parasitize people in such an appalling manner that many zoologists viewed reports of the candiru's behavior as yarns out

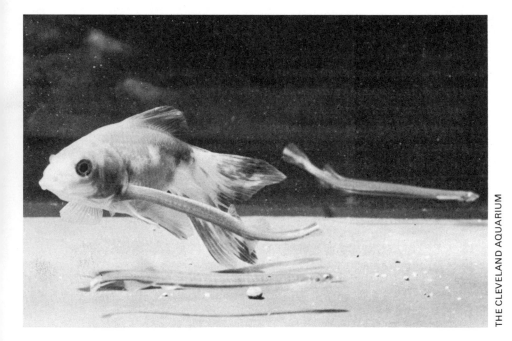

THE CLEVELAND AQUARIUM

BLOODSUCKER: This unusual photograph shows a candiru catfish feeding on a goldfish. With its head inside the gills of the goldfish, the candiru nibbles away at the gill tissue, draining the blood of its host. Two other parasitic candirus can be seen.

of the bush. Nevertheless the evidence accumulated that the candiru did indeed enter the human urethra, and sometimes the anus. During the early 1900s, Professor C.H. Eigenmann of Indiana University saw Indians in the Amazon don codpieces constructed of plant fibers before entering the water. Other Indian men merely tied the foreskin of the penis over the glans. The tribesmen told the professor that they took such precautions to protect themselves against the candiru. Indian women who had to enter the water wore a sort of G-string.

In 1922 Paul Le Cointe, director of the museum in Para', Brazil, reported three cases in which candirus had victimized people. He described an incident in which a catfish entered the urethra of an Indian woman while she sat in a river washing clothes with a group of friends. The typical position for such activity is to sit with ankles crossed and knees apart, a posture that makes the genital region easily accessible to the parasite. According to the story, the woman suddenly screamed and jumped to her feet, shrieking that she had been assaulted by a candiru. Her companions promptly grabbed her and wrenched the fish from her body before it gained substantial penetration. In the process they had to rip the candiru's spines from the flesh of the victim, causing considerable bleeding and doubtless a great amount of pain.

The existence of the candiru became widely known in 1930, when ichthyological bibliographer Eugene W. Gudger published a paper on the parasite entitled "The Candiru, the Only Vertebrate Predator of Man." Candirus, researchers had discovered, regularly attached themselves to the gills of fish, which are laced with blood vessels. Often, too, they had been found within the body cavities of dead fish, and it became apparent they were scavengers as well as parasites, and that they consumed offal as well as blood. Dr. Gudger's writing offered a complete review of what was known about the candiru, and it was well received by his colleagues. But, although it assurred acceptance of the candiru's existence in zoological circles, medicine had yet to be informed.

That was accomplished in 1941, when the *American Journal of Surgery* published a lengthy report on the candiru by two medical researchers, Kenneth W. Vinton and Hugh Stickler, of the Division of Schools, Panama Canal Zone. They had heard of the fish in 1936 from an adventurer who had visited candiru country, and again in 1938 from Indians while the researchers were collecting fish in the headwaters of the Amazon. They marveled at the remarkable adaptations by which the candiru survived, and, unlike Dr. Gudger, described first-hand experiences with the fish in its native waters. They collected candirus by leaving a bloody cow lung in the water, withdrawing it after several of the little bloodsuckers had collected on it. The candirus, bloated with blood and offal, clung to the lung even after it had been removed from the water.

Vinton and Stickler described several incidents in which people had been victimized by candirus. They cited a missionary, Edgar J. Burns, who during seven years in the Amazon knew of ten such incidents. Four of the victims were mature women, three were girls aged ten to sixteen years, one was an adult man, and two were boys, twelve and thirteen years old. In each case the catfish entered the body through the urethra. The man and one of the boys lost so much blood to the candiru that they passed out.

The researchers also described a method of ridding victims of the candiru that probably was much favored over amputation by males. Some Indians used a preparation concocted from the fruit of the jagua tree (*Genipa americana*), a 60-foot-high deciduous tree that grows in much of tropical America and produces an elliptical yellow-brown fruit about the size of an orange. The pulp of the fruit, which is covered by leathery skin, makes a sour but refreshing drink. Unripe pulp, mashed and mixed with water, was drunk by candiru victims, and within a few hours, the researchers reported, the candiru would relinquish its hold and slip out of its host.

Zoologists have speculated about what attracts candirus to the human genital region. The best bet seems to be that they are extremely sensitive to traces of urine in the water, for several victims reported encountering the candiru moments after they urinated, and the fish is said to be able to follow urine to its source. A sensitivity to urine may be common to a number of fishes; early in this century British medical researchers reported that some species of puffers in the East Indies were attracted by human genital organs to such an extent that they snapped at the testicles of men swimming naked in the water. Some researchers suggest that the current caused by the flow of urine in the water, rather than the urine itself, initiates the candiru's feeding pattern. The flow may be so similar to the flow of water from the gills of a fish that the candiru responds to it.

Once it has attached itself to its host, whether human or fish, the candiru rasps through its victim's skin—or, in the case of a fish's gills, the membranes that cover the blood vessels—using the long teeth that protrude from the middle of its upper jaw. All the while the horrid little creature sucks vigorously with its mouth, filling itself with the victim's blood, and its body thickens and grows turgid. The candiru preys not only on mammals and other fishes, but on reptiles as well.

James W. Atz of the American Museum of Natural History and William E. Kelley of Aquarium Systems, Inc., maintained four candirus in an aquarium for half a year, and they observed the reaction of the fish to various foods. The candirus ignored frozen brine shrimp (a popular tropical fish food), white worms, freshly killed goldfish, and even the blood of a goldfish which was offered by means of an eyedropper and a length of plastic tubing. As soon as a live goldfish was placed in the water, however, the candirus swam about searching for it, and quickly three of them attached themselves to gills of the goldfish and began to suck its blood.

Atz and Kelley observed that when a candiru attacks a goldfish, it first swims quickly about the victims head, touching it with its own, and then, swimming closely alongside the goldfish, it waits for a chance to slip its head under the moving gill cover of the host. Once the head of a candiru disappears into its host's gill cover, its belly rapidly swells with blood, while bits of gill tissue, rasped from the goldfish by the candiru, float away. Sometimes candirus used in the experiments were sated within half a minute after beginning their meal of blood, but at other times they clung to their host for as long as four minutes. After feeding, the candirus dropped to the bottom and lay there, swollen with blood. The goldfish did not try to resist the candirus that parasitized them. Though some small goldfish died after the candirus finished with them, large goldfish played host to the parasites many times.

Mammoth Man-Eating Catfish

At the other end of the size scale from the tiny candiru are several very large catfish of South American rivers, some of which are more than 10 feet long and may be capable of swallowing men. Theodore Roosevelt's writings refer to large South American catfish that attack people. The giant of South American freshwater fishes, however, is not a catfish but the arapaima (*Arapaima gigas*), which possibly attains a length of 20 feet and a weight of more than 500 pounds. Despite its size and its huge mouth, the arapaima feeds on small bits of organic matter and threatens little else. In fact, this huge creature often serves as food for Indians, who regularly fish for it. I know of only one instance of an arapaima causing even minor harm to a man—although certainly Indian fishermen must at

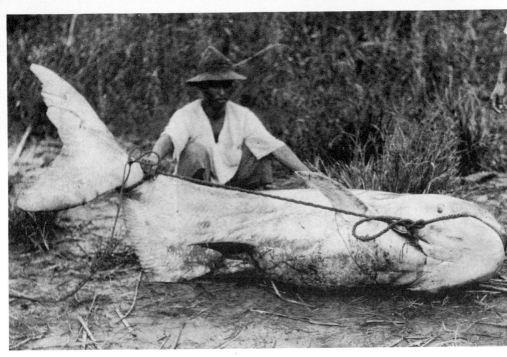

MONSTER CATFISH: Pla Biik, *(top), the giant catfish of Indochina, grows larger than a man but is dwarfed by the even larger* wels, right, *a huge catfish of eastern Europe, which is known to have killed several people in the Danube.*

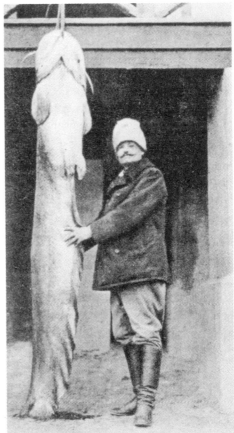

times be batted about by their giant catches. It occurred when a 6-foot arapaima at the London Zoo slapped a keeper with its tail as the water in its tank was being lowered.

Several related species of large fish inhabit the rivers of India and Southeast Asia, and some of them might be dangerous given appropriate circumstances. The goonah (*Bagarius bagarius*) of India, a hulking catfish with a massive jaw, grows to a length of 5 feet and weighs almost as much as a man. The Mekong River and other streams of Indochina provide a home for the monstrous catfish pla biik (*Pangasianodon gigas*), a dozen feet long and weighing 500 pounds. Whether these giant freshwater fishes endanger humans is open to question, but certainly their size and the voracious feeding habits of catfishes in general should make one wary of them.

One species of catfish *is* a known man-eater, and it lives not in some tropical wilderness but in the rivers of eastern Europe, including the Danube. From medieval times the sheatfish, or wels (*Silurus glanis*), has been reputed to gulp down humans as well as the frogs, fish, worms, dogs, lambs, and waterfowl that constitute the greater part of its varied diet. As much as 15 feet long and weighing up to 700 pounds, the wels indeed is capable of swallowing a child whole, if not a large man. A child was reported eaten by a wels near Pressburg, Hungary, in 1613; and in 1754 one of these great catfish was caught and opened and was found to contain the corpse of a seven-year-old child. A wels caught in 1558 had a right hand and two rings in its stomach, and late in the 18th century, the body of a woman was discovered in a wels caught in Turkey. Another report from Turkey in 1793 tells of two girls having been devoured by a wels. It could be argued that the human remains found in these giant catfish were victims of drowning or other mishaps and were scavenged by the fish, but it is just possible that among people reported missing in some of the rural regions of Europe down through the years are poor unfortunates that died horribly, swallowed alive by a wels.

Of the North American catfish, only the shovelhead (*Pilodictis olivaris*), also known as the yellow cat, reaches a size large enough to menace humans, but it seems not inclined to do so. Big shovelhead catfish can be 5 feet long and weigh 100 pounds. Another fish of North American lakes and streams that would seem to be the very personification of a fish that men should fear is the muskellunge (*Esox masquinongy*), so-called tiger of the north. Looking for all the world like a freshwater barracuda, with its underslug jaw, wicked teeth and a form like a slim torpedo, the muskellunge almost matches the barracuda in size. Some of these fish are more than 5 feet long and very possibly weigh of more than 100 pounds, although one that weighs half that is considered a prize catch by anglers. It is entirely carnivorous, even cannibalistic, but it generally leaves humans alone. The muskellunge ranges from the Great Lakes, the upper Mississippi Valley, and northern New York State into Canada. Animals as large as waterfowl and muskrats end their lives in the grip of the muskellunge's jaws. Men who fish for them know that those jaws can inflict a severe gash in the hand that carelessly removes a hook from them.

Often inhabiting water less than 15 feet feep, the muskellunge probably would come more in contact with human swimmers were it not that many of the regions in which it lives are sparsely populated, and that its waters tend to be cold. If so inclined a large muskellunge could surely mutilate a swimmer, but I can find no record of that ever happening. However, Arthur A. Oehmcke, a district director of the Wisconsin State Department of Natural Resources and an acknowledged expert on the muskie, says he has heard of several occasions when a muskellunge has bitten a foot that someone was dangling in the water from a pier. He adds, though, that he has not been able to verify those stories.

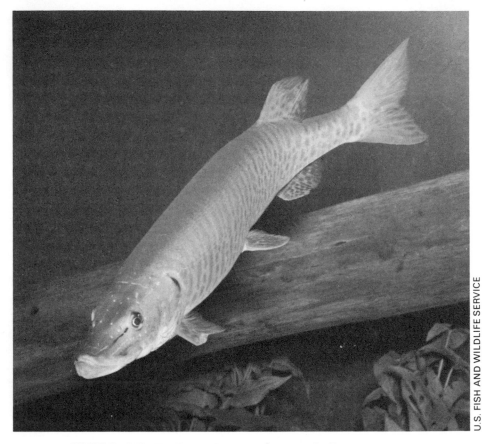

U.S. FISH AND WILDLIFE SERVICE

TIGER OF THE NORTH: The muskellunge, most awesome freshwater gamefish, is known to have attacked a swimming dog that came too close.

A hint that an aroused muskellunge might harry an adversary the size of a man is contained in an account, told to me by Oehmcke, of a one that ripped into a 120-pound St. Bernard dog that was swimming in Pine Lake, near Rhinelander, Wisconsin. The incident was witnessed by a conservation warden, Harley McKeague. According to Oehmcke, "The muskie harassed the St. Bernard, forced it to swim in circles, and then

106

slashed the flank of the right hind leg. The muskie caused such serious injury that the dog thrashed about for several minutes and had to be rescued by its owner in a rowboat."

Probably no one ever has been killed by a muskellunge. But at the same time it is not certain that no swimmer has felt the teeth of this fierce predator and, perhaps incapacitated by the fish's savage attack, drowned unheeded in the cold waters of some northern lake.

Of North American freshwater fishes, the most likely candidate for the title *man-eater* is not the muskellunge, but the enormous alligator gar (*Lepisosteus spatula*) of the lower Mississippi Valley and the Rio Grande. A survivor of a particularly ancient line of fish, the alligator gar is armored in the fashion of fishes that lived before the dinousaurs. The heavy, scale-like plates that cover its body are almost as impervious as metal. The alligator gar grows to at least 10 feet, and some fishermen claim that individual gars reach twice that length, although such claims are doubtful.

Like smaller species of gars, the alligator gar has a long, flattened snout lined with large, sharp teeth. Slow-moving, looking for all the world like a floating log, the alligator gar explodes into action when in reach of prey, slashing sideways with its jaws to seize the unfortunate fish, duck, or muskrat that has ventured too near.

Townsend, the New York Aquarium authority, once quoted fishermen from the area of Lake Charles, Louisiana, as saying that alligator gars and American alligators sometimes fight, with the alligators usually the victors over their namesakes. That may be true, as alligators habitually prey on smaller species of gar,—but should an alligator engage an alligator gar of comparable size in combat, the struggle probably would be a nip-and-tuck affair. Townsend, who called the alligator gar the freshwater counterpart of the shark, wrote in 1920 of receiving a letter from a man who was mauled by a giant gar while bath-

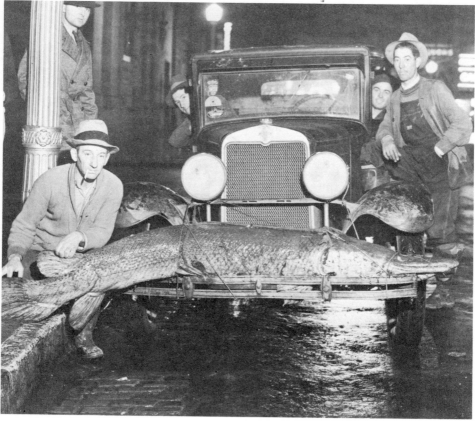

COURTESY OF THE AMERICAN MUSEUM OF NATURAL HISTORY

AMERICANA: Alligator gar and captors in Little Rock, Arkansas, circa 1928.

ing in a Louisiana lake. The fish seized the bather's arm, tearing it badly. (Louisiana fish and game biologists have told me of gars in the breeding season snapping at bather's legs.) Townsend did not say whether he believed the gar was attempting to devour the swimmer or was merely acting defensively.

Swordsmen of the Deep
(Swordfish, Needlefish, and Marlin)

Several species of fish that in no way can be considered man-eaters have taken human lives, often because of provocation. Among them is the swordfish (*Xiphias gladius*), which has killed a number of men with thrusts of its bill. The bill of the swordfish is flattened, whereas various species of marlin have a bill that is tapered like a lance or spear. Both extend from the upper jaw and snout. Although these unusual adaptations are deadly as defensive weapons when wielded against an adversary, their primary function is to streamline the fishes that possess them. Swordfish and marlin, known as billfish, travel at tremendous speeds through the water; both have been clocked at more than 50 miles an hour.

Swordfish generally have a mild reputation, but the history of seafaring abounds with stories of swordfish attacking men and penetrating the hulls of vessels. Not all of those attacks occurred in days long past, for as recently as 1967 the ramming of a vessel by a swordfish made world headlines. The vessel was the *Alvin*, a deep-sea research craft of the Woods Hole Oceanographic Institution. The attack happened at a depth of 1,800 feet on the floor of the Blake Plateau southeast of Charleston, South Carolina. The *Alvin* had been dispatched on a geological survey of the area, which contains significant mineral deposits, when a 200-pound swordfish slammed into the side of the research craft. The fish struck with such force that its weapon pierced the glass fiber skin of the *Alvin* and lodged there, causing a leak. With the swordfish attached, the *Alvin* headed for the surface, where repairs were made and the swordfish was converted into steaks.

Swordfish and marlin are pelagic, ranging the open sea far from land. The swordfish is almost global in its range, inhabit-

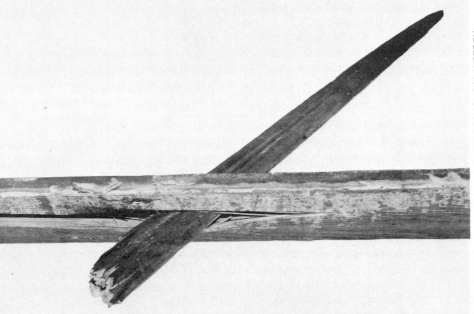

EVIDENCE: This chunk of the sword of a swordfish, lodged in a piece of wood from a dory, testifies that billfish sometimes attack vessels. The attack in this case occurred off Montauk Point, New York.

ing even the Black Sea. The various species of marlin are much more restricted. Both kinds of fish grow to immense size. Swordfish caught by sportsmen generally weigh about 300 pounds, but specimens weighing well over 1,000 pounds have been recorded. The black marlin (*Makaira nigricans*) of the Pacific is slightly larger than the swordfish, and the blue marlin (*Makaira ampla*) and the striped marlin (*Makaira mitsukurii*) are at least as large. Three California fishermen joined forces to land a blue marlin weighing 1,805 pounds off Hawaii in 1972. These colossal fish begin life as larvae so tiny that several of them could swim in a teaspoon. A larval blue marlin found by University of Miami scientists in the Bahamas measured only an eighth of an inch long. Because of their size large, swordfish and marlin have few predators, with the possible exception of very big sharks and killer whales. Seafarers have witnessed many battles between billfish and sharks. Small swordfish have been extracted from the stomachs of large sharks, and sharks sometimes bear scars and wounds from the weapons of billfish. Two fishermen off the Isle of Jersey once watched a swordfish dispatch a 25-foot-long shark after the two creatures had fought for a half hour.

Billfish use their weapons to procure food, which consists of smaller fish and squid. Swordfish flash through great schools of mackerel and menhaden, and even schools of large fish such as bonito, slashing back and forth with their swords, leaving mangled and stunned victims floating in the water. After a few such passes, the swordfish returns to pick up the pieces. Swordfish and marlin do not school, but sometimes they concentrate in numbers to bask upon the surface of the ocean.

While basking, billfish make an easy target for harpooners, and they have been taken that way at least since classical times. Strabo (63 B.C.-21 A.D.), in writing about the swordfishing industry in the Straits of Messina, tells how fishing boats were manned by an oarsman and harpooner, while a third man watched the swordfish from the shore. Keeping an eye on a harpooned swordfish makes sense, for it is likely to stab back. Pliny wrote that "The swordfish has a beak or bill, sharply pointed, with which he will drive through the side and planking of a ship."

Powered by several hundred pounds of fish lunging at high speed through the sea, the weapon of a billfish strikes with tremendous force. The book A *History of Fishes* notes that if a 600-pound swordfish swimming at 10 miles an hour collided with a wooden ship traveling at the same speed in the opposite direction, the force administered by the point of the

111

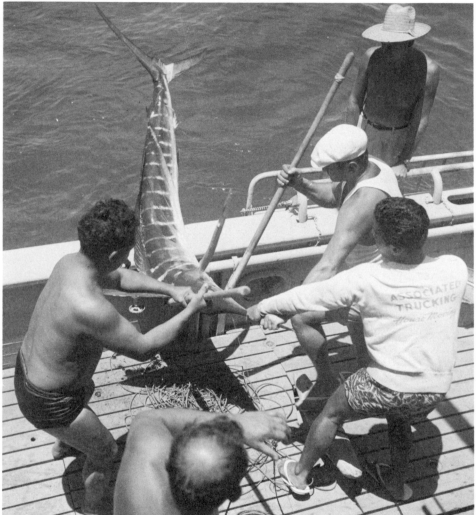

HUGH M. SMITH, U.S. FISH AND WILDLIFE SERVICE

BIG BILLFISH: Crewmen aboard the U.S. Fish and Wildlife Service ship land a struggling striped marlin off Kona, Hawaii. The bill of a marlin can pierce the side of a ship, and has done just that more than once.

112

sword be more than 4 tons. This sort of impact enables swordfish to impale even the hulls of modern vessels, and to penetrate quite deeply into wooden-hulled ships. A ship's timber in the British Museum contains a swordfish bill that has been thrust 22 inches into it, and in the College of Surgeons of Great Britain is a chunk of wood, from the bow of a whaler, into which a bill has penetrated more than 13 inches.

Many collisions with swordfish were reported by seamen in the days of sail, and often they were not provoked. A Danish vessel was struck by a swordfish in the Indian Ocean on July 30, 1719. Two years later, when the keel of the vessel was overhauled, workers discovered a 15-inch-long length of sword embedded in it. When the British ship *Leopard* was overhauled in 1725, workmen found that a fish had driven its sword through inch-thick metal sheathing, 3 inches of planking, and more than 4 inches of stout timber. In 1871 a swordfish being played on hook and line from the yacht *Redhot*, out of New Bedford, plunged its sword into the ship and sank it. The Glouster schooner *Wyoming*, sailing to Georges Bank in August 1875, almost suffered a similar fate after a swordfish broke off its bill in the vessel's side. More recently the Japanese fishing vessel *Genyo Maru* was hit by a swordfish, but with no serious effects.

Marlin also attack ships, and sometimes the damage they do is attributed to swordfish. Such may have been the case in the curious legal proceedings between the owners of the ship *Dreadnought* and the insuror, Lloyd's of London, during the last century. The ship had been insured for £3,000 against all risks of the sea. The crew hooked a billfish as the *Dreadnought* plied the Indian Ocean en route to London from Colombo, Ceylon. The fish, in its battle to escape, hammered into the hull of the *Dreadnought*, poking a round, inch-wide hole in the ship's copper sheathing and planking. After the fish, in its struggles, pulled free, the *Dreadnought* began leaking and was forced back to Colombo for repairs.

When the ship's owners demanded payment for the damage caused by what they claimed was a swordfish attack, the insurance firm maintained that while an attack by a swordfish might be considered a common risk of the sea, there was no previous record of a fish withdrawing its bill after striking a ship. When experts testified that the fish might have punctured the ship, then wriggled until it yanked free, Lloyd's paid the vessel's owners. From the circular configuration of the hole, the fish responsible for the matter probably was not a swordfish but a marlin.

Another billfish, also in all likelihood a marlin, punched a hole 4 inches deep in the wooden hull of an 18-foot motor launch off Woody Head, New South Wales, in 1938. The four men aboard the launch kept it afloat by plugging the hole with a cloth bag. The year before, off Bimini, a 400-pound blue marlin shoved its bill 9 inches into the boat of a fisherman who had hooked it. Another blue marlin rammed the 65-foot yacht *Frielands* on March 17, 1938.

Seemingly unprovoked attacks on vessels by billfish present something of a mystery, but probably they occur accidentally as the billfish speed after smaller fish that try to hide under the ships that are struck. Swimming at full speed, the billfish may not be able to swerve in time to avoid collision.

Fatalities that have resulted from billfish attacks on ships likewise seem accidental in that the victims probably were not the targets, although their vessels may have been. A tragic case occurred on August 19, 1886, when Captain F.D. Langford of the Massachusetts schooner *Venus* went with another man in a dory to bring back harpooned swordfish. The swordfish turned and charged the dory, plunging its bill through the craft's bottom and knocking the captain down. The sword pierced him as he tried to rise, but, in agony, he bravely declared, "We've got him, anyway." Three days later he died of peritonitis. Equally unusual is the case of another man, who suddenly was struck and killed in the back by a swordfish as he sat on the gunwale of a sailboat off Sierra Leone. Much more recently, in Australian waters, a 500-pound marlin that had been boated speared the fisherman in the chest, and escaped.

Some fishermen still harpoon swordfish today. Willis Blount, the young skipper of the 68-foot stern trawler *Ruth Frances*, out of Newport, Rhode Island, is one of the men who continues this ancient practice. Blount says he knows of several harpooners who have been stabbed in their dories by harpooned swordfish. Usually, the fish stabs through the bottom of the boat, so most of the injuries are to legs and feet—although experienced harpooners take refuge on the seats of the dory when the swordfish charges. Blount never has been injured, although one swordfish he had harpooned charged his boat and hurtled itself out of the water only a few feet from the Rhode Islander.

A number of people also have been transfixed by the sharp, pointed snouts of needlefish (Belonidae). Needlefish, some of which are known as silver gars or houndfish, reach a maximum length of about 5 feet. Exceedingly slender, they sometimes leap from the sea and hurtle through the air like silver lances when chasing prey or trying to escape predators. For some reason, a light shining over the waves in the darkness attracts leaping needlefish, a form of behavior that sometimes brings death in the night.

The *Malayan Nature Journal* of May, 1968, reported a tragedy of this type that took place on the night of November 13, 1966, during a dispute between Malaya and Indonesia. A Malayan customs vessel from Singapore had intercepted a small sampan with seven Indonesians aboard and was taking the sampan in tow. Amidst the barking of orders and the flashing of spotlights, one of the Indonesians suddenly screamed and collapsed, his neck gushing blood. He died quickly, and when his body was examined at the Singapore General Hospital, doctors found a bone from the jaw of a needlefish lodged in his neck. Apparently the lights and commotion had either attracted the fish or frightened it, and the creature had launched itself like a gleaming missile into the air, impaling the unfortunate Indonesian.

An article in *Collier's* magazine in January 1948 described the death of two men who were spearing fish in shallow water near Acapulco, Mexico, when needlefish turned the tables on them. And in 1936 a man who had been struck in the neck by a needlefish in the Miami Beach surf was saved from joining the list of needlefish fatalities by a lifeguard who stopped the flow of blood.

The most bizarre weapon carried on the snout of a fish is the great toothed saw of the sawfish (Pristidae). Because their gills open beneath the body, rather than on either side of the head as in sharks, sawfish are classified as rays—although the sawfish is much more elongate than any other ray. Sawfish grow to a truly monstrous size. Large individuals are as much as 35 feet long, including 6 feet of saw, and they weigh up to 2 tons.

Like the swordfish, the sawfish swings its weapon to and fro as it plows through schools of prey. The saw cleaves even large victims to pieces and impales smaller fish on its teeth, which are modified denticles. Despite their large size, sawfish show no inclination to harm people—but a man struck by the saw stands a good chance of being halved.

Harmless Giants (Manta Ray and Sunfish)

Another gigantic ray that is inoffensive as far as man is concerned is the manta (*Manta birostris*). Sometimes called the devil ray, it has an exceedingly sinister reputation, one that is

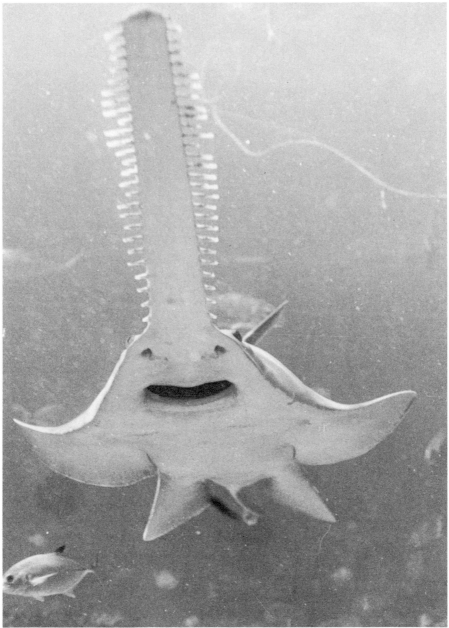

MIAMI SEAQUARIUM

VICIOUS WEAPON: The saw of a big sawfish can slice a man in two, but fortunately sawfish are not aggressive towards man unless provoked.

totally undeserved. The only satanic characteristics about this immense beast—it can span 22 feet from wing tip to wing tip —are the fleshy projections resembling horns on either side of the head. The manta ray sweeps through the water, scooping up multitudes of small fish and crustaceans in its cavernous mouth. Occasionally, for unknown reasons, they leap from the water and crash back with a thunderous impact that can be heard for a considerable distance. Although they are the villians of countless sea stories, manta rays leave swimmers alone and molest boats only if they themselves are harried. If a manta is harpooned or netted, it can smash a small boat to pieces.

Diver Robert Fabbri, writing in the November-December 1971 issue of the magazine *Sea Frontiers*, notes that although mantas have a foul reputation, he has been able to approach and even touch them. Fabbri describes how he watched the birth of a manta pup from below, as he was diving in the Red Sea. A huge ray had passed over him, launched itself from the water, and slammed into it again. After the ray had re-entered the water it began to give birth. When the young ray, wings folded, had emerged from its mother's uterus, the mother swam off, leaving the new-born manta resting on a reef with its wings still folded.

Another fish whose huge size belies its harmlessness is the massive ocean sunfish (*Mola mola*). This truly queer fish looks as if it is all head, an impression fostered by the fact that its gross, oval body is deeper than long, and its tail is short and stubby. A single high dorsal fin atop the body, and an anal fin of similar shape below, give the creature somewhat of a half-moon appearance. Large ocean sunfish sometimes measure 10 feet long and 14 feet from the tip of the dorsal fin to the tip of the anal fin, and they can weigh a ton or more. When it hatches, however, the larval ocean sunfish is but a fraction of an inch long. The larvae are covered with protective spines, but adult ocean sunfish have no protection against predators. Their teeth are fused into a beak-like structure adapted for feeding on jellyfish and other small animals. Ponderous and clumsy, the ocean sunfish moves slowly and seems incredibly dull and stupid. I once came nose-to-nose with one while investigating a kelp bed off southern California. Leaning over the side of a small motor launch, I pushed aside the kelp with a short pole and saw the insipid eyes of a sunfish staring up at me. For a moment it just stared, then melted into the blue-green water.

Some people have claimed that because of its size, the ocean sunfish is a menace—but this simply is not the case. Divers have poked them with gaffs and fishermen have prodded them with oars, and seldom has there been more than minimal response. Townsend wrote of seeing a large ocean sunfish basking at the surface, paying no attention to the gunshots fired at it by members of the crew of a passing steamship

A Y.M.C.A. diving instructor from New Jersey, Eugene Geer, told me of an unnerving experience with ocean sunfish, but it involved no hostile moves on the part of the fish. Geer, an electrical engineer who is active in the American Littoral Society, was scuba diving on the wreck *Mohawk* eight miles off Mantoloking, New Jersey, in September 1972. He had left the bottom and was swimming for the surface at a depth of about 60 feet, when an immense but vague gray form appeared at the edge of his vision. To his dismay, Geer perceived that the huge shape was coming right at him. "I decided it was a whale or an awfully big shark," he remembers, realizing he could do little but to turn and face whatever it was. As the shape closed with Geer it resolved itself—to his relief—into an ocean sunfish, which halted about ten feet away and regarded the diver dully. "We just looked at each other for a while. Then I saw another sunfish a short distance away," Geer says. After a few moments both fish swam off, one following the other in a de-

119

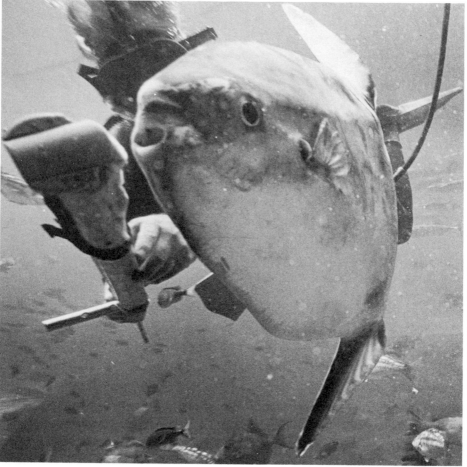

MARINELAND OF THE PACIFIC. BOB NOBLE

FUSSY EATER: The big ocean sunfish does not eat well in captivity so divers at aquariums must feed them by hand. A diver at Marineland of the Pacific swims close to a sunfish so he can pump a prepared food mixture into its mouth.

termined fashion. Geer, who is 6 feet, 4 inches tall, says the sunfish closest to him was at least as deep as he is tall. He has no idea what the two fish were doing, but he suggests that they may have been breeding.

Groupers: Jaws of Death

The giant groupers and sea basses of the family Serranidae are comparable to the ocean sunfish in size, but unlike the sunfish they are curious and aggressive. With their gaping maws, they actively prey on animals of considerable size, even sea turtles. The grouper or sea bass captures prey simply by opening its mouth and gill covers, thereby creating enough suction to sweep the prey between its jaws. Large groupers and sea basses easily could close their jaws over a man, for some members of the family are big enough to weigh more than 1,000 pounds. The giant grouper (*Epinephelus itajara*), which ranges from Florida to South America, weighs more than 700 pounds, and the Queensland grouper (*E. lanceolatus*) of the Indo-Pacific and the California black sea bass (*Stereolepis gigas*) approach a half ton in weight. The size of groupers and sea basses seems to increase with the depth at which they live, so it would not be surprising if individuals weighing almost a ton skulked in some of the deeper holes around the rocks and reefs that these creatures inhabit.

The tendency of groupers and sea basses to lurk in the dark recesses of reefs and old wrecks makes them especially dangerous to divers. It is easy to imagine a diver entering the black water in the hold of an ancient wreck and suddenly being engulfed in the jaws of a monstrous grouper. Pearl divers of the Indo-Pacific are said to fear big groupers and sea basses more than sharks, and around the waterfront of San Juan, Puerto Rico, people tell stories of groupers waiting beneath the wharves to snatch up youngsters from the streets who some-

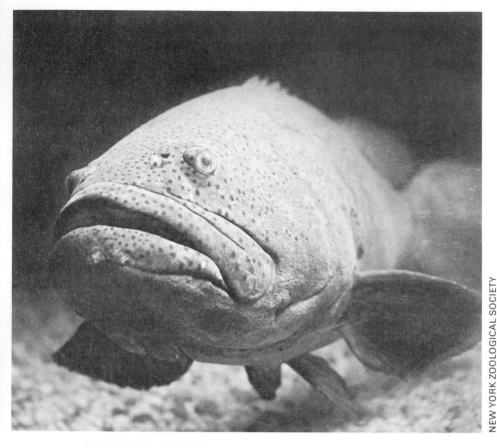

NEW YORK ZOOLOGICAL SOCIETY

MASSIVE BRUTE: Large groupers and sea basses—such as this giant grouper shown above, can pose a serious hazard to divers. A big grouper can suck a diver into its huge jaws.

times dive and swim there.

Nixon Griffis, president of the American Littoral Society, told me of an account he had heard of a Navy lieutenant who was diving with scuba and was swept into the maw of a giant grouper. The lieutenant escaped only because his bulky air tanks prevented the fish from swallowing him. William J. Cromie, oceanographer and science journalist, wrote in *The*

Living World of the Sea that a pearl diver was swallowed by a giant sea bass in Australian waters and escaped through one of the fish's huge gill openings.

That groupers and sea basses have a variety of weapons capable of harming divers was demonstrated at Marineland of the Pacific a few years ago. John Prescott, who before he assumed the directorship of the New England Aquarium in 1972 was Marineland's curator, told me of a Marineland diver who was stabbed with the spines of a sea bass's dorsal fin. The fish, which weighed more than 350 pounds, was to be moved from one tank to another, and the diver sent into its tank had cornered it. As the diver neared the big fish, it turned over on its side and backed into the man, thrusting its huge dorsal spines into him. He was injured so seriously that he was rushed to a hospital.

The Goosefish: All Mouth

When it comes to gaping maws, not even the groupers and sea basses can top the goosefish (*Lophius americanus*), a flaccid, flabby creature that probably rates as the world's most repulsive fish. The goosefish, which inhabits the Atlantic, belongs to the group of fishes called anglers because they utilize various tabs and other appendages of flesh as living fishing poles to lure smaller fish within reach of their jaws. The body of the goosefish, which can be more than 4 feet long, seemingly lacks structure when taken from the water, but in its own element it tapers back from the huge, rounded head like the tail of a tadpole. The huge mouth of the goosefish dwarfs the rest of its body. It is located almost on the top of the creature's head, and the mouth of a large goosefish can close over a soccer ball. The lower jaw juts so far beyond the upper that the bottom teeth stick out even when the jaws close.

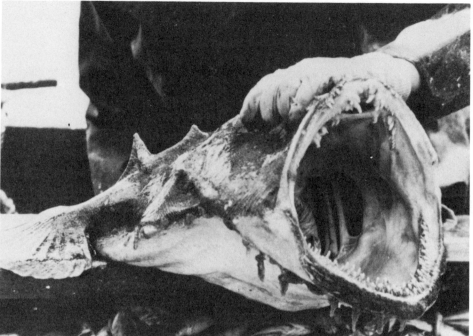

NATIONAL MARINE FISHERIES SERVICE

BIG MOUTH: The gaping maw of the goosefish can close over fish almost as large as it is. Goosefish eat large sea birds, but despite their name, as far as is known, they do not prey on geese.

Lying on the bottom, at depths from 1,000 feet to close inshore, the goosefish waits for cod, dogfish, skates, flatfish, and other creatures to come near its huge mouth. A 26-inch-long goosefish caught in Britain had swallowed a cod only 3 inches shorter than itself. Goosefish regularly prey on ducks, loons, grebes, and other sea birds, but despite their name they are not known to take geese.

A goosefish 3 or 4 feet long presents little danger to humans, but if the foot of a diver or swimmer was seized by one of these ugly creatures, the person might find himself in a serious situation, especially if the fish held fast. Furthermore, there are reports of goosefish reaching a length of 6 feet, and if a goosefish 2 feet long can swallow a cod of almost the same size, a 6-foot specimen might prove disagreeable indeed.

Fish That Shock

Of all the vertebrates, only fish are capable of producing enouch electricity to stun or even kill a man. About 250 species of fish cause electrical discharges, which in the various species serve for defense, navigation, obtaining prey, and possibly communiction. Only two kinds of electric fish generate enough electricity to seriously affect humans, however. They are the electric eel *(Electrophorus electricus)* of South America and the marine electric rays, which belong to the family Torpedinoidae.

How animals generate prodigious amounts of electricity poses something of a riddle for scientists, but the nature of the electrical discharge is not at all mysterious. All animals—including men—produce electricity in their bodies. To better understand how electric eels and rays generate enough electricity to stun other creatures, consider for a moment how electricity plays a role in the nerve messages that are flashing through your body even as you read this.

Historically, the fact that the stuff of which we are made produces electricity began to be known in 1791 when Luigi Galvani, a professor of anatomy at the University of Bologna, discovered that the nerve and muscle tissue in the leg of a frog conducts electricity. Gradually scientists learned that the impulses which carry messages along the body's network of nerves are electro-chemical in nature. Simply, nerve messages result from a movement of ions, charged particles, across the nerve cell membrane. When resting, or inactive, the membrane has a negative potential due to the build-up of negatively-charged ions on its interior. Among the ions of both positive and negative charge outside the cell are those of sodium, which are positive. When the nerve cell fires, the membrane reverses its polarity and sodium ions flood across it into the cell, making the potential of the membrane positive.

Normally, sodium ions are excluded from the cell by an unknown mechanism, which scientists call the sodium pump because it is believed to literally pump sodium ions out of the cell.

The sodium pump stops functioning when a nerve cell transmits a message. Sodium and potassium ions attract one another, discharging the potential and equalizing the charge on both sides of the cell membrane. Minute discharges sweep along the nerve fiber that extends from the cell, sending electric currents into the surrounding tissue and fluid. The message, or nerve impulse, travels along the fiber until it arrives at the point where the fiber branches into fingerlike projections called nerve endings. These reach across a minute void to the next nerve cell. This void, or space between nerve cells, is called a synapse.

A nerve impulse that is headed for a muscle eventually reaches a synapse with a muscle-cell fiber on the other side. This meeting place, known as a neuromuscular junction, performs a critical role in the production of electricity in electric fishes. The arrival of a nerve impulse at a neuromuscular junction causes the release of a chemical agent called acetlycholine at the nerve endings. As the acetlycholine diffuses across the tiny gap between nerve and muscle, it transmits the impulse to the muscle fiber, depolarizing it and producing an electric discharge. (Scientists believe that acetlycholine has the additional task of obstructing the nerve cell's sodium pump, permitting ions to move across the cell membrane.)

Normally this process signals a muscle to contract, resulting in various actions carried on by the body's muscles. However, some of the muscles in electric fishes have lost the ability to contract. The nerve endings that extend towards these muscles at the neuromuscular junction have massed in large concentrations, and the muscle fibers themselves have swelled, forming a living electroplate.

The electric organs of fish such as the electric eel and electric rays consist of several electroplates. When all of them discharge, they generate an electric current of great power. The discharge is controlled by nerves which, in the electric eel, stem from the spinal cord, and in electric rays, from the brain.

Electric rays, which inhabit both temperate and tropical waters, can generate a pulse of more than 50 volts, enough to kill the fish and crustaceans on which they prey. An electric ray resembles a flexible flapjack with a long but chunky tail. When the animal hunts, it flings itself upon its prey and envelops it with its "wings," each of which contains an electric organ. As the ray embraces its victim, the organs discharge, stunning the prey.

The largest electric ray, *Torpedo nobiliana* a 6-foot-long, 200 pounder that inhabits the North Atlantic, can generate an output of 200 volts, enough to stun anyone who happens to be nearby in the water when the ray strikes. The effect of the discharge is magnified by the fact that water is an excellent conductor of electricity.

The electric ray was the subject of considerable speculation during classical times, when people believed that the ray's appearance in a dream portended misfortune. The Greeks and Romans knew that the ray emitted some sort of strange power, which, since electricity was unknown, was believed to be a drug. Classical accounts told how rays that had been snagged on bronze hooks produced a force that eventually reached the hands of the fisherman and congealed his blood. At the same

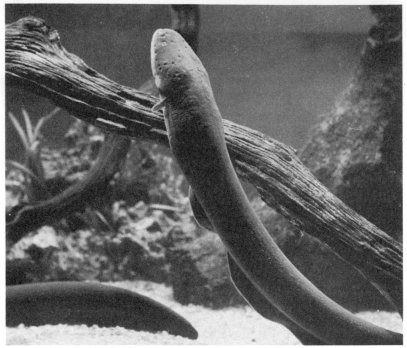

HIGH VOLTAGE: Electric fishes inhabit both marine and fresh waters. The fish capable of the strongest electrical discharge, the electric eel, top, can generate enough power to stun a horse. The electric ray, bottom, wraps its "wings" around its prey and stuns it with its discharge.

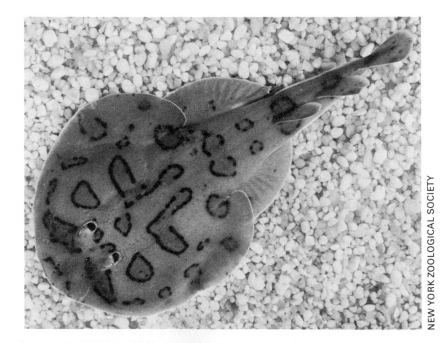

time, the ray found a place in classical medicine, in a primitive sort of shock treatment. Physicians plopped small rays down on the heads of patients suffering from headaches and other ailments, believing that the ray would provide a cure.

The electric eel generates several times the voltage of even the largest rays. It can discharge more than 650 volts, enough to kill a person in the water nearby. Not really an eel but a relative of the knifefish, the electric eel is a river dweller. It has three electric organs that take up four-fifths of its body, which in large specimens can be 9 feet long and is as thick as a man's arm. Only a fifth of the total body length contains the organs involved in respiration, digestion, reproduction, and other vital functions.

The waters in which the electric eel lives often lack oxygen, but that makes little difference, for the eel has become adapted to using atmospheric oxygen as well as that in the water. Numerous small blood vessels in its mouth take up oxygen from air that the creature gulps at the water's surface.

Although young electric eels can see, the eyes of adults degenerate. Their blindness does not matter, however, for vision would be of little use to them in the dark and muddy waters in which they usually live. When searching for prey, the eel generates weak discharges of about 40 to 50 volts, using these pulses to locate the small animals on which it feeds. Electric eels also may be able to receive one another's electricity, for several of the creatures will gather around one that has discharged and immobilized prey.

Electric eels do well in captivity, and aquariums often exhibit them, usually in displays that are wired to demonstrate their power-generating ability. Positive and negative electrodes linked to a strobe light or to an ordinary light bulb are installed in the eel tank. Small fish or bits of fish are put into the water to stimulate the eel, and when the animal discharges, the light is illuminated. Electric-eel exhibits also can be wired with amplifiers that broadcast the sound of static that accompanies a discharge.

Handling electric eels in aquariums can be ticklish. A keeper at the London Zoo's aquarium was jolted severely while feeding an eel. Another staff member was carrying an eel in a metal box and had to put the box down when the eel began to discharge. Although a man almost has to step on an eel to die from its shock, in the eel's native habitat there exists a very real danger of being stunned from a distance and drowning, or at least suffering repeated shocks while helpless in the water.

For more than a century biologists and physicists have pondered the electric eel's generating capacity, and during World War II, research on electric eels took a martial direction. The United States had been in the war for two years when 200 electric eels, collected in South America, were shipped to the Bronz Zoo and housed in 22 wooden tanks in the basement of the lion house. The eels had become involved in research on nerve gases, which, by stopping the transmission of nerve impulses, can halt the heartbeat, breathing, and other vital functions of the body. Essentially, nerve gases prevent the breakdown of acetylcholine after it inhibits the sodium pump in normal nerve functioning. Normally, immediately after acetylcholine completes its task, it is broken down by a chemical process that depends on the action of an enzyme called cholinesterase. Nerve gases obstruct the action of the enzyme.

The electric organs of the electric eel contain cholinesterase of extra high potency and quality, and the eels shipped to the Bronx Zoo furnished the enzyme for scientists studying nerve gases. Until the war ended, few members of the zoo staff knew the real reason why so many eels were kept in the lion house basement.

Among the creatures of the sea, the fishes are but a small minority. The invertebrates, those animals lacking the benefits of a backbone, far outnumber them. This vast assemblage of creatures includes the smallest motes of animal life in the ocean, and very nearly the largest, and by all accounts some of the deadliest as well.

Many motion pictures and romances of the South Seas have pictured the giant clam (*Tridacna gigas*) as a living death trap, ever ready to trap the foot of an unwary diver. Actually, the giant clam feeds on plankton and lacks the awesome strength so often attributed to it, although it can have a shell 4 feet wide and can weigh 500 pounds. No case of a diver drowning in the grip of a giant clam has ever been documented, but even authoritative publications as the Navy's *Science in the Sea* warn that the clam presents a hazard. Rather than holding on to a diver, a clam that found something as large as a human foot in its interior would more likely open up and try to rid itself of the object.

Many-Armed Mollusks: Octopus and Squid

Hidden in the fortress of its shell, the clam seems not even closely related to the octopus and squid, those active, many armed predators of rock, reef, and open water. Yet the clam, the octopus, and the squid are all mollusks. The octopus and squid are members of the class Cephalopoda. The class is of venerable age, for Cephalopods swam in the seas more than 400 million years ago. Squid and octopuses, like the giant clam, terrorize the heroes, anti-heroes, and heroines of many a sea story—but in their case the horror, although often exaggerated, can be real.

The term cephalopod means "head-footed," a reference to the arms—and in the squid's case, arms and tentacles—that sprout from the head of these mollusks. In the midst of the wriggly appendages is a parrot-like beak. The body, which is soft like that of other mollusks, has a mantle of thick skin that shields the internal organs. The molluskan shell of cephalopods is internal, although it consists of limy material secreted by the mantle just as in clams and oysters.

When a cephalopod breathes, its mantle expands and draws in water through openings at the base of the head, where the mantle ends. The water passes over the gills, located between the mantle and the body, and then is expelled in the direction it came from, but this time through a tube that pokes out from beneath the mantle. Normally a cephalopod expels water gently, but when it needs to move quickly, its mantle expands and contracts powerfully, jetting a stream of water that propels the animal through the water at speeds up to 20 miles an hour.

Most cephalopods are as harmless as a clam, or nearly so. Many make good eating. (Two of the most memorable dishes I have eaten were the squid in tomato sauce that my grandmother cooked for the traditional Italian Christmas Eve dinner, and an octopus creole prepared by a part-time chef in a small restaurant in southwestern Puerto Rico.) Some cephalopods, however, are among the most dangerous creatures known. Frank W. Lane, in his notable book *Kingdom of the Octopus*, writes of his belief that cephalopods indeed have killed people and that some have dragged small boats to the bottom. Lane notes that a man weighing 200 pounds, unless he struggles, can be held under the water by a pull of 10 pounds, considerably less than the force exerted by a cephalopod of only medium size.

The most terrifying of all cephalopods is the giant squid (*Architeuthis princeps*), the existence of which has been asserted by sea farers, particularly from northern Europe, since medieval times, but which failed to gain the acceptance of scientists until the last century. Squid have eight arms as well as two tentacles, which extend beyond the arms and have paddle-like tips. The arms and the tips of the tentacles are studded with suckers. The arms of a giant squid can reach as far as a dozen feet, and the tentacles 50 feet. When a squid attacks its prey, it seizes the doomed animal in its tentacles and draws it toward the embrace of the arms which hold it so the hooked beak can commence its grisly work.

The beak of a squid is quite powerful. The big Humboldt Current squid (*Omnastrephes gigas*), which lacks the bulk of the giant squid but nevertheless is a large, ferocious creature, has been known to bite hunks from a heavy wooden gaff. Humboldt Current squid will swarm over bait tossed into the water, slashing with their beaks, their oddly human-like eyes— which have eyelids, an iris and a pupil, and a moveable lens for focusing at distances—gleaming in the night.

A large squid is a frightening antagonist. Newspaper reports from the 1920s, noted in *Kingdom of the Octopus*, tell of a squid a dozen feet long that was dropped by a wave aboard the liner *Caronia* during an Atlantic gale. The brute grabbed the ship's carpenter, who, helped by others on board, battled for his life with an iron bar until after a struggle of several minutes the squid died. And after the troopship *Britannia* was sunk on March 25, 1941, one of the survivors was clinging to a piece of wreckage when a pair of tentacles reached from the sea and pulled him, screaming, to his death.

The giant squid, which reaches a length of at least 60 feet, probably was the animal described as the monster Scylla in Homer's *Odyssey*. Scandinavian literature from the Middle Ages groups the squid with other types of *Kraken*, or sea monsters, although the name now refers only to the squid. Not until the second half of the 19th century, when for some reason large numbers of giant squid were found floating dead on the sea or stranded ashore, did the world at large grasp that such colossal and terrifying beasts actually roved the sea.

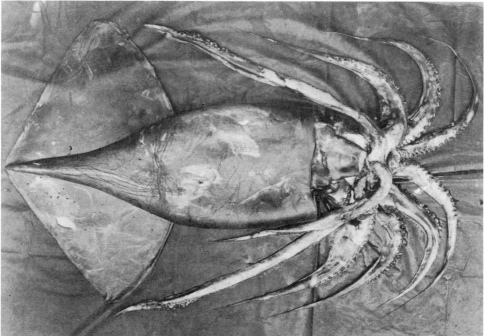

U.S. FISH AND WILDLIFE SERVICE

HORROR FROM BELOW: The giant squid shown here, a small specimen probably about 6 feet long, was boated and photographed aboard a research vessel in the late 19th century.

Not all of the squid that appeared in the late 19th century were dead when found. On October 26, 1873, three fishermen in a small boat found themselves in a life-and-death battle with a giant squid in a Newfoundland cove. The fishermen had seen a floating object, of no definite shape, and closed with it for a better look. When one of the trio jabbed it with a boat hook, the shape erupted in a flurry of arms and tentacles, gripping the boat and starting to pull it under. The boat was saved, with its occupants, when one of the party, a twelve-year-old boy, attacked the squid with an axe and sliced off an arm and a tentacle. The squid gave up the battle and the fishermen made for

134

shore. The fragment of tentacle chopped off by the youngster remained in the boat. When measured, it was found to be 19 feet long. The next month, in a bay not far away, four fishermen hauling in nets aroused a giant squid that was 32 feet long. One of the men killed it with a knife thrust between the eyes.

A deed of incredible bravery, or foolishness, was performed by three fishermen who tracked and killed a giant squid in April 1953 off Connemara, Ireland. The fishermen, in a curragh, sighted a squid about 60 feet long basking at the surface, and although armed only with a knife, they took after it. As the curragh drew alongside the huge beast, one of the fishermen slashed off an arm, whereupon the squid made for the open sea with the fishermen in pursuit. Several miles at sea they caught the beast again and followed it for two hours, slashing off a piece of tentacle or arm whenever they could. Finally only the animal's body and head were left. The fishermen removed the head and returned to port.

The existence of a giant squid longer than 60 feet never has been verified, but plenty of evidence exists that considerably larger specimens emerge now and then from the depths. The most frightening testimony, from newspaper reports of 1874, involved the steamer *Strathowen*, which was sailing from Colombo to Madras. According to the reports, the steamer came within sight of a small schooner, the *Pearl*, becalmed on a smooth sea. Then, in a scene that assuredly never was forgotten by any of those on the *Strathowen* who witnessed it, a monstrous squid arose from the glossy sea, snaked its arms and tentacles about the *Pearl*, and dragged the schooner into the depths.

The captain of the doomed ship was rescued by the steamer and later told his story. While the *Pearl* was becalmed, he said, the crew had witnessed a combat between a squid and a sperm whale. The struggling leviathans passed from view,

135

but soon afterward the captain noticed a huge form rising from the water about a half mile away. The form turned out to be a giant squid perhaps 100 feet long. It came closer, and the captain fired at it with a rifle, whereupon the squid hurtled towards the *Pearl*, rammed it, and dragged it down its cold embrace.

A much less disputable story was told by Frank Lane in his *Kingdom of the Octopus.* He quoted a report published in *Naturen*, the journal of the Bergen Museum, in Norway. The article, by Commander Arne Groenningsaeter of the Royal Norwegian Navy, described how giant squid several times attacked the 15,000-ton tanker *Brunswick* during the 1930s in its runs between Hawaii and Samoa. Lane corresponded with the naval officer for addition details, which are described in his book. The pattern of the squid attacks was the same in the three cases that Lane describes: a squid would overtake the *Brunswick* and strike her toward the stern—but each time, the squid would slip off and be killed as the ship's propellor chopped it to pieces. Lane wonders why the squid attacked in this manner and whether they mistook the *Brunswick* for a whale. If so, it would mean that squid sometimes turn the tables on whales, and prey on them. Indeed, in July 1966, South African journalist Lyn Freeman reported in the *New York Times* that a giant squid dragged a 7-foot-long whale calf to its death after a 90 minute struggle, during which the calf's mother circled the scene but failed to help her youngster.

Squid usually range in offshore waters, and octopuses inhabit the depths as well. They have been sighted as deep as 17,000 feet. But they come to the very edge of the sea, too. Octopuses are said to creep out of the water to capture rats and other prey, and while many zoologists dismiss the idea that that can happen, at least one octopus at a public aquarium has been found out of his tank, strolling across the aquarium grounds.

136

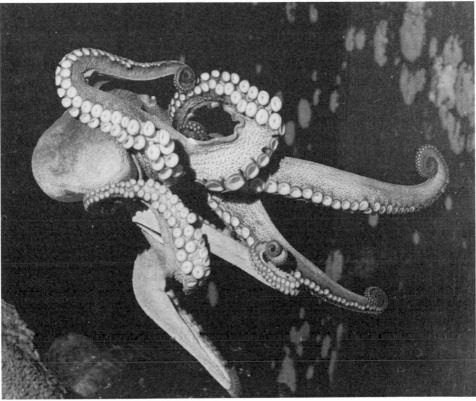

BIG GRASP: The giant Pacific octopus, which can grow to a span of 32 feet, is quite common in waters off the northwestern coast of North America. It is essentially a creature of cold waters.

Though often maligned, the octopus cannot be classified as a predator on man. Victor Hugo deserves much of the blame for the octopus's ill fame. In his book *Toilers of the Sea* he describes the octopus as "a disease embodied in monstrosity." Generally, the octopus preys on crabs, lobsters, and other crustaceans, whose shells it punctures with its hooked cephalopod beak. Modified saliva glands in the octopus produce a venom that, introduced into the prey by the bite of the beak, begins to digest the victim even before the octopus sucks up the softer parts.

Few species of octopus have the power to out-wrestle a grown man, although a number of people have been grabbed around the leg or foot by an octopus in shallow water and have had to batter and prod the beast into letting them go. In 1940, James Atz, now of the American Museum of Natural History, noted in the *Bulletin of the New York Zoological Society,* that in a few rare instances, octopuses have held on to people in the water until they drowned. The large Pacific octopus (*Octopus hongkongensis*) weighs more than 100 pounds and can spread out to a distance of 32 feet across its arms. Conceivably it could kill a man, but like other octopuses it is not especially aggressive. Perhaps the greatest danger from an octopus is the chance that the creature might wrap its arms around a man's face, causing suffocation—but only a large octopus could keep its hold if a man tried to dislodge it.

The most dangerous of all octopuses is the smallest, the blue-ringed octopus of Australian waters. It can.fit in a man's palm, but its venom is so toxic that people nipped by this miniscule creature have died within a few minutes.

CHAPTER 3

The Sting
of the Sea

The tiny blue-ringed octopuses, of the genus *Hapalochlaena,* creep among the rocks along many Australian beaches. They produce a venom so potent that a trace of it in the water with a crab convulses the crustacean and paralyzes it. Normally, an octopus intent on eating a crab envenoms its prey by biting it, but scientists, in laboratory experiments with venom extracted from the blue-ringed octopus, have demonstrated its toxicity in water. The venom of the blue-ringed octopus wrecks the functioning of the human neuro-muscular system. It blocks the conduction of nerve impulses, thereby halting the body's voluntary muscular action and preventing the victim from breathing.

When the animal's hooked beak tears into a victim, salivary glands near the octopus's brain secrete the venom, which flows through ducts that open at a single orifice near the tip of the tongue. The venom dispatches a crab in seconds, and humans bitten by the blue-ringed octopus have died, painfully, within an hour or so. As far as is known, the blue-ringed octopus—there are at least two closely related species—is the only octopus that kills people with its venom. That is not to say that, unknown to science, some of the larger octopuses may have venom of equal or even greater toxicity.

Although the beak of the blue-ringed octopus is powerful

141

enough to rip into a crab, people who have been nipped by the octopus rarely have felt its bite. Often a person's first realization that he has been bitten is when he begins to feel dizzy.

The fact that the blue-ringed octopus is potentially more deadly than a cobra was not even known until the 1950s, when the first human fatalities were recorded on Australian beaches. So little was known of the animal that as late as 1954, an experienced Australian diver, Kirke Dyson-Holland, died after being bitten by one that he had plucked from a tidal pool.

An Australian government study has revealed that the blue-ringed octopus inhabits the waters of at least 20 holiday resorts on Port Phillip Bay in Victoria. In the April 1972 issue of *Animal Kingdom*, the curator of fishes at Sydney's Taronga Park Zoo, U. Erich Friese, reported that in only one year a dozen specimens were collected on beaches near Sydney and delivered to the zoo's aquarium.

Small enough to be held in the hand, the blue-ringed octopus has a gem-like quality. Speckled rings of blue stand out against a brown-orange background and blaze with deep intensity when the animal is excited. Because of its compelling color, and because it lives in shallow water where it spends the day in crevices, under rocks, and even in discarded beer cans, this liliputian killer often attracts bathers. Some of them pick it up, with dire consequences.

Such was the case one day in June 1967, when a young soldier noticed a small octopus as he and two companions walked along some rocks off Cape Cove Beach near Sydney. The soldier picked up the octopus and put it on the back of his left hand. He left it there for about 10 minutes, when suddenly he felt dizzy. Realizing that the octopus must be responsible, the soldier tried to remove the creature—but the octopus clung fast until one of his companions ripped it away. Before anyone fully realized the severity of the situation, the soldier collapsed and stopped breathing. He was rushed to a nearby army hospital where physicians tried to revive him, but he failed to regain consciousness. Ninety minutes after he had discovered the octopus on the beach, he was dead. The only wounds that could be found on his body were two tiny bruises on the second knuckle of his left hand.

A teen-age boy in Australia suffered a similar fate after he had picked up a blue-ringed octopus on the beach to frighten his girl friend. The little creature slithered up his arm to the back of his neck and pecked the youth lightly. Within two hours he was dead.

Borgias of the Sea

The blue-ringed octopus shares a venomous nature with a surprisingly wide variety of marine animals. The venoms of some sea dwellers, in fact, rank among the most toxic known. Still other marine creatures are highly poisonous when eaten. There is a technical difference between being venomous and being poisonous, and some creatures are doubly deadly in that they are both. All venoms are poisons, but animals that are toxic when ingested are classified as poisonous, whereas those that transmit poison by a sting or a bite are said to be venomous. Venom is concocted in a gland or a specialized group of cells, and usually it flows through a duct to a sting or a fang. The system that produces and delivers the venom is called the venom apparatus.

The variety of venom apparatus, and of venoms and poisons themselves, seems devilish enough to engender envy in a Borgia. They are in no way fiendish, however, but are merely natural manifestations of adaptation in its many forms. Nevertheless, one cannot deny that most creatures with these adaptations seem to be peculiar in that they are either eerily beautiful or supremely grotesque.

143

Every phylum of the animal kingdom except the birds includes poisonous or venomous species. More than a thousand such species live in water, and they range from microscopic one-celled organisms to highly developed vertebrates. This great assemblage of creatures includes the sea wasp, a tropical jellyfish whose delicate tentacles are armed with stingers that can kill a man within half a minute after they brush against him. Also included is the stonefish, a reef dweller smaller than a football but more deadly than a huge shark, and the cone shell, a snail with a venom-tipped harpoon that has claimed many human victims.

Although poisonous and venomous animals live throughout the ocean, and in some places constitute a sizeable proportion of the fauna, they by no means represent a universal threat. In fact, Western science failed to show more than a cursory interest in this biologically important group of sea creatures until World War II sent servicemen into the Indo-Pacific region, where poisonous and venomous marine animals flourish in number and variety. It seems incredible that until so recently the scientific establishment should have overlooked such a fascinating and it now appears significant, part of biology, especially considering the fact that scholars of many ancient cultures recognized the unusual properties of these creatures.

For example, in the Fifth Dynasty of Egypt's Old Kingdom, in 2700 B.C., artists inscribed hieroglyphics depicting poisonous puffer fish (*Tetradon stellatus*) on tombs. Just as long ago, Oriental scholars wrote of the puffer and the poison it contains. The first known Chinese pharmacopoeia, the Book of Herbs, which was written between 2838 B.C. and 2698 B.C., refers to puffer poisoning; and an Egyptian papyrus of about 1500 B.C., which describes more than 800 prescriptions for treating human ills, carries instructions for dealing with intoxications caused by marine animals.

The Bible contains an apparent reference to poisonous and venomous animals of the sea in the Book of Deuteronomy (14:9-10), which was written about 1450 B.C. The passage instructs the Israelites: "These ye shall eat of all that are in the waters; all that have fins and scales shall ye eat; and whatsoever hath not fins and scales ye may not eat; it is unclean to you."

Researchers who study marine biotoxins believe that this passage was a primitive public-health provision aimed at eliminating poisonous and venomous aquatic animals from the diet of the Israelites. This belief represents more than romantic speculation, for the fact is that many fish whose flesh and organs are poisonous, and many of those with venomous spines, do indeed appear scaleless or finless. During World War II, American military authorities in the Pacific followed the example of the Old Testament writer when they issued warnings to troops in the region to avoid eating fish that seemed scaleless.

Another book in the Old Testament describes quite accurately another form of marine poisoning, the so-called red tide, which results from population explosions of microscopic organisms in the water. The Book of Exodus (7:19-21), written about 1500 B.C., relates: "And the Lord spake to Moses, Say to Aaron, Take thy rod and stretch out thine hand upon the waters of Egypt, upon their streams, upon their rivers, and upon their ponds and all their pools of water, that they may become blood . . . and all the waters that were in the river were turned to blood. And the fish that were in the river died; and the river stank, and the Egyptians could not drink of the water of the river; and there was blood throughout all the land of Egypt."

Aristotle, perhaps the Western world's first zoologist, described the venomous scorpion fishes in the third century B.C., and the Greek poet-physician Nicander (275-135 B.C.) described venomous aquatic animals in a poem. He believed, as many people do today, that moray eels are venomous; and he also believed that, spurred by desire, they would creep up onto dry land and copulate with serpents.

Dioscorides, a Greek physician who served with the Roman army during the first century A.D., collected different types of venomous aquatic animals from European waters, and Pliny the Elder, in his book *Naturalis Historia*, attributed considerable powers to the stingray. He asserted that it could kill a tree and corrode armor with its spine. He also believed that if the spine was burned and its cinders brewed with vinegar, the resulting preparation could cure a headache. Attached to the navel of a pregnant woman, the spine assurred an easy childbirth, according to Pliny, if it had been taken from a live stingray that had then been released in the sea.

Today, biologists, ecologists, biochemists, and scientists of many other disciplines have been drawn to the study of marine biotoxins. The field is so broad and new, however, that workers have yet to define most of the basic properties of the chemicals that interest them. A pioneer in marine-biotoxin research is Dr. Bruce W. Halstead, director of the World Life Research Institute in Colton, California. In *Poisonous and Venomous Marine Animals of the World*, a massive three-volume technical study compiled for the United States Government, he declares: "The fact that the pharmacology and chemistry of fish venoms are for the most part unknown is a regretable commentary on the state of knowledge of this subject. Moreover, the basic chemical structure has never been determined for a fish venom."

Scientists have traced some tantalizing links between various marine biotoxins. They have found, for example, that animals of the same phylum have similar venoms. And venoms that are adaptations for predation have certain common properties, as do those used in defense, even in unrelated creatures. However, the toxins of venomous animals differ considerably from those of poisonous animals, even among members of the same class. The toxin of the puffer fish, which is poisonous, and that of the stingray, a venomous creature, have nothing in common, even though both animals are fishes. On the other hand, the poison of the puffer fish is identical with that of a certain West Coast salamander, an amphibian.

The venoms and poisons of aquatic creatures produce a ghastly range of symptoms: convulsions, heart stoppage, respiratory collapse, paralysis, hemorrhage, searing pain, and breakdown of the nervous system. Some of the toxins of marine animals surpass the lethality of war gases by a factor of 3,000.

Because the chemistry of marine biotoxins is largely uncharted, scientists cannot even group them with reasonable accuracy. The state of the art today is explained by George Ruggieri, S.J. director of the Osborn Laboratories of Marine Sciences, a New York Zoological Society research institution that is a center for investigation of marine biotoxins. He says: "Because we lack detailed information on the chemical structures and the biological activities of marine biotoxins it is difficult to group them in a meaningful way. And although these toxins often are reported to be neuro-toxic, or nerve poisons, the fact is that since the whole toxin is a mixture of several components, they often elicit several biological activities." Some neurotoxins, for example, are cardiotoxic, and vice-versa.

Drugs from the Sea: Promise and Reality

Compared with the study of toxins from terrestrial organisms, research on marine biotoxins remains in the Middle Ages. It even may be that only a small proportion of the existing marine biotoxins have been discovered. There is substantial practical motivation for studying them, for, like other toxins, they are highly active in a biological sense and therefore useful in biomedical research. Because some marine biotoxins are so selective in their effects, they can be used as molecular probes; that is, they can be used experimentally to alter the functioning of tissues and cells to find out how they work. Some marine biotoxins already have limited use in medicine. For example the poison of the puffer fish, reduced in toxicity, is used in Japan as a pain killer.

During the 1960s some marine scientists, or more properly their public relations people, hailed the dawn of the era of drugs from the sea. Marine biotoxins, they claimed, would be developed into wonder drugs, much as toxins from soil microorganisms have furnished raw materials for antibiotics. The enthusiasm was premature for it takes decades in most cases to develop a drug. Few substances of significant value in treating human ailments have been developed from marine biotoxins to date, but this by no means says that the potential is not there. Several chemicals derived from poisonous and venomous marine animals have shown exciting results when used experimentally against cancer cells, tumors, and viruses, and as antibiotics.

The study of marine biotoxins has resulted in the development of an agent that kills human leukemia cells. In 1950 researchers found that a certain species of Caribbean sponge was rather unique. Its nucleic acids, the so-called building blocks of life, contained the sugar arabinose, instead of the sugar ribose, which in almost all organisms is the key ingredient of nucleic acids. Based on what they learned from the study of the sponge's nucleic acids, researchers synthesized a number of compounds that contained arabinose instead of ribose, one of which, produced in 1959, was cytosine arabinose. After a decade of perfection and testing, cytosine arabinose was licensed by the federal government. What it does, essentially, is substitute arabinose instead of ribose in cancerous

148

cells, curbing their growth and eventually killing them. Cytosine arabinose works in a substantial portion of the cases in which it is used, and although it is not fully effective, it may be the basis on which still more effective compounds are developed.

Scientists engaged in research on drugs from the sea now explain that it is unrealistic to expect them to turn up wonder drugs overnight. Dr. Ross F. Nigrelli of the New York Zoological Society, founding director of the Osborn Laboratories, and perhaps the leading authority on the subject, points out that the subject of marine biotoxins is so complex that relatively few poisonous and venomous sea creatures have been studied with any thoroughness. The problem, Dr. Nigrelli explains, involves much more than finding a useful chemical in a marine animal and then making it available. Once a promising form of chemical activity is observed, large numbers of the animals that produce the chemical must be collected. But first the animal's relationship to its environment must be studied so that it can be collected without harm to the ecological balance. The entire process may well involve a major expedition.

After they are collected, the chemical must be extracted, tested for biological activity, and purified, and its chemical components must be identified. For it be useful to humans, the chemical may have to be synthesized in a form somewhat different from its natural state. Eventually, if the agent still seems promising, it undergoes further testing and re-testing, and then, possibly, it will be put into use. The development of a drug in this fashion is a lengthy process that costs a great deal of money. It took millions of dollars, Dr. Nigrelli notes, to turn penicillin into a practical drug after its biological activity had been observed experimentally.

The first conference on drugs from the sea was held at the University of Rhode Island in 1967, during the initial flush of enthusiasm about the subject. Researchers optimistically applied for grants from government agencies and private industry, and many were approved. A flood of optimistic press releases appeared hinting, among other things, that great discoveries "potentially active against cancer cells" were just around the corner. Journalists snapped at the bait and in most cases swallowed it. Perhaps many of those involved were carried away with the glamour that seems to go with exploring the ocean. In any event, only a few scientists cautioned against excessive optimism.

Meanwhile, leading pharmaceutical companies initiated tentative steps toward full-fledged drugs-from-the-sea projects. mong the firms involved were Lederle Laboratories, a division of American Cyanamid Company, and Hoffman-LaRoche, a giant of the industry. Less than a year after the Lederle program began, however, it seemed as if interest was waning. The program's director, J.J. Denton, was quoted in the newsletter of the New England Marine Resources Information program in this fashion: "What we plan to do is skim the surface and gather up the most easily used organisms. We're not planning to get any more involved than that. We hope that by the time a lot of other people get around to this kind of marine research, we will already have been in and out of the sea."

This statement may have heralded the crash, for by 1972 many of the research programs that had seemed about to flourish were languishing as scientists sought vainly for continued funding. With surprising lack of foresight, funding agencies began to back away from research into the nature of marine biotoxins. Of the total 1972 budget of $21 million for the National Oceanographic and Atmospheric Administration's sea grant program, only $1.3 million went for research on drugs from the sea. The University of Rhode Island conference on drugs from the sea that year was a glum affair. The scientists who attended it held out little hope for any sudden achievement that might renew the enthusiasm of only a few years before. Lederle Laboratories revealed that it had closed down its sea research program, explaining that their investigators had turned up enough interesting substances to keep them busy, but at the same time admitting a lessening of interest in the entire subject.

The situation has not lacked some signs of hope, however. An extremely realistic approach to the use of marine biotoxins in bio-medicine was taken by Edward Miller of Hoffman-LaRoche, co-chairman of the 1972 Rhode Island conference. Quoted in the September 11, 1972 issue of *Chemical and Engineering News*, Dr. Miller predicted that the sea probably would be the initial source of biologically active compounds but not of raw materials for production of drugs. In other words, chemists might find useful drugs in chemicals produced by marine animals, but once identified, the drugs would be synthesized rather than derived from the animals in which they originated.

In 1973 the harvesting of one form of sea life for the production of a promising new drug drew the fire of conservationists. The Upjohn Company had discovered that the sea whip *Plexaura homomalla*, a gorgonian related to the corals, produces a form of prostaglandin similar to the forms derived from mammals. Prostaglandins are chemicals which exist in almost every tissue of the body and play key roles in an astounding variety of metabolic processes. Isolated initially from the seminal vesicles of sheep, these chemicals promise to be useful in controlling fertility, inducing labor in pregnant women, regulating gastric secretions and blood pressure, and many other forms of treatment. The tissues of few mammals contain prostaglandins in sufficient supply to be useful to scientists, however. Therefore the Upjohn Company had concluded an arrangement with the government of Grand Cayman Island to harvest sea whips form the island's waters. Environmentalists criticized the idea, claiming that the harvest would destroy the sea whips

151

and mar the beauty of the reefs. But Upjohn claims to have perfected a method of pruning the smaller branches of the sea whips, leaving at least 25 per cent of the larger branches intact so the colonial organisms can regenerate.

The Spines of Death: Stonefish

Venomous animals, which may strike without warning, are more feared than poisonous animals, for the latter can be avoided by simply not eating them. At least 220 species of fish are known to be venomous, and probably there are many more. Many venomous fishes are slow-moving, even sluggish, which is not surprising in terms of evolution, for creatures that can protect themselves with venom need not be particularly agile or swift.

The most dangerous family of venomous fishes is unquestionably the Scorpaenidae, the scorpion fishes, which range from temperate to tropical waters. At least 80 scorpion fishes possess venom, and most can be identified by their chunky, stubby form and the profusion of warts and other protuberances that cover their slimy bodies. Scientists divide the scorpion fishes into three main groups, which are distinguished from one another by the structure of the venom apparatus.

The most notorious of the three is the group comprising the stonefishes (Synaceja), reputed to be the world's deadliest fishes. They have accounted for numerous deaths. The three closely related species all bear 13 thick spines on the back. At the base of each spine is one gland at each side of the needle-like protuberance, which is concealed almost completely in the stonefish's warty skin. Sharp and strong enough to puncture even the thick rubber sole of a tennis shoe, the spines can penetrate deeply into flesh. When a spine is depressed, the venom sacs squirt their contents down a groove along either

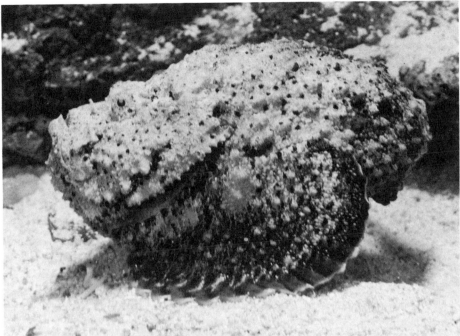

NEW YORK ZOOLOGICAL SOCIETY

WORST OF THE LOT: The stonefish, most venomous fish of all, so resembles a stone or hunk of coral that barefoot waders step on it unawares and are sometimes killed by its vicious dorsal spines.

side. They resemble hypodermic needles in their penetrating ability and their capacity to inject fluid.

Native to the Indo-Pacific region from the east coast of Africa to Australia, stonefishes frequent reefs where they lie in wait for prey. The stonefish is a superb example of natural camouflage. The warts and growths on its body conceal its shape, and even its mouth hides behind a fringe of tissue. Lying on a reef, a stonefish looks for all the world like a weathered chunk of coral or stone. Its foot-long body is almost impossible to detect against a background of reef or coral. I have often watched visitors to the New York Aquarium pause before a tank holding two or three stonefish, and then walk away complaining that there were no fish in the tank.

When a small fish approaches a stonefish, the squat creature moves with blinding speed, lunging at its prey with its bulldog mouth agape. In an instant, the smaller fish vanishes within the jaws of the stonefish, which immediately returns to its rigid pose at the bottom. The venomous spines serve the stonefish not for catching prey, but to protect it against sharks, rays, and other predators as it lies quietly on the reef.

The natural camouflage and defensive spines of the stonefish evolved long before man was around to step on it. However, these adaptations make the stonefish a menace when man enters the water, especially barefoot. Merely the prick of a spine can induce torturous pain, and often death. A woman was wading on an Australian reef several years ago when but one spine of a stonefish poked through a hole in her shoe. She spent 12 hours in agony and barely survived.

Many victims are less lucky. The venom of the stonefish can kill in minutes. A 15-year-old Indian boy was stung by a stonefish in March 1956 as he bathed near a beach in the Seychelles Islands. While swimming toward some rocks, the youth touched the sandy bottom with his foot and felt a stab of pain knife up his leg and radiate through his body. A stonefish had been resting on the bottom, and three of its spines had jabbed into the boy's foot. He managed to reach the rocks and crawl out of the water, while friends came for him in a boat. They put him aboard and headed for shore, but even before they got there the youth was frothing at the mouth and had turned blue. He died in a car on the way to a hospital.

In September of the same year, two men were fishing over a reef five miles from the Pinda Peninsula of Mozambique. They had left their canoe in shallow water and were wading across the reef, fish spears in hand, when one of the men suddenly collapsed. Before he lost consciousness, he mumbled one word to his companion: *sherowa*—the local term for stonefish. Within an hour the man was dead. He had been stabbed once in the second toe of his right foot.

Both of the deaths described above were reported by the South African icthyologist J.L.B. Smith, who himself once felt the pain of a stonefish's sting. Dr. Smith recorded his agony with precise scientific detail in a remarkable paper published in the journal *Copeia* in 1951. Accompanied by an assistant, Dr. Smith was collecting fish on a reef off the Pinda Peninsula in August 1950. He collected a stonefish and gave it to his assistant to place in a special container, rather than on a cloth-covered tray that the assistant carried to hold non-venomous specimens. Some time later Dr. Smith went to place more specimens on the tray, which his helper had balanced on his head. As Dr. Smith reached up to place the specimens on the tray, he felt his thumb stabbed to the bone. He thought he had jabbed himself on a hypodermic needle that was on the tray, but to his horror, when he examined the wound, he found two punctures instead of one. Within seconds he felt pain stabbing through his hand.

"With foreboding," Dr. Smith wrote, "I made the boy bend over. I lifted the cloth, and there was a stonefish . . . in the tray."

Tying a tourniquet of string around the thumb, and slashing the wounds to drain the venom, Dr. Smith headed for a nearby lighthouse, where he had been living. Meanwhile another assistant ran to summon Mrs. Smith.

"Before reaching the beach, only five minutes away," wrote Dr. Smith, "the pain was spreading through the hand . . . and was of an intensity [that I had] never before experienced." He describes the half-mile trip to the lighthouse as "a grim battle to remain conscious." All the while he resisted a desire to try to alleviate the pain by rolling on the ground.

155

Some of Dr. Smith's helpers, meanwhile, had summoned a local witch doctor, who soon arrived with his wife. While the bush physician cut the wounds and sucked the venom, his wife chewed a batch of green leaves; and then, when the witch doctor was finished, she placed the chewed leaves in the wounds. She then rubbed the injured thumb with a red stone, assuring Dr. Smith that the pain would diminish within six hours. All the same, Mrs. Smith doused the wound with disinfectant.

The pain increased, however, and morphine injected under the skin did no more to halt the scientist's agony than had the leaves and red stone of the witch doctor's wife. After four hours of torture, Dr. Smith found that he could diminish the pain by plunging his throbbing hand into hot water. After he soaked the hand for four hours, the pain had lessened enough so he could remove his hand from the water. By the next morning his thumb was swollen, black, and numb, and his lower forearm was sensitive to touch. Later, blisters formed on the thumb, which had become infected and required treatment with penicillin. Three months after the incident, Dr. Smith's hand and thumb were still sensitive and weak. "Having been stabbed by an eagle ray," Dr. Smith asserted, "It is possible to say that *Syaneceja* is in a class by itself."

Researchers from the University of Southern California and from the Commonwealth Serum Laboratories in Australia have discovered that stonefish venom disrupts both the circulatory and the nervous systems. By 1958, the Australian laboratories had produced a stonefish antivenin.

Another member of the Scovpaenidae is the zebrafish (*Peterois volitans*), also called the turkeyfish and lionfish. Like the stonefish, it dwells on the reefs of the Indo-Pacific. As gaudy as the stonefish is ugly, this foot-long creature is decorated with a wild assortment of spines, fins, and other appendages that make it look like a galleon under sail as it swims gracefully through the water. More than a dozen tabs of skin dangle over its head. Its pectoral fins are huge, and each has 15 separate rays that fan out at right angles to the body. The high dorsal fin is topped by 13 long spines, each with a flap of skin streaming from its tip like a pennant. The zebrafish is vividly striped in cream and maroon, making it as fine an example of warning coloration as the stonefish is of natural camouflage. Striking color and pattern in a wild creature often signals that the animal is particularly dangerous in some way—the skunk is a terrestial example of an animal with warning coloration. The zebrafish is dangerous, but not nearly so venomous as the stonefish. Unlike other venomous fishes, it will attempt to spear an opponent with its spines.

The zebrafish carries a total of 18 venomous spines, including the 13 on its back. Three of them extend beneath the fish, and there are two in the rear. The spines are grooved and largely filled with tissue that secretes venom. A single spine injects only a small amount of venom so, although the venom of the zebrafish is more toxic than that of many dangerous snakes, a wound from a single spine usually is not fatal. If more than one spine penetrates the flesh, however, the result can be critical.

When menaced, the zebrafish stands its ground, wheeling about in an attempt to drive its dorsal spines into its opponent. Many times I have tested the willingness of a zebrafish to stand and fight by reaching for it with a long stick. Each time the fish responded by turning and backing into the stick. John Prescott of the New England Aquarium reports that zebrafish react quickly to a paper cup if it is placed in the water with its open end toward the fish. Possibly, he suggests, the open end of the cup may look like the maw of a predator to a zebrafish.

Even young zebrafish seem ready to take on all comers. James Atz, icythologist and bibliographer, in *Animal Kingdom* (March-April 1962), described an occasion when adult zebrafish tried to gulp down young ones at the New York Aquarium.

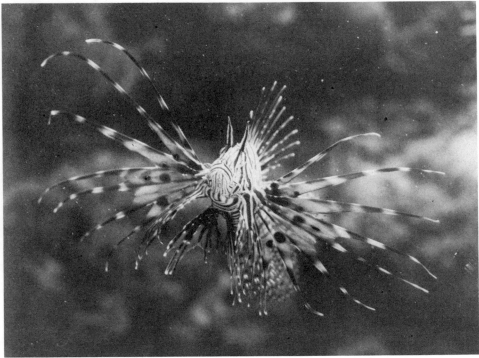

NEW YORK ZOOLOGICAL SOCIETY

DEADLY BEAUTY: This gorgeous cousin of the stonefish, the zebrafish, is one of the most beautiful creatures of the coral reefs of the Indo-Pacific. It is highly venomous but not quite as deadly as the stonefish.

The young responded by lowering their heads, erecting their spines, and preparing for battle, and the adults did not press the issue. Nixon Griffis, while diving off Mafia Island, Tanzania, found a zebrafish only an inch long in a tidal pool. Griffis says the venomous mite acted in the same pugnacious manner as a large zebrafish and seemed ready to oppose any adversary.

Although the zebrafish is said to be capable of killing humans, evidence is lacking that a human ever has died from a zebrafish sting. Edward Dols of the New York Aquarium, a former associate and diving companion of mine, was stung by a small zebrafish and, though he survived, suffered excruciating pain. One day in December 1957 he was cleaning a 100-gallon fish tank that, among other species, held three small zebrafish. One of the zebrafish, which had retreated into a corner as Dols reached into the aquarium with both hands to remove a large rock, suddenly raised its spines and jabbed him in the thumb.

Dols yanked his hand from the water and saw three small punctures in his thumb. "I had heard stories about zebrafish," he says, "but I thought they were exaggerated." He found out differently. Within a few seconds his hand swelled, and gradually it ballooned to twice its normal size. "It felt as if a fiery spike had been driven into it," Dols says. Within five minutes he could feel no sensation in the hand, even though cold water was run over it—but in another five minutes, on the way to the hospital, he barely could stand the pain. Like J.L.B. Smith after his encounter with a stonefish, Dols felt a strong urge to roll about on the ground. After he was treated at the hospital the pain subsided, but the area of the wound remained sore for several days.

Similar symptoms were reported by a professor from the Hebrew University of Jerusalem, who was stung by a lionfish in the Gulf of Aquaba. The pain, he reported, would not let him sit down. On the other hand, C. Lavett Smith of the American Museum of Natural History told me that he felt only slight pain when stung by a small zebrafish.

The third group in the family Scorpaenidae comprises the true scorpion fishes (*Scorpaena*). The venom of most true scorpionfishes lacks extreme toxicity, but that of the black vohu (*Emmydrichthys vulcanus*), which lurks near the lava-strewn shores of some South Pacific islands, is said to be highly dangerous. A scorpionfish with less dangerous venom stung astronaut-aquanaut Scott Carpenter on the left index finger in September 1965, while Carpenter was participating in the Sealab underwater habitat program.

Some species of the toadfish family (Batrachoididae) are venomous. One group of toadfishes (*Thalassophryninae*) has the most highly developed venom apparatus of any fish. The apparatus reaches its highest sophistication in species that inhabit South American waters. They carry two spines on the first dorsal fin and other spines on the gill covers. Unlike the grooved spines of scorpion fishes, the spines of South American toadfishes are hollow and hold the venom within, as do the fangs of a venomous snake. When the toadfish stings, venom glands at the base of each spine empty their dangerous contents directly into it, and the spine injects the venom into the victim.

Ichthyologist Albert Gunther first described the toadfish venom apparatus in 1864, and the following year, before the London Zoological Society, he described the effects of the sting as similar to that of a scorpion. Toadfishes have not been linked to any human deaths, however, and probably not all species are venomous. It is questionable, for instance, whether the oyster toadfish (*Opsanus tau*) of the Atlantic Coast of the United States is venomous, although this big-headed, thick-lipped creature bites viciously. Oyster toadfish often hole up in cans, old pipes, and other debris tossed into the water by the more slovenly members of our society, and whenever I see one of these small brutes glaring out at me while I am diving, I watch where I place my fingers.

Since ancient times, European fishermen have kept an eye out for the spines of weaverfishes (Trachinidae). The toxic nature of these creatures of the sandy shore were recognized long before that of most other venomous fishes. The spines of the weaverfish, carried on their dorsal fins and gill covers, inflict stings said to be as painful as those of the zebrafish. Severe stings can cause respiratory difficulty, convulsions, and some-times death. Weaverfish are sometimes caught as food fish, and most injuries from their spines occur when fishermen take them from nets, or fail to see them on the sandy bottom and step on them.

Every youngster who has fished for catfish knows they have spines that can sting. A sizeable number of the 1,000 species are venomous, and some are extremely deadly. Venom-ous catfishes usually bear spines on the first ray of the pectoral fins and in front of the dorsal fins. The venom is secreted by glands in the sheath of tissue that covers the spines.

The sting of most catfishes causes pain like that of a bee sting. But the marine catfish (Plotosidae) of the South Pacific is

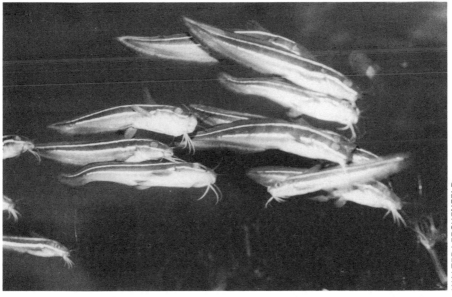

WALTER LERCHENFELD.
OSBORN LABORATORIES OF MARINE SCIENCES

WARNING COLORATION: The vivid stripes of the black-and-white marine catfish warn that this species is highly ven-omous. Venomous catfish often school in large numbers.

nearly as venomous as stonefishes. Slender fish about a foot long and vividly striped in black and white, they school in concentrations that sometimes measure several feet across. The schools, boiling with thousands of fish, take on the shape of large balls, and I cannot imagine a worse fate that being encompassed by one.

Dogfish and Rays

All the fishes discussed thus far are bony fishes, but among the cartilaginous fishes there are also species that are venomous. The spiny dogfish (*Squalus acanthias*), one of the most common venomous fishes of temperate seas, is a shark about 4 feet long that carries a short, thick spine before each of its two dorsal fins. Dogfish have a global range and often travel in schools of thousands as they swim through inshore waters, driving off cod, mackerel, and other fish of commercial importance. Dogfish schools also damage nets and other commercial fishing gear to the tune of several hundred thousand dollars yearly.

Tagging programs demonstrate that dogfish travel vast distances. In 1942, researchers tagged 300 dogfish off Newfoundland, and within four months one was caught 1,000 miles away off the Massachusetts coast. Five years later another of the tagged fish turned up off Virginia.

Sports fishermen as well as commercial fishermen consider dogfish great pests, for once a school has moved into an area, no other fish will be landed. While out for bluefish I have been frustrated by dogfish that have grabbed every line in the water, snatching bait, and worse, hooking themselves. The dogfish offers little sport, and removal of the hook is complicated by the presence of its venomous spines. The physical injury from the stab of a dogfish spine is severe and would hurt fiercely even if the spine had no venom. Some sources, including *Science in the Sea* contend that people have died after being stabbed by dogfish, but this is highly debatable.

Stingrays, which like sharks are cartilaginous, account for most of the injuries caused by venomous fish, not because they are especially aggressive but because they often lie half-buried in the sand in places frequented by bathers and fishermen. Stingrays injure about 750 people a year along the coasts of North America, according to Findlay E. Russell, director of the Laboratory of Neurological Research, University of Southern California. The world-wide toll of stingray victims probably numbers in the thousands, for these flattened cousins of the sharks live in inshore waters ranging from northern Europe, North America, and Japan to the temperate regions of the Southern Hemisphere. Like sharks, they also inhabit many large rivers in the tropics.

The weapon of the stingray consists of a sharp spine— sometimes more than one—at the end of a whip-like tail. The spine, derived from a structure similar to a denticle, is sheathed in tissue that produces venom. The venom affects the cardiovascular system, causing a loss of blood pressure and faster heart beat. Researchers now are investigating the possibility that the venom might contain an agent useful in treating high blood pressure.

Stingrays vary in size from midgets as small as a frying pan to gigantic *Dasyatis brevidaudata*, which is 6 feet wide and 12 feet long, with a tail as thick as a man's leg. This huge ray, which can drive its spine through the side of a wooden boat, weighs about 700 pounds.

The most dangerous stingrays belong to the family Dasyatidae. They favor shallow bays, estuaries, and river mouths near beaches. Another family, the Potamotrygonidae, live in fresh water. Until 1962, scientists believed they inhabited only the streams of South America, but since then these rays have

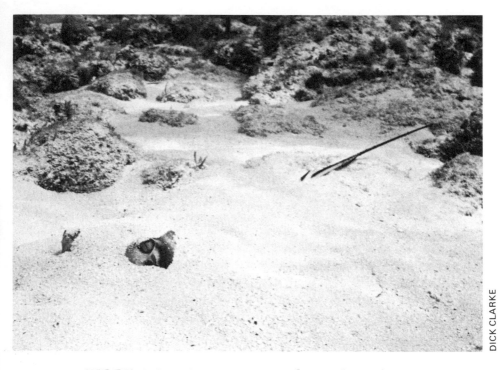

DICK CLARKE

HIDDEN DANGER: Lying in the sand amidst the coral off Grand Bahama Island, a venomous stingray is hardly visible. If stepped on, the ray will lash out with its barbed tail.

been seen in the rivers of central Africa and Indochina.

Most people are wounded by stingrays when they step on the creatures. A ray can lash out in any direction with its long, flexible tail, and anyone who steps on one of the animals is likely to be spiked in the leg. Most victims recover from wounds in the extremities, but if a ray manages to drive its spine into a person's chest or stomach, the results can be fatal.

Captain John Smith nearly missed his place in history because of a stingray. Six years before Pocahontas saved him from Indian war clubs and assured him a paragraph in the history books, he was jabbed by a ray in Chesapeake Bay. His ship had run aground on a shoal, and the captain decided to amuse himself by wading through the shallow water stabbing fish with his sword. One of the fish so transfixed stabbed back, driving its spine into Smith's wrist as the captain removed it from his sword. For the next several hours he writhed in agony while his men, anticipating his death, dug his grave. But gradually the pain eased, and by dinner time Captain Smith was hale enough to eat the fish that had caused his misery.

Others, struck in the trunk rather than on a limb, have not

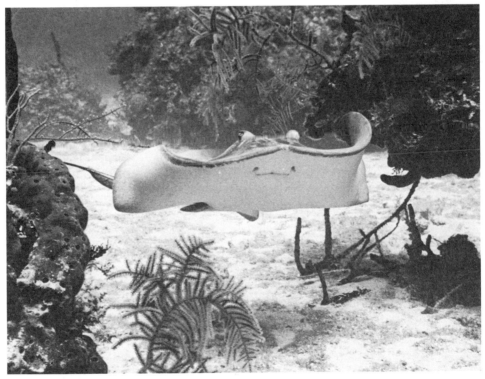

DICK CLARKE

UNDERWATER BALLET: With fluid grace, a stingray glides through a channel in between ridges of coral near the Hydro-Lab manned underwater habitat, off Freeport, Grand Bahama Island.

been so lucky. In 1955 a 12-year-old Mexican boy working on a shrimp trawler was lanced in the stomach by a large ray. He died in a few hours. Another fisherman, working on a tuna boat, was struck in the chest by a ray and died in five minutes.

Although stingrays strike at humans when stepped on, ordinarily they are no more dangerous than a guppy. I have flippered along with large rays, marveling at their fluid grace, without ever having to fear them. Even a ray lying on the bottom will not take a swipe at a swimmer unless approached within arm-length.

Only once have I been frightened by rays, and then it was a case of mistaken indentity. I was in the surf at Litchfield Beach, South Carolina, with my brother-in-law, James Hogan, who was standing about 20 feet away. As a large wave broke I noticed a long, dark form gliding toward us on the foaming crest. The form appeared sinuous, with its head biased horizontally, and I thought it was a hammerhead shark. As the form seemed to streak directly at my brother-in-law I yelled, "Shark!" He bolted for shore just as the shape in the water swerved to avoid hitting him. At that moment we saw that the shape was really two stingrays, one following the other so closely they appeared to be one animal. Still almost touching, the rays were swept back to sea with the retreating wave. I suspect that the rays were courting, for I cannot imagine these creatures playing in the manner of otters.

The Delicate, Deadly Coelenterates

Ironically, the deadliest animal in the sea, bar none, also is among the most delicate and fragile. The sea wasp (*Chirosalmus quadrigatus*) a small jellyfish of the Indo-Pacific region, has killed people in seconds after draping its tentacles over them. The sea wasp belongs to the phylum of creatures called coelenterates, or, as some people prefer to call them, cnidarians —the jellyfishes, corals, hydroids, sea anemones and their kin. All of these animals are venomous, though not all are so much so that they affect humans. Many of them rival flowers in delicacy and color, for superficially they resemble plants more than animals.

Coelenterates are among the simplest of animals. Most of them live in the sea, although a few of the 9,000 species in the phylum inhabit fresh water. Among the latter is the hydra, a tiny polyp that biology teachers often use as being representative of the entire phylum. Almost microscopic in size, the hydra nevertheless possesses the basic coelenterate structure. It has a sac-like body, or coel, with a wall consisting of two cellular layers—an outer skin and an inner lining of digestive cells —separated by a tough sheet called the mesoglea. The mesoglea gives the polyp a form whose central feature is a digestive cavity, or enteron. The enteron opens into the water through an orifice that is used both to ingest food and to eliminate waste, surrounded by a fringe of delicate tentacles armed with stinging cells.

Polyps have a considerable size range, some being barely larger than the period at the end of this sentence, while others are many times that big. Little more than hollow blobs of jelly with tentacles, the polyps that form coral are responsible for creating entire islands. In fact, they have built the largest single structure on this planet, Australia's Great Barrier Reef. Covering 80,000 square miles, the Great Barrier Reef was constructed bit by tiny bit during a million years or so.

Reefs flourish only in clear water because particulate materials suspended in the water settle on the coral, clog the polyps, and stunt their growth. Corals also need light, which is the reason coral growth diminishes at depths below 100 feet and vanishes before the water is 200 feet deep.

Each coral polyp sits within a tiny cup of limestone which

it builds by gleaning chemicals from the sea water and using them to produce a limey secretion through cells that line the exterior of its body. The base of the polyp's body is anchored to a substrate where the polyp lays the foundation of its cup. Most polyps have bright colors, but because they generally remain withdrawn in their cups during the day, the reef's true beauty is revealed only at night when the polyps emerge and splash the coral with brown, greens, oranges, and other hues. The only coral that is white is dead coral.

Coral polyps seem to produce very large reefs only when associated with mysterious little organisms called zooxanthellae which have characteristics of both plants and animals. Thousands of them live within each polyp and, since they are photosynthetic, assist their hosts by using the carbon dioxide the polyps produce as waste.

Polyps also receive other assistance in building a reef. A species of algae, *Lithothamnium*, grows in patches on the coral and secretes lime which adds to the reef. As it grows, the reef is covered with a skin of life, for the polyps live only on its outer surface. The matter beneath the surface is a mix of dead coral, shells, and detritus that has rained down on the reef for ages. This loose material congeals, partly through the action of huge concentrations of bristle worms that build tubes of sand glued together with their secretions.

All coelenterates have the basic polyp structure, although in the jellyfish the tentacles hang down around the rim of the gelatinous bell, which itself is a compressed version of the elongate hydra-type body. Coelenterates live either as individuals or in colonies, either as tubular polyps like the hydra, with one end open and the other attached to a substrate, or as a free-swimming medusa, like a jellyfish. Many coelenterates go through both stages.

Although coelenterates are simple biologically, they snare prey with a form of armament that is a masterpiece of natural engineering. Their tentacles are armed with structures called nematocysts, which when activated launch diminutive, venomous harpoons. Essentially a nematocyst consists of a round capsule, capped by a lid, containing a coiled, hollow thread bathed in venomous fluid. A hair-like trigger called a cnidocil projects from the capsule. When activated the cnidocil opens the lid and the tube, which is pointed, springs forth. The capsule actually turns itself inside out. The triggering of the cnidocil may be caused by chemical agents, rather than, as commonly believed, by brushing against it. Chemical activation of the cnidocil has been accomplished in the laboratory. Moreover, clownfish and other fishes that live in association with coelenterates certainly brush against the nematocysts without triggering them. If the point of the thread penetrates a target, the target is envenomated. (The name *cnidarian* comes from *cnidos*, the Greek word for thread.) A coelenterate may discharge thousands of nematocysts at a time, loading its victim with venom. The nematocysts of most coelenterates cannot penetrate human skin—but those that *can* present a serious hazard.

About 70 species of coelenterates have killed or injured humans. The gossamer-like appearance of coelenterate tentacles deceives, for their touch can feel like a lash of fire. The torment produced by the sting of many coelenterates probably results from a chemical called 5-hydroxytryptamine, a histamine in the tentacles that releases mechanisms in the skin sensitive to pain. The searing caress of a coelenterate's tentacles leaves the body scarred with vivid weals, and the effects of some of the more toxic venoms range from headache and nausea to respiratory failure and cardiac arrest.

Hydrozoa, the class of coelenterates that includes the little, harmless hydra, also embraces several highly toxic creatures. Representative of the class are the hydroids, polyps that live collectively in lush, branching colonies whose herbaceous appearance fools many people into believing them plants. Hydroid colonies in deep water sometimes stand higher than a man, but those that beard rocks and pilings at the seashore exist merely as fluffy growths an inch or so high. They are colored various shades of pink, purple, red, and other plesant hues. Most of the 2,700 species of hydroids are harmless, but a few sting with sufficient intensity to cause distress. The hydroid *Pennaria tiarella,* which sways in the undersea currents off California like a fern moving in the breeze, stings like a nettle and leaves a rash that lasts for several days. Few hydroid stings are more intense.

Much more painful are the venoms of the notorious "stinging corals," which are not true corals but are related to the hydroids. They consist of polyp colonies that build huge, branching, calcareous skeletons. The most dangerous of this group is the hydrocoral, *Millepora alcicornis,* which graces many coral reefs with an elegant form that often tempts people who see it to break off a piece. Giving in to the temptation is ill advised, not only because it mars the beauty of the reef, but because stinging corals also known as fire corals, sear those who touch them with white-hot pain.

A friend once told me of a victim of stinging coral who deserved his fate, if anybody ever has. My friend, an experienced diver, was accompanying a party of tourists on a skin-diving tour of a beautiful reef off northeastern Puerto Rico. Before they entered the water, the leader cautioned the party, as an aid in preserving the reef, not to remove chunks of coral as souvenirs. However, one man apparently decided he needed a souvenir more than the reef needed coral. After a short time in the water he swam back to the party boat, where his wife was sunning herself on deck. Boarding quickly, he surreptitiously reached a hand into his bathing trunks, produced a piece of the reef, and showed it to his wife. Minutes later he was rolling about the deck howling, and clutching his nether parts as if they were afire. His ill-gotten treasure turned out to be a piece of stinging coral.

Not all encounters with stinging coral are quite so painful. Dr. Martin Stempien, of the Osborn Laboratories of Marine Sciences, was examining a reef in the British Virgin Islands when he contacted a colony of them. He was exploring a crevice with his hand when it suddenly felt as if he had burned himself between the fingers. But the pain, Dr. Stempien says, was not very severe.

The graceful skeletons built by hydrocorals shelter myriads of polyps, which emerge through tiny pores that dot the colony's branches. There are two types of polyps in a colony, large individuals with wide mouths that gather small bits of food for the colony, and smaller ones, mouthless, that sting.

Quite unlike the hydrocorals and hydroids is the most infamous of the hydrozoans, the far-ranging Portuguese man-of-war (*Physalia*). It is thought by many people to be a jellyfish, but in reality it is a great, floating colony of hydrozoans. Within the colony live many different types of individuals, with different jobs to perform for the good of the aggregate. One polyp produces the bright blue, pink-crested float, the part of the man-of-war most evident from afar as it bobs over the surface, its glistening float pushed by the wind, the man-of-war cruises the sea. Beneath the float hang concentrations of other polyps, head down, and tentacles as much as 100 feet long that trail in the water. The tentacles, armed with batteries of nematocysts, resemble the ocean in color and thus blend into the background. When the tentacles contact an unwary fish, millions of nematocysts discharge their tiny harpoons, which inject a venom that paralyzes the prey.

The fate that awaits the fish is most unpleasant. The tentacles contract slowly drawing the paralyzed but still living fish toward the colony, where feeding polyps await it with

171

yawning maws. A sticky material and batteries of nematocysts rim the mouth of each feeding polyp, which, as the prey reaches it, clamps its maw over as much as 2 square inches of the fish's body. As the fully contracted tentacles, now bright blue, clasp the fish to the feeding polyps, they cover it so completely that the fish virtually disappears. With their guts everted, the feeding polyps digest the fish, absorbing nourishment for the entire colony. As the feeding polyps finish, they release their hold on what is left of the prey, and the few fragments that remain become part of the organic matter that constantly rains from surface waters to enrich the depths.

Ironically, one species of fish (*Nomeus gronovi*) takes shelter amidst the tentacles of the man-of-war. Whether it escapes the nematocysts by avoiding them, which seems impossible, or whether it is immune to the venom, remains a mystery. It may be that the fish has some quality that prevents nematocyst discharge. Occasionally, however, some of these fish do end up as prey of the coelenterate.

Bathers frequently encounter the man-of-war, which has stung many people but has only a handful of human deaths to its credit. Even if it has been washed up on a beach, the man-of-war remains dangerous and should be avoided. The result of a sting is an almost instantaneous pain which has been described as resembling an electric shock. Welts appear where the tentacles encountered the skin, and some victims experience fever, vomiting, and paralysis.

Nixon Griffis joined the list of man-of-war victims while diving in the Florida Keys. As he swam up from the bottom, he saw several men-of-war on the surface above him. He kept careful watch on the one nearest him but wandered into another, whose tentacles clung to his right arm. Griffis managed to get out of the water, but his arm throbbed with intense pain for five hours.

An editor of my acquaintance, Carol Sanders, told me of a

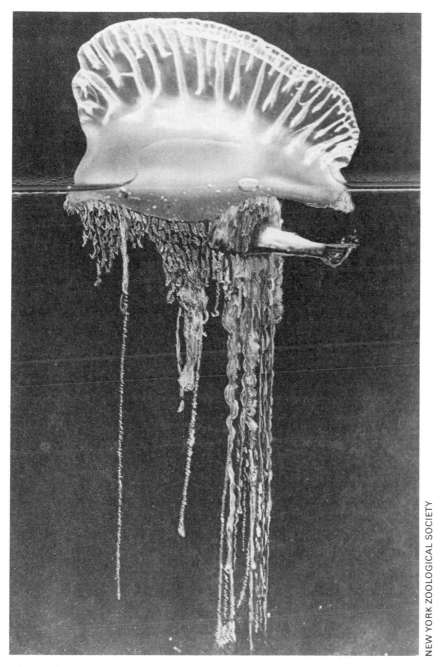

A COLONY OF FISHERMEN: Its tentacles contracting, a man-of-war draws in a fish to its maw where the prey will be digested. The man-of-war is not a single creature, but a colony of many small polyps.

painful experience she had with a man-of-war: "Swimming off Miami Beach in 1957, I saw what looked like a beautiful bathing cap floating about 75 feet offshore. I swam toward it, and when I was about 6 feet away I suddenly felt excruciating pain, like a burn combined with an electric shock in my arms and legs. To my horror I saw bright purple strands wrapped around them. I swam back to shore as best I could and knelt in the shallow water, trying to scrape the tentacles off on the sand. My actions and a plea for help attracted a curious but unhelpful crowd. For some minutes the tentacles clung tenaciously, as if they had a life of their own. Fortunately my cries for help did draw a friend down to the beach. With great presence of mind he pulled the tentacles off with a towel wrapped around his hand.

The pain persisted for hours, and for several days my arms and legs bore what appeared to be white scars, as if left by a lash. My fellow hotel guests, although unwilling to come to my aid on the beach, were geneous with advice afterward. They cordially urged me to sue the management for having ignored a city ordinance requiring that a picture of the Portuguese man-of-war be posted at the beach. Back in New York I regretted not having heeded their advice, for my encounter with the creature resulted five days later in so violent an allergic reaction that I required emergency medical treatment."

The true jellyfishes, which belong to the class Scyphozoa, are individual medusae, rather than colonies of polyps like the man-of-war. The bell, or umbrella, of the jellyfish is fringed with tentacles at its rim. As the bell, pulsing rhythmically, moves through the water, the tentacles enmesh fish that they contact. The fish are paralyzed, lifted to the hollow stomach on the underside of the bell, and digested. Jellyfishes capture and consume relatively large fish for their size. The largest of these coelenterates is the Arctic jellyfish (*Cyanea arctica*), a monster with a bell that measures 8 feet across and tentacles that trail for a distance of 200 feet. It never has been known to sting a human being, but, considering the relative size of the fish eaten by smaller jellyfishes, it is reasonable to ask whether a large Arctic jellyfish might entrap a man, sweep him to its bell, and engulf him in its stomach.

Smaller members of the genus *Cyanea* inhabit both coasts of the United States and other shores as well. Many sting painfully, and the venom of one species, the sea blubber, or pink jelly, (*C. capillata*), can cause loss of consciousness and is reported to have caused fatalities. Some scientists class this and the giant Arctic jellyfish as the same species. The white sea jelly, *Aurelia aurita*, also appears along our coasts. This creature, whose bell is a half-foot wide, can sting painfully.

The most venomous of the jellyfishes, and probably the deadliest creature in the sea, is the sea wasp, the terror of Australian beaches. It is about the size of a small balloon and can kill in seconds. The venom of this creature was isolated at the University of Queensland in 1966. Once the venom enters the human bloodstream it can reach the heart muscle, and if enough venom is involved, it can paralyze the heart in half a minute. The pain caused by the venom may be the most excruciating in the world. Dozens of people bathing in Australia have been stung, and many have died. One man brushed by a sea wasp died in less than 30 seconds. Another ran screaming from the water with a sea wasp clinging to his back and died in an hour. An eleven-year-old girl died within a minute after being stung on the leg while wading 30 feet from shore. A few years ago, at a beach near Cairns, Queensland, a father was teaching his young son how to swim when a sea wasp struck the child. Screaming with pain, the boy was rushed to the hospital, but he died a half hour after he had been stung even despite efforts by doctors to keep his heart beating.

The day on which the boy was stung was dull and calm. That sort of weather, coupled with an incoming tide, seems likely to bring sea wasps near shore. Beachwise bathers avoid the water on such days.

The third class of coelenterates, the Anthozoa, contains the least dangerous and also the most members of the phylum. Included are the sea whips, sea fans, corals, and sea anemones, which make some parts of the hydrosphere resemble a fairyland. Of this class, only some of the sea anemones and a few of the corals can harm humans.

The sea anemones and corals are closely related and constitute the subclass Zoantharia. Sea anemones, which range in size from hardly visible mites to creatures that would fill a mix-

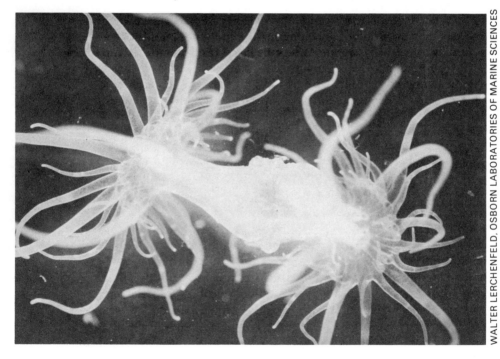

ANEMONE FREAK: This sea anemone has developed a freakish second "head." It was photographed at the Osborn Laboratories of Marine Sciences, Brooklyn, New York.

ing bowl, are named after the little flowers that dot the ground in woodlands, and, indeed, they are flowers of the sea. The polyps, which have a slit-like mouth, are mounted on long stalks and have tentacles that resemble delicate petals. They are brightly colored in shades of red, white, purple, yellow, and brown. Anchored to the sea floor, or to rocks or shells, sea anemones gracefully wave their tentacles in the water, like blossoms moving in the breeze.

Fish and other small creatures that come too near these flower animals encounter the nematocysts in the tentacles. As would happen with other coelenterates, the prey is paralyzed and brought to the anemone's mouth. A few sea anemones have stings powerful enough to harm humans. They include the rosy anemone (*Sagartia elegans*) of European waters and the sea anemone *Actinia equina* of the eastern Atlantic.

Corals, which build their great reefs only where the water temperature stays above 70 degrees F., are delicate polyps, each within its little cup of lime. I doubt if anyone who has spent time diving in the tropics has not experienced the painful cuts that result from carelessly rubbing against or banging into coral. Untreated, the cuts can become infected and ulcerated taking months to heal. A few corals sting painfully, however. The most well known of these is the elkhorn coral (*Acropora palmata*), whose branching structures reach out from reefs at depths of 5 to 30 feet.

The polyps that build coral reefs withdraw into their cups during the day, but at night they emerge to carpet the reef in yellow, green, and red. Seen at night with the aid of a light, the reef is more colorful even than during the day.

Sea Urchins and Cucumbers Researcher's Delight

Of the groups of marine animals that interest biomedical research, none holds more promise than the echinoderms—the sea urchins, sea cucumbers, sea stars, and their relatives. Of the 6,000 species of echinoderms, about 80 are venomous or poisonous. Many produce chemicals that have proved useful in the laboratory, if not in clinical medicine.

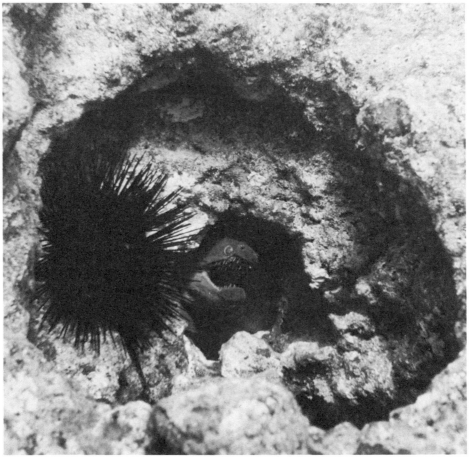

RON CHURCH. PHOTO RESEARCHERS

DISAGREEABLE DUO: A snaggle-toothed moray eel peeps out through a crevice in the coral around a sharp-spined sea urchin. Sensible divers will steer clear of both of them.

The sea cucumber looks for all the world like a slightly misshapen version of the garden vegetable from which its name is derived. Sea cucumbers crawl along the bottom in many parts of the sea, from depths of only a few feet to thousands of feet below the surface. One species, the Bahamian sea cucumber (*Actinopyga agassizi*) inhabits the clear waters of Bimini, site of the Lerner Marine Laboratory of the American Museum of Natural History. The brownish-red Bahamian sea cucumbers swarm over the bottom in some places, moving about on the tiny, suction-tipped tube-feet that characterize echinoderms. When menaced by predators, the sea cucumber has a particularly noxious way of defending itself. Its cloaca ruptures, and the animal spews its insides into the water, an act that surprisingly does not harm the sea cucumber. The predator that triggered the action finds itself in the midst of the sea cucumber's gut and assorted glop, including a pair of tube-like structures called the Cuvierian organs which tie in to the creature's respiratory system.

During the early 1950s, Ross F. Nigrelli was studying Bahamian sea cucumbers at the Lerner Laboratory. He discovered that when one of the animals spewed its guts into the water something in the odious mess killed fish. Investigating further, he found that the most toxic material was in the Cuvierian organs. When an extract was prepared, one ounce of it in 750 gallons of sea water killed fish in less than a half hour. Dr. Nigrelli named the chemical holothurin, because the sea cucumber is an echinoderm of the class Holothuroidea.

Since Dr. Nigrelli prepared holothurin extract, researchers have found that it has a host of interesting effects. It is a powerful nerve poison, blocking the action at the synapse without deteriorating the nerve. This means it has potential as a pain killer. The chemical also seems to supress the growth of tumors, at least in experimental mice. Natives of the South Pacific preceded Dr. Nigrelli in knowing that the sea cucumber

179

contained a toxic material. They have used the innards of this echinoderm to poison fish in enclosed lagoons since ancient times. Holothurin can also be extracted from sea stars and other echinoderms.

Some echinoderms are studded with spines which can inflict painful wounds. The crown-of-thorns sea star (*Acanthaster planci*), which during the 1960s began to chew its way through the Great Barrier Reef, carries a forest of spines as long as a man's finger on its platter-sized body. The spines puncture flesh deeply, and they possess a venom that irritates the wound and in some cases makes it very painful.

The worst offenders among echinoderms, however, are the sea urchins, of the class Echinoidae. The basic shape of sea urchins is globular. Aptly known as living pincushions, they are covered with spines except for a small region on the underside of the test, or shell. The test, which carries the spines in individual sockets, surrounds the soft parts of the urchin. The soft parts are mostly reproductive organs, which in some cultures are considered a gastronomic delicacy. Among the spines are pincer-like structures called pedicellariae, each of which consists of two or three fangs mounted on a flexible stalk. These pincers grasp and hold prey. Sea urchins nestle in almost every crevice and cranny of coral reefs. Moving on tube-feet and on their spines, they also travel over the rocks of temperate seas; in parts of the Arctic they literally carpet the sea bottom.

Urchins of the family Diadematidae, the so-called hatpin or black sea urchins, plague divers, swimmers, and waders on tropical reefs. Their hollow spines resemble knitting needles in size and shape, except that they are sharper and are filled with venom. The spines seem always in motion, like fencing foils feinting here and there, searching for an opening. When a shadow falls on an urchin, the spines swing around in the direction of whatever cast the shadow, presenting a front as prickly as a phalanx. The hand or foot that brushes against the spines comes away with their tips which release a violet-colored venom as they penetrate the skin. Stepping on a black sea urchin creates a sensation similar to treading on a red hot spike, and the burning pain lasts for several hours if the penetration is deep. Moreover, the spine tips in the wound increase the chance that it will become infected.

Countless people have been jabbed on the hands or feet by black sea urchins, but I have had the ill luck to be stabbed in the rump by one of the creatures. While free-diving over a Puerto Rican reef one time, I was treading water in a near-standing position when my flippered foot stepped on an urchin. Its spines drove through the heel of the flipper and into my flesh. Instinctively I bent in the water to grasp my foot, and the motion sent my body backward in a half circle. Behind me a few feet under the surface rose a shelf of rock that held another urchin. As I spun in the water I literally sat on the spiny creature. It was a toss-up whether the anguish caused by the spines was greater than the embarrassment of having to ask a friend to remove their tips from my posterior.

A sea urchin that lives in the Indo-Pacific region can cause truly agonizing pain with its sting. The urchin, *Toxopneustes pileolus*, possesses venom that attacks the nervous system. Persons stung by this creature in deep water risk death by drowning. Not only does the urchin have needle-like spines, but its extremely large pedicellariae seem to have a life of their own. Equipped with venom glands that open through ducts on the tip of the fangs, the pedicellariae hold on with a bull-dog grip; and if detached from the urchin while clamped in flesh, they continue to hold on, pouring venom into the wound.

Stinging Worms

There are many marine worms in the phylum Annelida,

which include the familiar earthworm. Some of the marine forms are capable of inflicting nasty bites, which some researchers regard as venomous. The clamworm (*Nereis*) allegedly can sink its pincer-like jaws into a finger, but I have used hundreds of them for bait and never have been bitten by one.

I am much more ready to believe that some of the other marine annelids are venomous and indeed quite dangerous. During the summer of 1972 one of the creatures caused me a night of extreme pain. I was diving in a shallow, rocky cove at Yabucoa, Puerto Rico, when I saw a worm of gorgeous color creeping across a patch of sand on the bottom. It was about half a foot long, and it had reddish-pink sides and bore white tufts of bristles along its entire length. It was a fireworm (*Hermodice carunculata*), a species described as capable of serious stings. Forgetting that I was not wearing gloves, as I normally do when diving, I reached for the worm to take a better look at it. I had barely picked up the creature when I dropped it quickly realizing that I was gloveless, but several of the bristles, as fine as spun glass slivers, had already stuck to the thumb and first two fingers of my left hand. I was out of the water within a minute, and already the pain had begun to spread through my fingers. It felt as if hot needles were penetrating my flesh, but I could see no marks to indicate where the bristles had entered.

My fingers felt as though they were afire, and at the same time they were numb. Within an hour the pain had radiated up my arm toward my shoulder. Although a physician treated the affected area with various pain killers, my discomfort continued. I remembered what Ed Dols had told me about his urge to roll on the ground after being stung by a zebrafish. Once or twice I had the same desire, but such moments were fleeting. I am sure that the pain was not as severe as that inflicted by the spines of a zebrafish. The pain in my arm gradually retreated until only my hand throbbed; and finally, after six hours, it began to leave my fingers—but they remained sore for a day.

Sponges: Aquatic Enigmas

Some of the most fascinating research on marine biotoxins focuses on sponges, animals so primitive that they were regarded as plants until the 19th century—although Aristotle long ago placed them in the animal kingdom. They lack sensory organs and, as adults, the power of locomotion. They are the only multicellular animals without a mouth. Instead of ingesting food through a single opening, the sponge filters tiny bits of organic matter from the water that flows through the pores, passages, and channels honeycombing its rigid structure. Sponges, which have been sidetracked from the main line of evolution, seem virtually ageless. They also seem indestructible; when strained through a sieve, sponges have been known to reaggregate and form a new animal. Many sponges appear to resist diseases, possibly because they protect themselves with chemicals that destroy disease organisms.

For several decades, researchers have known that various aquatic animals are killed by chemicals extracted from certain sponges and placed in the water. Recently, Dr. Stempien and other investigators at the Osborn Laboratories have discovered substances in sponges that display antibiotic activity in the test tube, but so far not beyond that point.

A few sponges can injure humans, but none cause serious harm. The most injurious is the West Indian fire sponge (*Tedania ignis*), which causes a burning sensation and a rash on contact with the skin. The symptoms may be caused by an allergic reaction to the sponge, however, not by a toxin.

183

Killer Snails

Somehow it is not difficult to conceive of mollusks such as the squid and the octopus as dangerous, but it surprises many people to learn that also among the mollusks are snails that have claimed human lives. The cone snails, of the family Conidae, have killed at least fifteen persons and have injured dozens more. Their weapons are venomous "darts" which have evolved from the radular teeth of normal snails.

A typical cone snail has a ribbon-like structure called a radula which is studded with fine teeth like those of a file. The snail uses the radula to rasp away at food. In the cone snails, the teeth have become modified into long, hollow darts, barbed near their pointed tips. They are stored in a sac within the cone like arrows in a quiver. When ready for use, each tooth contains a highly toxic venom, squirted into it by a muscular bulb. The cone uses its darts to kill prey such as fish and other mollusks. New ones are produced to replace those used to shoot victims.

When a cone prepares to strike, it picks up a dart with the tip of its long, muscular proboscis—which it can extend several inches from its shell—and waits for a chance to stab it into its victim. I once watched a textile cone (*Conus textile*) ambush a periwinkle half its size. The cone lay buried in the sand with just the tip of its siphon protruding above the surface. Water that flows into the cone through the siphon passes over a special organ called the osphradium, which senses chemical clues to the presence of prey. When the periwinkle drew within two inches of the textile cone, the cone rose from the sand with its maw agape, and its long proboscis snaked toward the periwinkle. For several seconds the cone played its proboscis over the periwinkle's shell as if fingering it for an opening. As I watched, the proboscis lingered for a moment at the periwinkle's operculum, or lid, then rippled, flexed, and jabbed a dart into the victim. As the cone struck, a wisp of smoky white fluid drifted in the water, and the periwinkle, now limp, oozed out of its shell. After killing its prey, a cone stretches its mouth and either swallows the prey whole or digests it part by part.

The cone also uses its venomous darts to defend itself, and at least 8 of the 500 species of cone snails can kill humans. Most cone stings have occurred in the South Pacific, and in almost every case the victim had picked up the cone; most species have gorgeous shells.

One cone, in fact, ranks among the most prized of shells. The glory-of-the-seas cone (*C. gloriamaris*), has brought prices as high as $2,000. There is a story of an 18th-century French aristocrat who owned a glory-of-the-seas and believed that there was only one other such shell in a collection—one belonging to a Danish shell fancier. The Frenchman managed to buy the Dane's shell at an auction, and immediately he threw it to the ground and pulverized it with his foot, asserting that now he owned the *only* glory-of-the-seas. (Several other people did own shells of the glory-of-the-seas, but the French collector was unaware of the fact.)

The first known fatality attributed to a cone shell, reported in 1705 by a Dutch naturalist, involved a woman slave on the Indonesian isle of Banda. The woman was skining fish when she noticed the shell and picked it up. She did not realize that the cone had stung her, but suddenly her hand felt as if it was being tickled, and the sensation spread throughout her body. Within a few minutes she died.

In 1968 Dr. Halstead, the marine biotoxin authority, and researcher Reginald D. Rice described in the journal *Toxicon* the death of a Filipino man from a cone sting. In August 1964 the man was diving on a reef off Guam when he picked up a cone shell and placed it in his left shirt sleeve. For a while he continued diving, not knowing he had been stung, but after an hour or so he began to feel numb and weak. An ambulance was summoned and the Filipino was taken to a hospital, but on the way his breathing failed and he died.

Like other marine biotoxins, cone venom is little understood. Scientists believe it acts against nerve and muscle functioning, and indeed respiratory failure and heart arrest are among the most serious symptoms. Some cone venoms seem no more harmful than the sting of a bee, but because others can cause rapid death, all cones should be treated as if they were dangerous.

CHAPTER 4

The Poisoners

The puffer fishes, of the family Tetraodontidae, contain a nerve poison that is 150,000 times more potent than curare. It is one of the deadliest poisons known. Yet in Japan, diners flock to special restaurants that serve puffer in elaborately arranged dishes. Called *fugu*, it is considered a great delicacy. Specially licensed and trained chefs serve *fugu* in several ways, sometimes with slices of ray puffer delicately shaped into petals and arranged in the representation of a flower or flying bird. Flesh, fins, skin, ovaries, livers, and testes of the puffer find their way to the table. Puffers are said to be especially tasty from November to February, although the complete puffer season lasts from October to May.

Fugu disciples claim that the dish tastes like chicken, but it may have more of an enticement than its effect on the palate. Many people eat *fugu* regularly—it is something of a fad among the wealthy—and they seem to experience a mild high. After eating the dish, they feel flushed with warmth and oddly exhilarated, while their lips and tongue tingle with a strange numbness. This sense of euphoria may indeed be the reason why *fugu* remains a popular dish, despite the fact that about 100 Japanese die annually from consuming it.

Puffer poisoning is more deadly than any other form of fish poisoning. Victims have been known to succumb in min-

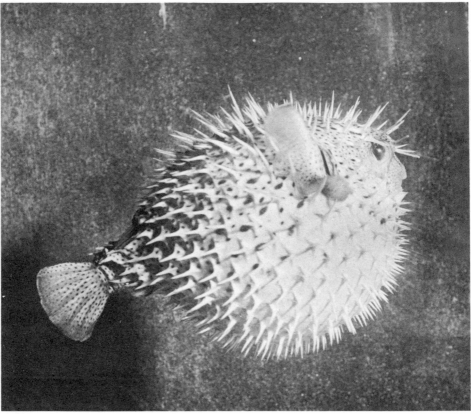

LIVING BALLOON: A porcupine fish, a cousin of the puffers, inflates itself with water when threatened. Like the puffers, its flesh is poisonous to eat.

utes. However, many fishes other than puffers—and in fact several aquatic invertebrates as well as the fishes—are highly poisonous. Some are poisonous in will-o'-the-wisp fashion, which makes them all the more dangerous. People who eat *fugu* generally realize they are gambling with their lives, for there is no question that puffers contain poison—but some other fish poisons are highly erratic: fish that never before have been poisonous in a given locale may suddenly turn toxic almost overnight.

190

The problem of fish poisoning gains in importance when one considers how drastically many nations of the third world need protein for their malnourished populations. The United Nations and other international organizations have suggested that fish-protein concentrate might supplement the protein-poor diet of people in many parts of the world. Researchers say, however, that such a concentrate, in the form of fish meal or fish flour, probably could be produced in quantity only in the more technologically advanced nations. Suppose that such a program were initiated: imagine the political ramifications, aside from the human suffering, that would ensue should a batch of poisonous concentrate manufactured in a Western nation be distributed in an African, Asian, or South American country.

Fugu: The Potent Puffer

Puffer poisoning, although the most severe type of fish poisoning, promises not to become a major international problem, for puffers are regarded by most people as unattractive and unpalatable. However, one species of puffer has begun to appear on tables in the United States, its identity disguised by the appealing but deceiving name *sea squab*. Perhaps sea squab it must be, for few people lick their chops at the thought of eating the common blowfish (*Sphaeroides maculatus*), that small puffer that irritates fishermen by stealing bait meant for more desirable fish.

Sea squab would be more accurately called blowfish tail, for only the tail of the fish is eaten. At least one death in the United States has been attributed to poisoning from eating blowfish—a 65-year-old woman died in March 1963 in Homestead, Florida. Bruce Halstead, in the U.S. government publication *Poisonous and Venomous Marine Animals of the World* cites this death and states: "Undoubtedly more deaths will occur in the United States as puffers grow in popularity and authorities fail to instruct people in proper preparation of these fishes."

Puffers are so named because their bodies contain air sacs that they can inflate when menaced, making them larger and more impressive to enemies. Almost all puffers, as well as their relative the ocean sunfish, are suspected of containing a poison called tetrodotoxin, after their family name. Tetrodotoxin is present in the skin, flesh, intestines, and sexual organs of the puffer, especially during the breeding season, indicating that the production of the poison relates to sexual activity.

Tetrodotoxin is unusual among fish toxins in two ways: unlike most, it is not a protein; and its chemical structure has been determined. Tetrodotoxin obstructs the flow of nerve messages by somehow changing the nerve-cell membrane's permeability to sodium. The poison acts so selectively that while the passage of sodium is blocked in both directions across the membrane, potassium continues to permeate the membrane in normal fashion.

Because tetrodotoxin stops the transmission of nerve impulses so selectively, it has excellent potential as a pain killer. In fact, low concentrations of tetrodotoxin are marketed in Japan as an analgesic. Orientals have used tetrodotoxin for a long time to treat a variety of ills, including asthma, headaches, coughs, spasms caused by tetanus, and even some of the symptoms of leprosy.

One of the major discoveries in research on biotoxins was that tetrodotoxin and a neurotoxin produced by a newt native to California are chemically identical. During the 1930s an embryologist at Stanford University, Victor Twitty, discovered a very toxic poison in a newt he was using as the source of embryonic tissue for transplants in the amphibians known as mole salamanders. The transplants paralyzed the salamanders, indicating that the poison involved was neurotoxic. The newt poison was isolated by Stanford scientists a few years later and named tarichatoxin. Then, after World War II, Japanese scientists succeeded in purifying tetrodotoxin. By the 1960s, researchers on both sides of the Pacific realized that tetrodotoxin and tarichatoxin were chemical duplicates, even though they came from animals of different phyla. Since amphibians are one step above fishes from an evolutionary standpoint, comparison of the genesis of the two chemicals and of their physiological roles may increase understanding of the evolutionary links between the two groups of animals.

Tetrodotoxin can send a person to his eternal reward very rapidly. Among the first symptoms is a tingle or numbness of the mouth, like the sensation felt by the people in Japan who eat *fugu*. If enough tetrodotoxin is ingested, the sensation creeps through the rest of the body within a short time, accompanied by pain and sometimes diarrhea or vomiting. Death usually occurs because respiration ceases when the muscles involved in breathing fail to receive nerve impulses.

The muscular paralysis caused by tetrodotoxin differs from that caused by tetanus, which makes the muscles convulse. Tetrodotoxin causes a *lack* of muscular function because the muscles, instead of contracting, simply slacken.

Puffer poisoning has been the subject of scientific curiosity for centuries in Japan, where more than 300 years ago one researcher tried to determine the toxicity of puffer flesh and viscera by feeding them to prisoners. Oddly, his subjects showed no ill effects from their hazardous meal. Europeans became curious about puffer poisoning during the 17th century, when Western traders began to visit the Orient in substantial numbers. Engelbert Kaempfer, a physician at the Dutch embassy in Japan during the 1690s, wrote that the puffer could balloon itself "into the form of a round ball." Several puffers were deadly poisonous, Kaempfer reported, but the Japanese readily ate them after tossing away the head, gut, and bones, and carefully washing what remained. Soldiers, according to the Dutch doctor, were forbidden to sample the puffer, and if a soldier died from puffer poisoning, his son forfeited his post, which under the rigid Japanese caste system, would have gone to him. One form of puffer was so deadly, according to Dr. Kaempfer, that no amount of cleaning lessened its toxicity, and people bent on suicide chose this fish for their last meal. Another physician, Peter Osbeck of the Swedish East India Company, reported that Cantonese law banned the sale of puffers under severe penalty.

The first recorded puffer poisoning in the New World took place in 1706, when four Spanish soldiers caught a puffer in the Gulf of California and ate its liver. One soldier lived but a half hour after he consumed the liver, and another died a short time later. The other two lived, but only after suffering acute symptoms.

Captain James Cook seemed to have considerable trouble with poisonous fish during his second global voyage, in 1774. A week after sixteen of his men were sickened from eating puffer, Cook himself suffered a severe attack of poisoning.

Puffer poisoning makes victims comatose, a fact that is responsible for a few macabre incidents. One man, during the 1880s, was poisoned by eating puffer and fell into a coma so deep that he appeared dead. In preparation for burial, his body was put into storage for a week. Shortly before his scheduled interment, however, the man suddenly arose as his coma broke. He reported that although paralyzed, he had possessed his full intellectual faculties and had feared greatly that he would be buried alive. There are stories of other puffer victims, also in a comatose state, who have jumped up as they were being carted to the graveyard—an action that certainly must have unnerved those present.

In his study of poisonous and venomous marine creatures,

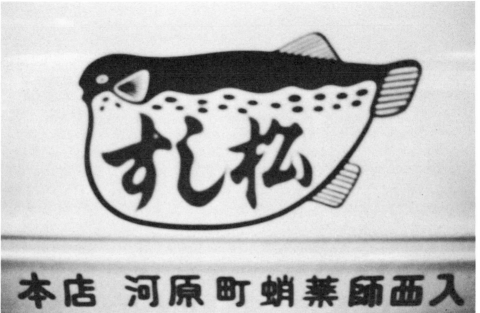

FUGU LICENSE: The Japanese characters on this restaurant sign tell diners that "this restaurant is authorized by the City of Kyoto to serve Fugu." Unless properly prepared, fugu *can be deadly to eat.*

Dr. Halstead published a survey of the incidence of puffer poisoning in Japan based on information received from Japanese health officials. During 1886, the first year covered, 86 persons were poisoned and 74 of them died. In 1892, 219 persons were poisoned and 141 died. Of 164 persons poisoned in 1963, 82 died.

In trying to reduce the toll from puffer poisoning, Japanese authorities have used a variety of legislative controls, including, in some places, an outright ban on the sale of the fish. In most cases the legislation prescribes standards for training and licensing *fugu* chefs and licensing only certain restaurants to serve the dish. *Fugu* chefs must have sound health and

195

eyesight, and they must undergo a stringent examination on their knowledge of puffers. They must be able to identify the different species by scientific name, and they must know the relative toxicity of the different parts of the fish. And in case they should ever err while preparing *fugu*, the chefs must pass a test on first aid for victims of puffer poisoning, although there is little one can do for a victim but to induce vomiting.

Shellfish Perils

The effects of tetrodotoxin resemble those of another poison sometimes ingested when eating marine animals. Saxitoxin, the agent responsible for paralytic shellfish poisoning, also may interfere with the passage of sodium across the cell membrane. This idea is speculation, however, for the nature of the poison remains mysterious. Paralytic shellfish poisoning is a global problem. It is not related to the stomach distress caused by eating shellfish contaminated by bacteria, but is an intoxication that acts upon the nervous system.

Laboratory tests suggest that the toxin accumulates in the tissues of shellfish that feed on certain tiny organisms belonging to a group called the dinoflagellates. Of microscopic size, dinoflagellates of various kinds constitute a major part of the base of the marine food chain. At times they undergo sudden population explosions called blooms, reproducing so quickly that they turn the water syrupy with their numbers. Blooms of some dinoflagellates cause the ill-famed "red tides," and also, scientists believe, outbreaks of paralytic shellfish poisoning.

Clams, mussels, and other shellfish filter dinoflagellates from the water. If the dinoflagellates are toxic, the poison accumulates in different organs of the shellfish, such as the gills, siphon, or digestive system, depending on the species of shellfish involved. Non-toxic shellfish placed in aquariums with certain species of dinoflagellates become toxic in a matter of days.

Dinoflagellates pose a biological puzzle in that they have characteristics of both plants and animals. They are tiny blobs of life that trail whip-like appendages, and some species produce their own nourishment through photosynthesis, like plants. Others prey on their fellow micro-organisms, and some species feed in both ways. Actually, whether one regards dinoflagellates as plants or animals depends on one's scientific orientation. Zoologists tend to look upon them as animals, while botanists view them as plants.

Dinoflagellates were not linked to paralytic shellfish poisoning until after a serious epidemic swept the San Francisco area in 1927. Concerned, California health authorities, along with fish and game officials, lent their support to an investigation by scientists at the University of California to determine the reasons for the epidemic. The scientists turned their attention to micro-organisms in the waters around San Francisco, and in 1932, when shellfish became exceedingly toxic, they noticed that one dinoflagellate, *Gonyaulax catenella*, had bloomed vigorously. They found the cause of the shellfish poisoning by testing this organism on shellfish in the laboratory. Since then, other species of dinoflagellates have been linked to outbreaks of shellfish poisoning elsewhere. Poisoning by dinoflagellates is not the same as caused by man-made pollution, in which pathogenic micro-organisms—germs—accumulate in shellfish and can sicken the person who eats them.

Indians of the Pacific Northwest certainly understood the relationship between blooms of dinoflagellates and outbreaks of shellfish poisoning. Coastal tribes knew that the appearance of large areas of discolored water signalled that shellfish would be toxic. They stationed sentries on the shore to watch for changes of color in the sea during the day and for extraordinary luminescence of the waters at night.

Dinoflagellates, like fireflies and some of the deep-sea

fishes, are often bioluminescent, capable of producing light biologically. Not all dinoflagellates have this power, but those that do, when disturbed, spark with living light. Although they are only about 1/500 inch across, vast numbers of them can make the sea look as if it were afire. It is the presence of dinoflagellates, rather than phosphorus, that makes the sea phosphorescent at night.

Researchers have discovered that during a bloom, *Gonyaulax* dinoflagellates amass in such numbers that there may be 40 million of them in a liter of sea water. Once a bloom peaks, however, the dinoflagellates almost vanish from the water. This phenomenon may be the work of other micro-organisms that are drawn to the bloom and feed on the dinoflagellates.

Paralytic shellfish poisoning has occurred on many shores, from northwestern North America to Japan and New Zealand, and from Europe and South Africa to eastern North America. As with other types of marine biointoxications, it has struck down members of exploring parties. One of the first recorded outbreaks, in June, 1793, sickened several crewmen of explorer George Vancouver's vessel on the coast of what now is British Columbia. Vancouver's men were exploring a channel in a small boat. They stopped for breakfast on the shore of a cove and ate some mussels they found there. Soon afterward the men sickened and felt lightheaded, and numbness spread through their limbs. One man, named Carter, died and was buried on the shore of a little bay. The others recovered.

Since the 18th century only about 600 persons have been victims of paralytic shellfish poisoning, but some of the outbreaks have been particularly severe. A hundred Aleut hunters died on Sitka Island in one such outbreak after eating mussels. More than 100 persons were sickened in the San Francisco outbreak of 1927 and a half dozen of them died. In 1898, 23 of 59 persons who were poisoned by clams and mussels in Maysuye, Japan, failed to recover.

The dinoflagellate *G. tamarensis* caused shellfish poisoning in northeastern Canada during 1945 and along the New England coast in 1972. The latter outbreak sickened more than a score of persons, although none died. The outbreak hit hard at the New England shellfish industry, and government authorities declared the region a disaster area so fishermen could collect unemployment insurance. The New England outbreak was labelled a red tide, although it was not caused by the same organisms that cause the notorious red tides of Florida.

Red Tides and the Burning Sea

The red tides that so often wash the beaches of western Florida are the result of blooms of the dinoflagellate *Gymnodium brevis*, a saucer-shaped, tailed organism that whirls through the water in a series of barrel rolls. Actually the term *red tide* is a misnomer, for dinoflagellate blooms turn the water any of a variety of murky colors—including red, yellow, brown, and milky white.

Outbreaks of paralytic shellfish poisoning do not invariably follow the red tide. In fact, the red tides of Florida have never caused this form of poisoning. But outbreaks of the red tide are noxious events, with serious implications for the tourist industry of the coasts they strike. Red tides like those of Florida turn the water into a stinking soup that closely matches the description in the Book of Exodus when the waters of the Nile turned red. Fish die by the thousands in the discolored water, and, washed ashore, they litter the beach and rot in the sun. Red tides also sometimes produce odious gases. People who live by the sea have had to seek cover, reeling with the stench of decaying fish in their nostrils and irritation caused by the gases in their eyes.

Since the mid-1940s, red tides have become almost commonplace on the west coast of Florida. The first major outbreak of this period began in November 1946 and lasted until August 1947. It killed an estimated half-billion fish, as well as bottle-nosed dolphins, sea turtles, and various other sea creatures. The magnitude of the 1946-47 red tide attracted droves of scientists to Florida's west coast. Two researchers, Carl S. Miner of the Miner Laboratories in Chicago, and J.N. Darling, former chief of the United States Bureau of Biological Survey, were on the scene at the onset of the outbreak and recorded it carefully.

Fishermen off Naples, Florida, first began to notice discolored streaks in the sea during November 1946, and toward the end of December, one party of sports fishermen sighted a patch of yellow discoloration 300 feet wide and 500 feet long about 21 miles west of Fort Myers. Thinking the discoloration resulted from a school of fish near the surface, the anglers sailed their boat into it. They found fish in the yellow water, but the fish gasped for air at the surface, giving every indication of great distress. When the mustard-colored liquid from the sea entered the boat's bait well, live fish that had been stored there began to gasp for air as well, and soon some of them died.

The fishermen took a sample of the yellow water to Miner, who examined it under a microscope and found it alive with whirling dinoflagellates. Miner observed that the dinoflagellates were speckled with yellow granules which reddened when the organisms died, an indication of why the color of the water changes during red tide outbreaks.

By January, hordes of dead fish had begun to drift ashore. In the days that followed, seamen reported seeing miles of sea covered by dead and dying fish, and seaside residents wheezed and coughed as the wind carried the stench in off the water. There was gossip that the fish kill had resulted from the dump-

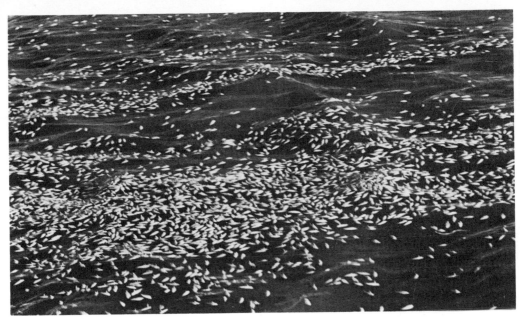

DEADLY TIDE: *The organism* Gymnodium brevis, *shown in a drawing magnified 4,200 times in the bottom photo, caused the red tide that killed the fish shown floating in the sea, above, off Sanibel Island, Florida. After a red tide, dead fish and horseshoe crabs litter a sandy beach at Pass-A-Grille, Florida.*

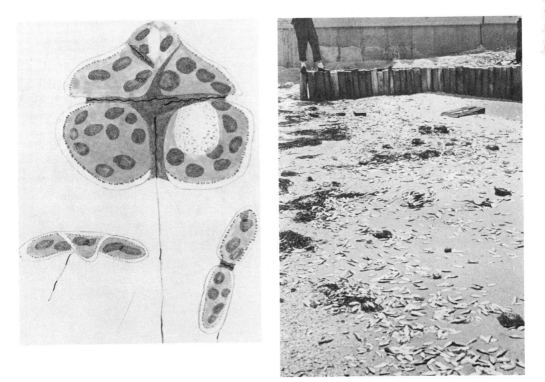

ing of surplus war munitions. At that time it was not known that *G. brevis* produces an irritant that distresses the respiratory tract.

The plague ceased in a few weeks, but in April it began once more, blighting the coast as far as Key West. Beaches that should have glistened in the summer sun were buried under tons of rotten fish—small species such as menhaden and even big jewfish weighing several hundred pounds. Workers buried 60,000 dead fish on one 200-foot-long stretch of beach, and scientists who walked the beach at Fort Myers counted 150 dead fish per foot.

Just what agent in the red tide kills fish is uncertain, but researchers at the University of Miami have found that sheepshead minnows placed in sea water containing red tide organisms die within a few minutes. Doubtless the organisms produce a toxin, but they also may kill fish mechanically, by clogging their gills and suffocating them, or by using up oxygen when they decompose.

G. brevis, found thus far only in Florida waters, caused other red tides in the 1950s. From 1952 to 1954, thousands of fish died along the west coast in repeated outbreaks. The tide struck the west coast again in the summer of 1971 when the *St. Petersburg Times* headlined the catastrophe "A Blood Bath in Tampa Bay." There was a horrendous smell from the tons of dead fish that littered the beaches and clogged the creeks leading to the bay. A year later, still more red tides struck the west coast of Florida.

The serious effect of the red tide on tourism, fishing, and other human activities has prompted a new effort to piece together the conditions responsible for dinoflagellate blooms. In 1972 the Mote Marine Laboratory, on the west coast of Florida in Sarasota, initiated a concentrated effort toward that end.

Scientists believe that among the ingredients of the

witch's brew that stimulates blooms of dinoflagellates—which reproduce by cell division—are increased temperature, lowered salinity, and an increase in nutrients, particularly vitamin B-12. This vitamin is produced by bacteria and algae that thrive in salt marshes. It washes into the sea in large quantities after heavy rains, which also lower the salinity of the water. In addition, upwellings of water from the depths carry nutrients that promote the growth of dinoflagellates.

Not all dinoflagellate blooms discourage tourism. On the contrary, in a few places dinoflagellates are responsible for major tourist attractions. In a very few bays and coves scattered through the tropics, conditions permit the constant bloom of bioluminescent dinoflagellates in such quantity that they illuminate the water at night. The most famous of these so-called phosphorescent bays is only a 20-minute boat ride eastward from La Parguera, a tiny fishing hamlet on the southwestern coast of Puerto Rico. Considered a hideaway for people knowledgeable about out-of-the-way places, La Parguera nestles between a mangrove forest that fringes the sea and the hot, red hills of Puerto Rico's desert country. Boats from the village leave for the bay in the evening, if the tourist trade warrants a trip.

The boats set out from the waterfront at dusk, when the twilight has cooled the barren hills and dimmed their rusty color to dead brown. Over the darkening sea, cattle egrets sail silently through the twilight like white ghosts. They are returning to their roosts on mangrove islands from the fields where they have stalked frogs and insects all day.

The entrance to the bay is hardly visible from the sea, for two great arms of mangroves almost enclose this unusual body of water. As soon as a boat enters the bay, the water's bioluminescent quality comes alive with startling beauty, as the wake of the boat glows with a cold, ghostly fire. As the boat churns into the heart of the bay it frightens barracuda, half-beaks, and other fishes, which streak through the water like meteors trailing liquid golden streamers. Overhead, glittering stars and flashes of heat lightning mirror the living light emitted by the tiny organisms in the water.

Ciguatera Will-O'-The-Wisp

The marine poisoning that is most puzzling to public health officials is one called ciguatera, which occurs in a wider variety of fishes than any other. It is known in more than 300 species of fish. Ciguatera can strike without warning almost any place within a belt that encircles the globe between 35 degrees north and 34 degrees south latitude. Most common in the South Pacific and Caribbean, it almost always involves fish that dwell on and around coral reefs, usually in less than 200 feet of water. The name of the poison originated from the name of a snail rather than a fish. The snail, called *cigua* in Cuba, was said to prompt indigestion when eaten, and eventually it lent its name to the more widespread and severe form of poisoning.

Ciguatoxin is a clear, light-yellow oil which attacks the nervous system. Among its most severe symptoms are numbness, nausea, pain in the muscles and joints, weakness, lack of coordination, and, oddly, reversal of the sensations of heat and cold. A classic ciguatera story describes how a Navy officer who had been poisoned was blowing on his ice cream as if to cool it.

Usually ciguatera intoxication lacks the severity of puffer poisoning, but at its worst it can cause muscular paralysis, convulsions, and death. The symptoms begin from three hours to more than a day after the victim has eaten ciguatoxic fish. Stomach pain usually initiates the ordeal, and sometimes sensory disturbances develop rapidly. The effects of ciguatera are as varied as its occurrence. Death can result, or the victim can be on his feet within a day. I had a mild case of the poisoning after eating a meal of various reef fishes caught by some friends in Puerto Rico. About two hours after I had eaten, cramps wrenched at my stomach and I became so weak that I could only lie on my back and suffer. Two days passed before I felt well again.

There is no way to distinguish fish with ciguatera from harmless fish except by laboratory analysis or by feeding the fish to animals and watching for a reaction. The problem is compounded by the fact that many fishes that are commonly ciguatoxic are important food fishes. Prominent among them are snappers (Lutjanidae), groupers, and jacks (Carangidae).

An exasperating fact about ciguatera is that it can occur suddenly in a species of fish that the day before was perfectly harmless, and no one knows why. A team of scientists from the University of Tokyo, headed by the noted Japanese authority on marine biotoxins Yoshiro Hashimoto, interviewed 93 ciguatera victims in the Ryukyu and Amami islands. The victims reported a great individual variation in toxicity even among the fish of a given species at the same fishing ground at the same time. This finding gives an idea of the capricious nature of the poisoning.

Wake Island had never had a reported case of ciguatera until May 1963, when fish that previously had been fit for consumption suddenly became toxic. The Line Islands, south of Hawaii had not experienced a ciguatera outbreak for more than a century, but at the end of the 1930s the region experienced an epidemic of ciguatera poisoning. Scientists tested 60 species of reef fishes collected in the Line Islands during 1954 and found that 45 were ciguatoxic, but by 1967 only one species of shark and the moray eel remained so.

Moray eels generally are regarded as highly poisonous, but experts do not agree on whether the ill effects are caused by ciguatoxin or by some other agent. Whatever the nature of their toxin, the animals never should be eaten. Fifty-seven Filipinos feasted on a large moray eel caught off Saipan in May 1949, and almost immediately they suffered ciguatera-like symptoms. Many had convulsions, several became comatose, and two died.

Some of the reef fishes that are ciguatoxic also have been involved in a highly unusual form of poisoning called Ichthyoallyeinotoxism, which causes severe hallucinations. Many victims feel that someone is sitting on their chests, and they suffer extreme depression, nightmares, and an unnatural dread of death. The symptoms may persist as long as 24 hours.

Mackerel, tuna, and other members of the family Scombridae can be poisonous under certain conditions, particularly if left in the sun after they are caught. These fishes contain a chemical that, in sunlight, is changed by bacteria into a histamine that causes stomach sickness, a rash, and other allergic symptoms. Sharks also are poisonous under certain circumstances. They may contain several different toxins, including that responsible for ciguatera.

The largest outbreak of ciguatera in history changed the course of a small war in 1748, when British troops were preparing to invade Mauritius, an island in the Indian Ocean. Stationed at Rodrigues Island, east of Mauritius, the British dined on ciguatoxic fish, and 1,500 men were put out of action by the poison and the invasion was a total failure.

Barracudas can be highly ciguatoxic, especially if large. Ciguatoxin is persistent, and large fish accumulate more of it than smaller ones do. In May 1956, five guests at a rooming house in Fort Lauderdale, Florida, sat down to eat a six-and-a-half-pound barracuda, and in due course they were very sorry. Within two hours all who had eaten the fish were ill. Three were hospitalized, and one did not recover for four months. And five persons had to be hospitalized for ciguatera after they ate a fifteen-and-a-half-pound barracuda caught off Key Largo in December 1960.

Scientists are baffled as to why the same species of fish can be highly ciguatoxic along one coast of an island and harmless on another, and why an outbreak suddenly takes place where ciguatera had been unknown for years. Since the early 19th century, they have suspected that the agent responsible for the poisoning must be in the immediate environment of ciguatoxic fishes.

An ancient legend of the Marshall Islands asserts that ciguatera comes from the body of a leper who had been thrown into the sea. Natives of other areas where the poisoning is common have placed the blame on certain types of algae which some fish consume. Scientists today have considerable confidence in this idea theorizing that the algae are pioneer species that establish themselves after an ecological upheaval has destroyed a resident plant community. This theory may explain why ciguatera outbreaks seem to follow earthquakes,. violent storms, the dumping of debris, dredging, and other disturbances that eliminate existing plant communities on reefs. Ciguatera probably moves up the food chain through herbivorous fishes to those that prey on the algae eaters.

Clupeoid Poisoning

Until a few decades ago, intoxication caused by eating fishes of the family Clupeidae—herrings, anchovies, tarpon, and their kin—was thought to be ciguatoxic in nature. But unlike most of the ciguatoxic fishes, clupeiforms feed on plankton, so researchers now believe that herrings and their relatives can cause a different type of intoxication, which has been designated clupeoid poisoning.

Like ciguatera, clupeoid poisoning is something of a mystery but is believed to stem from an agent in the food chain that is probably algal in nature. The symptoms are a metallic taste while consuming the food, dryness of the mouth, stomach distress, and often paralysis, coma, sometimes followed by death. Five persons died from the poisoning on Fiji in 1955, and in 1962 one died from it on Tarawa. The toxin that causes the symptoms acts so quickly that some victims have died with a piece of the fish that killed them still in their mouth. It is fortunate that, with a mortality rate of 40 percent, this form of poison is not too common.

CHAPTER 5

Seagoing Mammals

A few hours before dawn on April Fool's Day, 1968, a huge killer whale on a flatbed truck rode down New York City's Belt Parkway from the John F. Kennedy International Airport to Coney Island. It is understandable if anyone who might have been abroad that early thought a monumental prank was under way, or went straight home and vowed to keep off the sauce for life. The red flashers of a police escort played upon the glistening, black-and-white bulk as the strange procession moved slowly along the road. Finally the vehicles turned off the parkway and proceeded along the deserted streets of Coney Island to the New York Aquarium.

After the truck entered the aquarium grounds, and halted, a construction crane, its hook dangling at the end of a steel cable, rumbled into place alongside the vehicle. The whale was resting in a king-size canvas sling which hung from a large, steel yoke. With its hook attached to the sling, the crane hoisted the massive beast into the air. Weighing 5,800 pounds and 18 feet long, the whale was then the largest in captivity. Together with Ed Dols, the aquarium keeper whose encounter with a zebrafish was described earlier, I rode the sling into the air. Our job was to brace ourselves against the sides of the sling, keeping them apart so they would not constrict the whale. Slowly the crane lifted the whale and eased it over the

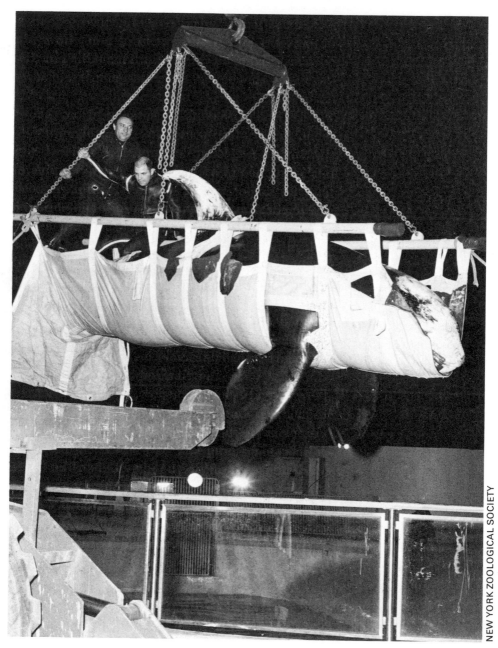

AIRBORNE WHALE: The author, right, and keeper Ed Dols ride a sling with a huge killer whale as it is transferred to its new home in a tank at the New York Aquarium.

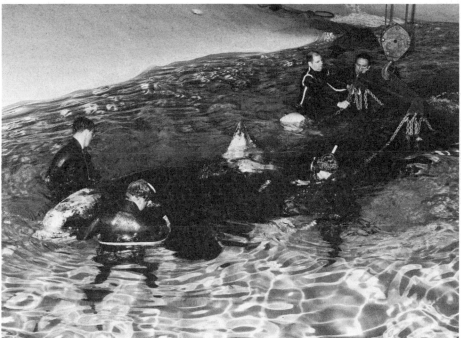

WALKING A KILLER: The author lends a hand as the killer whale is eased off the sling and walked about a pool after arriving at the New York Aquarium.

pool that was to be its home.

The sling and its cargo descended a few feet at a time into the cold water, which had been lowered to a depth of three feet to receive the whale. Waiting in the water were three aquarium keepers, clad in wetsuits as were Ed Dols and I. After the whale, a female captured in Puget Sound, had been lowered, the keepers eased her out of the sling and began to walk her around the pool. By moving her through the water, they forced her to use muscles that had stiffened during a transcontinental flight from Seattle, Washington aboard a DC-8 jet freighter. The whale looked far more imposing in the water than she had in the sling. I stood by her flukes, which together made her tail as wide from tip to tip as I was tall.

At her other extremity—the business end—were jaws that, could have closed over any one of us. In those jaws were 40 teeth of white ivory, as long as my index finger but more stout. I had been close to other whales before, but never close to a killer. As I stood in the 55-degree water in the half-light of an April dawn, I became totally engrossed in the creature, whose kind supposedly are the fiercest creatures in the sea.

Whale Family Tree

Unquestionably rapacious, seemingly fearless, butcher of seals, sharks, sea lions, penguins, and just about anything else that it encounters when hungry, the killer whale (*Orcinus orca*) combines a highly predacious nature and brute power with the remarkable intelligence of a dolphin. That, in fact, is what the killer whale is—the largest member of the dolphin tribe.

The names dolphin, whale, and porpoise sometimes are used interchangeably, and all three are basically the same type of animal, members of the mammalian order Cetacea, which left the land for the water millions of years ago. Porpoises and true dolphins differ in several respects. Dolphins have conical teeth, while those of porpoises are spade-like. The head of a porpoise is blunt; dolphins are beaked and generally larger than porpoises. Cetaceans have adapted to life in the hydrosphere almost as well as fish, particularly in terms of form and locomotion, although of course they still must breathe atmospheric air.

Two other groups of mammals have forsaken the land for a fully aquatic life. Dugongs and manatees, of the order Sirenia, inhabit the warmer fresh and marine waters of the world; and seals, sea lions, and walruses, of the Pinnipedia, live along most seacoasts, especially in the higher latitudes.

The sirenians are dull, slow-moving vegetarians that harm

no other animal, but both the cetaceans and the pinnepeds include species that can be extremely dangerous to humans. It is ironic that, among the many creatures in the hydrosphere that are alien to humanity, some of the most ferocious are our mammalian cousins.

Of the three orders of aquatic mammals, the cetaceans are the largest in terms of both size and number of species. There are ninety species of cetaceans, and all of them superficially resemble fish. But they differ physiologically from fish in ways that other mammals do: as in humans, the body temperature is maintained within a narrow set of limits suited to the creature's way of life. And the young, like human babies, are born alive and feed on milk produced by the mother's mammary glands. In adapting to an aquatic life, the cetaceans, as mam-

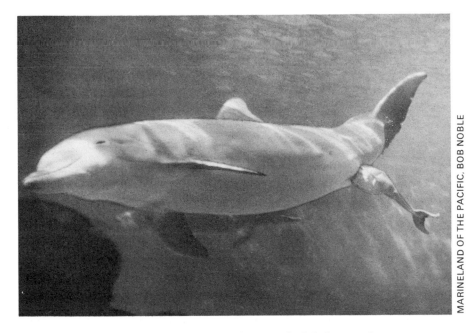

MARINELAND OF THE PACIFIC, BOB NOBLE

BIRTH OF A DOLPHIN: A bottle-nosed dolphin is born at Marineland of the Pacific. It emerges tailfirst. If it emerged headfirst it might drown.

215

mals, had to overcome several problems, not the least of which were quenching their thirst in sea water and holding their breath during deep dives.

The ancestors of cetaceans were terrestrial creatures closely related to the progenitors of cattle, sheep, and camels. The relationship is evident from an analysis of the biochemistry of the animals. In whales, sheep, cattle, and camels, eleven percent of the proteins are identical, whereas only two percent of the proteins of these animals are the same as those of other mammals.

The evolution of this unusual group of mammals is blurred by the millions of years that have elapsed since the ancestors of modern cetaceans took to the water. By 45 million years ago, however, modern forms of whales were swimming in the sea, together with a group of whales whose line dwindled out of existence after more than 20 million years of aquatic life. The two suborders of living whales, the Odontoceti, or toothed whales, and the Mysticeti, or baleen whales, have existed almost from the beginning of cetacean history. A third suborder, the Archaeocetes, is the group that became extinct. They will be discussed in Chapter 6. Baleen whales are named after the great plates of fibrous material called baleen that hang down from their upper jaw. Baleen was used for many years to stiffen women's corsets. There are sometimes as many as 300 plates in a single whale. Arranged so their bristly fringes overlap, the baleen plates strain out tons of plankton as the whale moves through the water. It is plankton, acquired this way, that feeds the largest creature ever to live on earth, the great blue whale (*Balaenoptera musculus*). This enormous animal can be 100 feet long and can weigh 150 tons. The toothed whales, on the other hand, have teeth adapted for grasping and tearing prey. This suborder includes the sperm whale (*Physeter catodon*), the killer whale, and the curious, playful beluga, or white whale (*Delphinapterus leucas*).

The main reason why whales have developed into creatures of such great bulk is that, being supported by water, they require far less muscular and structural support than do large terrestrial animals. When the ancestors of whales and other cetaceans first ventured back to the sea, they were four-legged and looked nothing like the streamlined creatures of today. But, as they evolved, they developed a fish-like shape and a pair of flukes, horizontally biased rather than vertically, as in fish, to propel them through the water.

One can imagine the flukes evolving, over countless ages, from an ordinary mammalian tail. The proto-cetaceans that were more likely to survive were those whose tails helped propel them more rapidly. As they reproduced, the characteristics that shaped their tails were refined and reinforced. Their hind legs were of little use, however, and in cetacean adults today, they are represented by only a few vestigal bones deep within the body. (Embryonic cetaceans have tiny flaps remniscent of rear limbs, but they vanish before birth.) The front limbs evolved into flippers which enable the cetacean to maneuver. The flippers still contain five digits but they are concealed by muscle and skin.

Even the structure of the cetacean's sex organs contributes to its streamlining. The penis of a male whale may be several feet long, but it is withdrawn into the body except when needed. Whales copulate gracefully, the male swimming belly up beneath the female. Sometimes when two males are kept together in an aquarium, the dominant cetacean repeatedly attempts to serve the other in this fashion.

Why Whales Spout

Because their mammalian respiration ties them to the atmosphere, cetaceans must use oxygen extremely efficiently to

217

cope with their aquatic environment. Before a cetacean dives, it fills its lungs to capacity, carrying as much oxygen as possible into the depths. The metabolism of cetaceans is relatively slow, so their bodily processes exert a minimal demand on the oxygen in the bloodstream. At the same time, their blood holds oxygen in relatively large quantities. This combination of conditions enables cetaceans to make the most economical use of their oxygen supply. Some whales can stay underwater for one or two hours, and the sperm whale dives to a depth of more than a half mile. During deep dives, bodily functions unrelated to diving slow down or even stop completely, so that a maximum amount of oxygen is conserved. There is a constriction of blood vessels serving parts of the body that are not active in diving—the digestive system, for instance—so blood that usually supplies those areas is shunted to the brain and other organs that must continue to function at a high level.

When a cetacean dives, the air in its lungs becomes saturated with moisture from its blood. On surfacing to breathe, the cetacean expels this compressed air which expands in the lower pressure of the atmosphere. The sudden expansion cools the air and condenses the moisture in it. The condensation forms a cloud, which is what makes cetaceans appear to spout water when they breathe.

Cetaceans breathe through a blowhole in the top of the head. In toothed whales the blowhole has one opening, and in baleen whales it has two. The blowhole is an adaptation of the nostrils, which very early in the evolution of cetaceans moved upward from the snout. Unlike other air-breathing vertebrates, whose nasal passages and throat share a common channel, the cetacean has separate conduits for each. Thus the cetacean can breathe even though its mouth and throat may be full of water.

A muscle sheet of many layers, called the maxillonasolabial muscle, controls the action of the blowhole. This muscle is formed from a fusion of the many small muscles that in humans produce facial expressions—so, in effect, the cetacean has sacrificed the ability to smile in order to breathe through a hole in the top of its head. The trade is a good one in terms of survival, for the cetacean can breathe through its blowhole with almost all of its body hidden beneath the surface. When it dives, it clamps the blowhole shut by means of a muscular lip that encircles it.

Many whales, as almost anyone who reads newspapers must realize, are nearing extinction because the whaling industry has displayed an abysmal ignorance of sound wildlife management and common sense. Cetaceans cannot be discussed without mention of the threat to the larger whales that have been slaughtered so remorselessly that some species may no longer exist in sufficient numbers to continue their kind. By killing the whales on which it depends, the whaling industry is committing suicide, a fact which it does not seem to comprehend. The United States, among other nations, has acted in behalf of whale conservation by banning whaling and the use of whale products, but a number of other countries continue to permit hunting of whales with little regard to their conservation. The blue whale population once numbered more than 100,000 individuals, but today there are no more than 1,000 of them left. There are now so few blue whales, that not enough of them may be able to get together to breed and perpetuate the species. Thus far, the slaughter has been directed mainly at the larger whales, but as these disappear, the hunters doubtless will turn their explosive-tipped harpoons on smaller and smaller species.

Ways of the Killer

The killer whale, although a big animal, by no means compares in size with some of the larger whales. Even so, it occasionally preys on them. Killer whales hunt cooperatively, in packs, or pods, of a few dozen to 40 animals—mother, young, and bulls together. The largest bulls can be more than 30 feet long and weigh more than 10,000 pounds.

Divers who have observed packs of killer whales in the sea say that the bulls seem to patrol the edges of the group, shielding the females and young. So close are the bonds between these creatures that a female once was observed for three days swimming around the spot in Puget Sound where her calf had been killed. Observers also have counted up to 30 killers surging through the sea in response to distress calls from one of their species.

The organized structure of the pack permits complex group hunting procedures, highly cooperative and well ordered. Big bulls sometimes patrol offshore while smaller bulls and youngsters range in loose packs through the shallows, casting about for prey. When killers attack a large whale such as a baleen they assault it from every direction, but they focus their slashing charges on the head and lips. Ripping at the lips, they eventually expose the tongue, which they tear out and consume. Occasionally, however, a big baleen will win a battle royale and drive off its tormentors.

Killers habitually prey on big animals. John Prescott once saw a killer whale leap from the water, holding in its jaws a bull sea lion that must have weighed 600 pounds. Dr. Ross Nigrelli has told me of seeing killer whales attacking schools of giant tuna off Bimini and tossing specimens weighing 300 pounds or more high into the air. The stomach of one killer whale, 21 feet long, contained the remains of thirteen porpoises and fourteen seals.

Other cetaceans and seals will flee before the approach of killer whales. In October 1971, recordings of killer whale vocalizations, broadcast under the water, were used to frighten belugas away from salmon that were returning to Alaska's Kvichak River to spawn.

The proclivity of killers for attacking injured whales and for hunting prey close by the shore has permitted excellent observations to be made of predation by these fierce sea mammals. The following account was reported by Age Jonsgard in *Norsk Avalfangst-Tidende*, the Norwegian Whaling Gazette. A Norwegian whaling vessel had sighted a dead bottlenosed whale off northwestern Sptizbergen. Several killers were feeding on the carcass while two killers, one on each side, supported it. As the vessel approached, the killers sounded and the bottlenose sank—but later the killers once again pushed the dead whale to the surface and resumed feeding. Another incident described in another issue of the same journal tells of an attack by killers on a bottlenose that had been harpooned but not killed. Three killers swept down upon the injured whale, which was about the size of a killer, and quickly bit off its flippers and one fluke, leaving it helpless.

In May 1964, David Hancock, a Canadian biologist, bush pilot, and film maker, observed an attack by killers on a minke whale (*Balaenoptera acutorostrata*) in Barkley Sound off Vancouver Island. He recorded what he saw and later published it in the *Journal of Mammalogy*. Hancock told me how while boating on the sound with two other men, he noticed the minke swimming into a small bay, about 30 feet deep and 150 yards wide, through a channel that permitted access only at high tide. Swimming rapidly, the minke surfaced every 100 to 200 feet. The reason for its haste became evident as Hancock noticed three killer bulls, with two females and two calves, entering the bay perhaps 600 yards behind the minke. Hancock followed the killer pack across the bay to its western edge where he saw that the bulls had attacked the minke. While the bulls carried on their gory task, mostly under the surface, the females and calves stayed to one side.

A half hour after Hancock first sighted the minke, it thrust its body vertically out of the water, raising its head 8 feet above the surface, then submerged. It repeated this maneuver 10 minutes later—the last time Hancock saw it. He spotted no killers near the minke on either occasion, but it died after the second time it shoved itself above the surface. Females and calves then joined the males as the killers continued their repast. Pieces of flesh floated to the surface, but surprisingly there was no blood in the water, although it was filmy with oil.

The carcass, almost 29 feet long, was found the next day as it floated about four-and-a-half miles from the site of the kill. Its skin had been stripped off, although its flukes remained covered. The minke had been flayed so neatly that the blubber under the skin had not even been gouged. Tooth marks on its flukes hinted that perhaps the killers had finished it off by grabbing its flukes in their jaws and holding it under until it drowned. The minke may have been trying to breathe when it lunged above the surface toward the end of the grim episode.

In July, another minke was found dead in Barkley Sound, and it too had been stripped of its skin. In reporting these events, Hancock suggested that they may have been the first reports of killers skinning other whales and consuming only their skin.

Killer whales commonly are seen by people on the beaches of the West Coast. Sometimes killers even are seen preying on other whales. An attack by seven killers on three gray whales (*Eschrictius robustus*) was described in the *Journal of Mammology* by C. Victor Morejohn of the Moss Landing Marine Laboratories in California. Gray whales often pass close to the coast of California during their migrations. Morejohn and eight of his students were in the laboratory when they saw killer whales leaping about 400 yards offshore. A gray whale surfaced in the midst of the killers while two others appeared a short distance from the sleek black-and-white hunters. It soon became evident to the watchers that all three gray whales were under attack. One of the killers rolled on its side, biting the belly of a gray, and several times the grays raised their heads above the water. Suddenly a large gray with a calf veered toward the shore, swimming almost into the surf where the water was only about 10 feet deep. The killers did not follow, and the adult with the calf remained close to shore until the killers moved off, then headed back to sea.

Thirty miles from the site of the attack described above, and ten days after it occurred, Alan Baldridge of Stanford University's Hopkins Marine Station witnessed another assault by killers on gray whales. Dr. Baldridge, too, described what happened in the *Journal of Mammalogy*. The killers attacked a large gray and a calf outside the kelp zone that borders the beach. The killers concentrated their attention on the calf, harassing it by swimming over it, one at a time. Then the whales disappeared for several minutes. Finally the calf appeared at the surface four different times, either under its own power or bouyed up by the killers, which began to rip chunks of flesh from their victim. One killer was seen to be spinning around in the water, probably tearing loose a hunk of blubber.

Meanwhile another gray, probably the one that had been with the calf, eased its head barely above the surface in the midst of the kelp, several hundred yards from the carnage. When the killers paid it no heed, it slipped away, quietly moving through the kelp with only its blowhole exposed. About a week after this incident, a pack of killers again was seen attacking a gray whale, not far from the site of the attacks already described.

Man and Killer Whales

Because they range from one pole to the other, killer

whales hunt an extremely varied list of prey. In the Antarctic they regularly feed on penguins, including the 4-foot-high emperor penguin. When killer whales sight penguins or seals on ice floes, they sometimes swim under the ice and smash into it from below in an attempt to dump the creatures on it into the water.

As far as is known, killer whales never have killed a human—but a number of times they have rammed ice floes on which men have been standing. The most famous of these incidents occurred early one morning in January 1911, in Antarctica's McMurdo Sound. Captain Robert F. Scott's research vessel *Terra Nova* had anchored next to an ice floe in the sound, and the expedition's photographer, Herbert G. Ponting, was on the ice photographing a half-dozen killers that had surfaced not far away. Suddenly the ice under Ponting's feet heaved and shattered as the whales, acting in concert, attempted to break through the floe. Ponting ran for the ship, with the whales still trying to get at him until he reached safety.

Are killer whales in such instances aiming for human prey? Or does a man in heavy polar clothing look enough like a seal or penguin to initiate predatory activity in the whales? Perhaps only by chance is man not part of the diet of killer whales, or then again, possibly killers will not prey on humans except in cases of mistaken identity. I have talked with divers who have approached packs of killer whales under water. The killers, they say, seem hesitant to approach men wearing diving gear. Possibly, because no creature in the sea stands its ground before them, killer whales are confounded by the sight of a creature moving *at* them.

John Prescott has told me of falling into a holding pen for killers in British Columbia. None of the whales made an aggressive move toward him. Another time, Prescott and three companions were diving in California waters when, unknown to them—but witnessed by people in a nearby boat—four killers passed nearby.

In the booklet *Marine Mammals of California,* published by the California State Department of Fish and Game, marine biologist Anita E. Daugherty describes several instances when killer whales could have attacked humans but refrained. In 1960 three divers in the water off Anacapa Island were approached by nine killers, one of which swam to within twenty-five feet of the men. The divers were not molested, but they wisely retreated to their boat. An apparently curious killer whale once followed two other divers in a small boat off the California coast, and at Pismo Beach, killer whales followed incoming divers as far as the surf line. During a skin-diving contest at Leo Carillo State Park in 1962, a pack of killers swam past just outside the kelp that lay offshore, and one bull came close to the divers before leaving.

Two attacks on boats in California waters merit consideration. In March 1952, a 14-foot boat with two men aboard, 25 miles offshore near San Francisco, was attacked by a creature described as a killer whale. The men battled the sea beast with an oar and escaped to shore. Later, biologists examined the marks left by the animal's teeth on the oar and reported that they fitted the teeth of the great white shark. An authenticated attack did occur, however, when a collecting crew from Marineland of the Pacific roped a female killer whale as she uttered a high-pitched alarm call, drawing a big bull to the scene. Together they charged the boat but were killed by the crew.

Featured Entertainers

Killer whales became the chief attractions at public aquariums during the 1960s. The first one to be exhibited in an aquarium was Moby Doll, in 1964. Moby Doll, a 15-foot animal, had been harpooned so she could be converted into a display model. The wound was apparently superficial, so instead of being killed the whale was placed in the Vancouver (British Columbia) Public Aquarium. Moby Doll died within three months, however, reportedly from complications due to the harpoon wound.

Namu, the first killer whale to gain national attention in the United States, was captured in fishermen's nets near Namu, British Columbia, and in June 1965 was exhibited at the Seattle Aquarium. Namu lived for a year. At that time, that was setting a record length of time for the species to live in captivity.

In *The International Zoo Yearbook*, the bible of the zoo-aquarium field, Seattle Aquarium director Edward L. Griffin and assistant director Donald G. Goldsberry wrote "From Namu we learned that the killer whale is beyond all reasonable doubt friendly to man under almost every conceivable circumstance." Many persons entered the water with Namu, but not once did the whale act aggressively. In July 1966, Namu became ill and drowned in a pool at the aquarium.

As more killer whales joined aquarium collections, keepers refined their techniques of caring for the big animals. Aquarium visitors no longer gasped at seeing divers enter the water with the allegedly dangerous creatures. Killer whales even have been force-fed when off their diet and have displayed no dangerous tendencies. On the contrary, they seem to like people.

Lupa, the killer whale at the New York Aquarium, described at the beginning of this chapter, became a favorite of school children in the few months she was there, before dying of a respiratory ailment. As the youngsters crowded around the glass railing above her pool, Lupa would stop directly below them and exhale, sending a fine mist of condensation into the

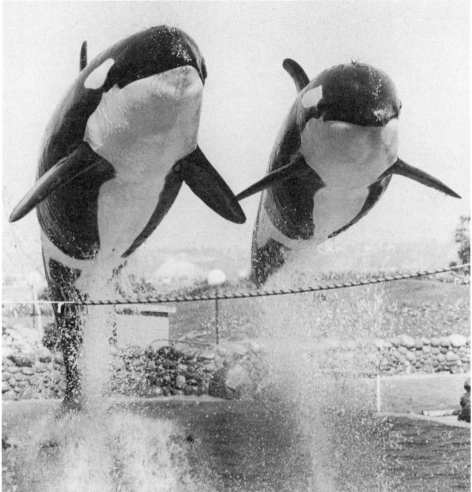

SEA WORLD

LEAPING WHALES: Two trained killer whales at Sea World Aquarium, San Diego, leap high in the air during their act. The whales weigh almost 2 tons each.

air. Her action invariably elicited yowls of delight. Lupa was not always docile, however. One time she sent her keepers scrambling from the pool. The water had been lowered to a depth of four feet so the pool could be cleaned. As the keepers moved around working, Lupa began to swim past them only a few feet away, snapping her jaws threateningly. The men wisely left the water.

Most of the killer whales originally captured and exhibited were young, and as the decade of the 1960s ended, aquariums that had successfully kept them found themselves with maturing animals on their hands. Some of the creatures, particularly bulls, began to play a bit more roughly with the trainers who put them through their paces in aquarium animal shows, and at some aquariums, bull killers fell out of favor.

A good example of how a killer whale's disposition can change as it grows older occurred at the aquarium of the Flamingo Park Zoo in Yorkshire, England. An 11½-foot-long killer was shipped there from Seattle in November 1968. The whale grew more than 3 feet in two years and had learned a repertoire of tricks. However, its play with divers become increasingly rough during the second year of its captivity—so much so that keepers had to clean the pool from the protection of a shark cage.

Cetaceans used in shows at aquariums are trained to complete a set of behavioral axticities to get a food reward. They connect their trainer, or anyone else working with them, with the behavior they must display to gain the reward. This type of training is perfectly safe with smaller cetaceans, but has created some problems with killer whales.

One of these whales is Orky, a bull that was about three years old when he arrived at Marineland of the Pacific in 1968. When captured Orky was less than 17 feet long and weighed 5,500 pounds. Within five years, Orky—well into sexual maturity—weighed 8,000 pounds and measured 23 feet in length. Orky had been trained to carry his trainer around a pool and then return the trainer to a platform in return for a reward. On one occasion Orky failed to return the trainer to the platform. When the trainer left the whale's back and started swimming towards the platform, Orky seized the man by the leg and dove for the bottom of the pool. He held the trainer there until the man almost had lost consciousness, and then released him. Marineland personnel believe that the whale was angered because the trainer had attempted to reach the platform himself, thus preventing Orky from receiving his reward. As of mid-1973, Orky was being re-trained, and under the new system of training is rewarded whether or not he returns the trainer to the platform.

A publicity stunt with a killer whale trained to receive a reward in return for retrieving objects very nearly ended in tragedy at Sea World, a public aquarium in San Diego, California. "We were contemplating having a female trainer in the show," explains William J. Seaton of Sea World. "An attractive young woman who worked at Sea World as a secretary, and who was a trained scuba diver, volunteered to ride the whale."

Newspapermen and television newsmen were invited to watch the shapely young woman ride Shamu, a killer whale female, around a large pool. A television cameraman recorded what happened on film, a print of which was shown to me by Sea World officials. Wearing a bikini bathing suit instead of the rubber wetsuit usually worn by the whale's trainers, the young woman climbed aboard the whale's back just in front of its high dorsal fin. As the whale circled the pool, the young woman waved and smiled, seemingly much at ease with the big animal. On successful completion of a circuit, she began a second ride, but this time as the whale circled the tank it turned quite sharply, and the young woman slid from the killer's back into the water.

Apparently confused, the whale seized the woman's left leg in its jaws and began to swim around the tank with the woman screaming and thrashing her arms in terror. The mo-

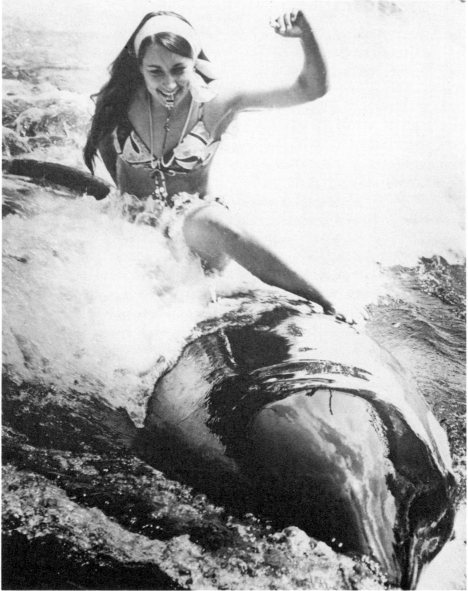

SEA WORLD

BEFORE MISHAP: Annette Eckis rides a killer whale around a pool at Sea World, San Diego, shortly before she is swept from the whale's back. The whale then grabbed Miss Eckis by the leg and refused to release her until it was quieted by keepers.

ment the woman had fallen into the water two scuba divers, stationed at the side of the pool, plunged and swam to her aid. Fortunately, the whale had not submerged and the woman was able to keep her head above water until one of the divers reached her, staying with her as the whale, still on the surface, continued to swim about the pool.

Meanwhile, attendants at the side of the pool thrust long poles towards the divers and the terrified young woman who, after several attempts, finally managed to grab a pole. Helped by the divers and attendants the woman got to the edge of the pool, but the whale, its great head thrust out of the water, continued to hold her leg. It is obvious from the film that the whale did not intend to injure the woman; it can be seen holding her leg in its jaws, rather than biting it. A killer whale, if it intended, could rip off a human leg in a split second.

As the divers, both of whom were whale trainers, soothed the whale, it released its grip on the young woman's leg, which had been cut by the whale's teeth, and then she was taken to a hospital by an ambulance. Some time later Sea World staged a "kiss and make-up" event between the young woman and the whale, but she later left the aquarium's employ and instituted legal action over the matter. Sea World officials theorize that the whale was attempting to retrieve its rider, and became confused.

At the Miami Seaquarium in Florida, another trained killer whale, named Hugo, starred in a show during which his trainer placed his head in the cetacean's huge jaws. Once, Hugo apparently misinterpreted a motion by the trainer as the cue to close its jaws, while the man's head remained between them. The trainer, Chris Christiansen, survived to tell the story: "When I remove my hands, that is the signal for him to close his mouth. One morning when my head was in Hugo's mouth, the audience started clapping and I removed my hands. Hugo was by that time doing part of the act with his eyes shut. Upon what he thought was the signal, he started to close his mouth with my head in there. I could see him open an eye and swivel it around on its turret. When he saw that my head was in his mouth he opened it immediately, but not before his teeth had cut into my cheeks. I took my head out, wiped off the blood, and went on with the show. Afterward I went to the hospital and had seven stitches taken in the cuts. The incident was my fault; I gave the wrong signal."

Hugo was paired with a female, Lolita, in June 1972. Eventually he became more aggressive, and Lolita took over his act. But Lolita can be aggressive, too, according to the whales' present trainer, Manny Velasco. Both killers have lunged at him, mouth open, as he has worked with them from the training platform, but Valasco says they continue the attack only if they detect fear on the part of the person against whom they are directing their actions.

One incident did frighten him, however. "When Lolita does the show," Velasco explains, "Hugo is penned in a section of the pool that is separated from the area where the show takes place. But one time Hugo broke out of the pen as I was riding Lolita. She never bucked, but she went down, and I was in the water with both of them. She came up beside me with her mouth open. I just tried to keep my cool. Luckily she didn't hurt me, and I got out of the pool without any trouble."

It is difficult to compare the behavior of an animal in captivity with its behavior in the wild. Captive behavior can be quite abnormal. But both in the wild and in captivity, the killer whale's attitude toward humans remains an enigma.

The Mighty Sperm Whale

The sperm whale, largest of the toothed whales, can at times display power and ferocity unmatched by any other creature on this planet. Seventy feet long and 50 tons in weight,

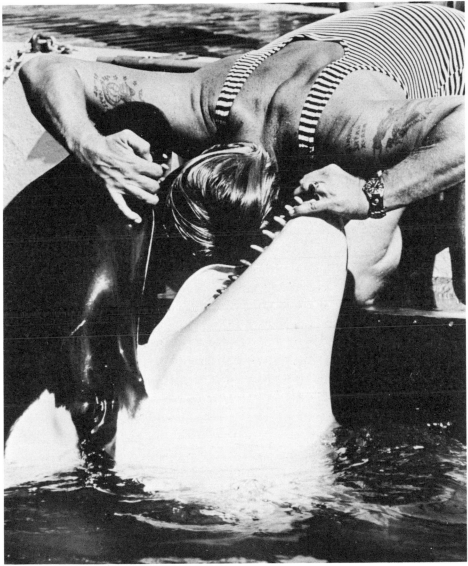

MIAMI SEAQUARIUM

DANGEROUS JOB: A trainer at Miami Seaquarium places his head in the jaws of a killer whale during a show at the aquarium.

233

the sperm whale has a massive, square head, with a toothless upper jaw. Its lower jaw, relatively narrow in shape, more than makes up for the lack of dentition in the upper. It is edged with 40 teeth, each 8 inches long, according to whale researcher Victor B. Scheffer, in his book *The Year of the Whale.*

Capable of diving to more than 3,000 feet—in 1932 a sperm whale was found tangled in a trans-oceanic telephone cable at 3,200 feet—the sperm whale preys on the giant squid. Battles between sperm whales and monstrous squid are the stuff of legends. The two colossal sea creatures sometimes engage each other for hours in clashes that range from the surface to the depths. The squid, slashing at the whale with its wicked beak, wraps its arms and tentacles around its adversary, while the whale tries to rend its adversary with its huge jaws. Usually the whale overcomes its prey, but if the squid happens to clamp an arm or tentacle over the whale's blowhole and prevents the whale from breathing, it can well become the victim.

Sperm whale bulls engage in similarly titanic battles with one another for the right to harems of females, ramming their adversaries with their mighty heads, and slashing at flukes and flippers with their teeth. It is the lone bull sperm whale that has caused some of the most spectacular maritime disasters of the 19th-century whaling industry. In each case the story is similar. A lone bull, often not even provoked by a harpoon, bears down on the small whaleboats, crunching them to splinters in its jaws, smashing the boats and men with thunderous whacks of its mighty flukes, and sometimes churning and turning to batter the mother vessel itself.

In 1807, the whale ship *Union* was sunk by a sperm whale. Thirteen years later, the vessel *Essex* out of Nantucket, was the victim of a sperm whale that punched a massive hole in the ship and sent it to the bottom. Often such disasters were the work of rogue bulls whose identities became known to

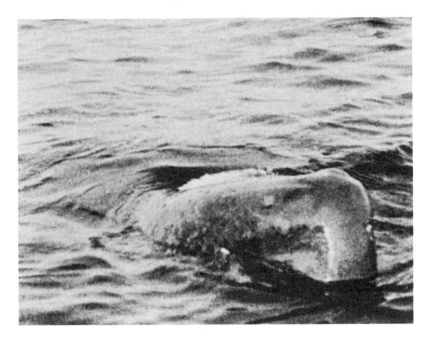

NANTUCKET SLEIGH RIDE: Old photographs from the days of the Yankee whalers show the hazards faced by whalemen who hunted the great sperm whale. A sperm whale pursued by whalemen surfaces (above), while in the other photo a whaleboat whose harpooner has struck a sperm whale is towed through the sea by the huge beast on what whaling men called a Nantucket sleigh ride.

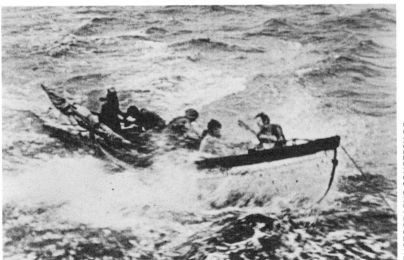

PHOTOGRAPHS COURTESY OF
THE AMERICAN MUSEUM OF NATURAL HISTORY

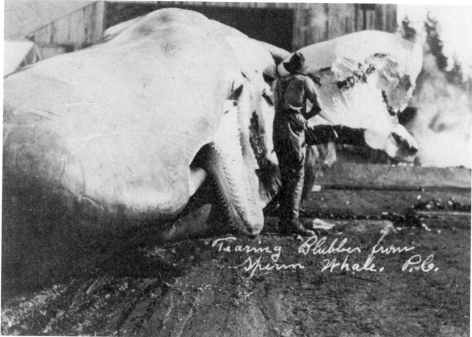

WHALERS AT WORK: This old photograph shows workers stripping blubber from a dead sperm whale at the Port Armstrong whaling station in Alaska. The whale's head faces the camera.

whaling men. The most feared of these was Mocha Dick, a white sperm bull said to be the basis for Herman Melville's *Moby Dick.*

Mocha Dick became the terror of the whalemen. In 1840 the beast thundered out of the sea to demolish the boats of the British whaler *Desmond* and of the Russian ship *Serepta,* and in 1842 a white whale, possibly Mocha Dick, rammed a coastal freighter off Japan and then turned on the boats of three whaling ships that came after him, chewing up boats and men alike.

The whaling vessel *Pocahontas* survived a ramming by a

big bull of Argentina in 1850, but the following year off the Galapagos Islands, another whaler, the *Ann Alexander*, was not so lucky. A sperm whale, after demolishing two of the *Ann Alexander*'s boats in its jaws turned on the whaling ship itself, bashing a huge hole in it, and sinking it. More recently, according to Victor B. Scheffer in his *The Year of the Whale*, a sperm male killed a man when it destroyed a fishing vessel off Sydney, Australia in 1963.

White Whales of the Arctic

None of the other toothed whales can be considered dangerous, but as animals of substantial size, even though not large for whales, they merit the respect of anyone who happens to be in the water with them. My favorite of all cetaceans is the beluga, or white whale, a toothed whale about 18 feet long that is milk-white when adult. Belugas range the sea around the top of the world, occasionally straying as far south as the northwestern and northeastern coasts of the United States. Belugas are also known as sea canaries because they produce underwater vocalizations that are highly audible. The beluga inhabits inshore waters, and even swims up rivers in search of fish and small squid. Sometimes gathering in herds of several hundred, belugas stand out against the dark sea because of their color and are easy to spot from the air.

When born, a beluga is not white but grayish black, a hue that lightens as the animal matures. Like other toothed whales, belugas have about 40 teeth which are adapted to holding their squirmy prey, and which become rounded with age and wear.

Several years ago I participated in an expedition to upper Hudson Bay to bring back a pair of female belugas as mates for the New York Aquarium's two males. The expedition was led by Robert Morris, then the aquarium's curator. The whales, collected near the tundra town of Churchill, Manitoba, were

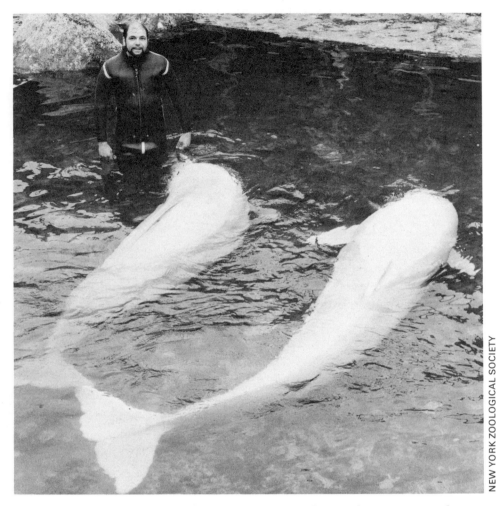

AT HOME WITH WHALES: The author visits with two friends, beluga whales, in the whale tank at the New York Aquarium.

loaded aboard the cargo compartment of an ancient World War II C-46 twin-engine aircraft on September 7, as the first bad storm of the season closed in with icy rain and chilling fog. We sat on rubber bags of aviation fuel in the cargo compartment, where the heat had been switched off for the benefit of our captured Arctic cetaceans. We bathed them regularly with cold water and ice cubes as they rested in wooden crates lined with foam rubber and plastic sheeting, which had been partially filled with water by the Churchill Fire Department.

When the females arrived at the aquarium, they were the only four belugas in captivity, and television celebrity Dick Cavett was persuaded to take a dip in the 55-degree water and visit them. It was my task to arrange the affair, and, in a sense, introduce Cavett to the whales. We outfitted him with a wet-suit and flippers, and explained how to enter the tank, soon he was cavorting in the water. An aquarium diver and I entered the tank, too, to be ready in case of emergency, but we remained out of camera range while Cavett gamely paddled about, trying to get close to his quarry. He managed to get within a few feet of the whales, but we warned him not to close in on the females because the larger of the males, Blanchon, was becoming quite possessive.

While belugas are inoffensive, and seem quite cuddly and playful to people watching them at an aquarium, one gains considerable respect for them on meeting them in their own environment. The underwater wake left by a beluga as it swims by is enough to tumble a person head over heels in the water.

As time went by, Blanchon focused his attentions on one of the females and would snap his jaws aggressively at any diver who approached her. Peter Fennimore, a keeper who regularly worked with marine mammals at the aquarium, recalls that once as he went into the whale tank to make repairs, Blanchon repeatedly swam between him and the female, clacking his jaws and becoming increasingly aggressive. Finally he snapped at Fennimore's air tank, and after a while he grabbed Fennimore's leg, which fortunately was clad in a wetsuit. Fennimore remembers feeling only a slight pressure from the whale's jaws, and afterward he found small indentations in the rubber of the wetsuit that apparently had been left by Blanchon's teeth.

Grabbing a leg seemed to be Blanchon's way of telling people to stay out of his territory. He used the same tactic on me when I entered the pool with another diver to observe him and his potential mate. After watching the whales underwater we surfaced and talked for a moment while treading water. I had turned away from my companion and was about to swim for the side of the tank when I felt a pull, steady but brief, on my leg. Thinking my companion was playing tricks, I turned around—but he was several feet from me. Then I saw Blanchon swimming away. Afterward I discovered the marks of his teeth in the leg of my wetsuit. I am sure the whale was not attempting to bite me, but was merely warning me that he was tired of our presence.

The Baleen Whales

The Mysteceti, which include the largest whales, also are inoffensive—but when they or their young are menaced, some species can be formidable because of their immense bulk and power.

William Scoresby, a 19th-century Scottish scholar and son of a whaling captain, and later a captain himself, wrote poetically about the way the female whale protects her young in his book, *An Account of the Arctic Regions*. While defending her calf, the female "loses all regard for her own safety" and "dashes through the midst of her enemies, despising the danger that threatens her."

Nixon Griffis, who in 1971 accompanied a New York Zoological Society expedition that filmed southern right whales (*Eubalaena australis*) off Patagonia, tells of an encounter he had with a large female. Right whales reach a length of 50 feet, and one big female came up under Griffis's rubber boat, lifting it from the water. The boat, 10 feet long, slid over the

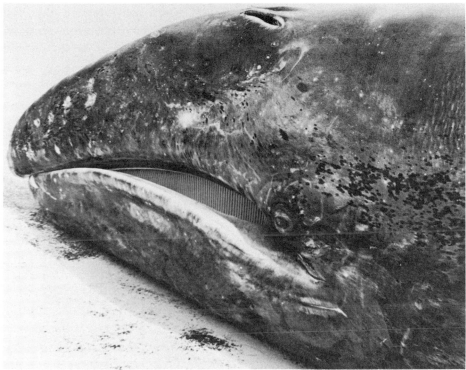

SEA WORLD

SUPER STRAINERS: The baleen plates in the jaws of whales like this gray whale strain small organisms on which the whale feeds from the water. The whale's blowhole also is visible atop its head.

whale's back and tail and into the water once more, and the sea mammal made no attempt to upset it. Expedition leader Roger Payne, writing in the October 1972 issue of *National Geographic*, tells of similar encounters between whales and other members of the party. He speculates that the behavior of the whales was possibly their way of gently easing people away from their calves.

It is an eerie experience to have a large whale pass under

your boat, especially if the craft is not very large. I have had that experience with gray whales off the California coast. Silently, a great gray hulk, perhaps 50 feet long, approaches on the surface from a distance of several score yards. Then it slides noiselessly beneath the surface, leaving small boils in its wake. A shadow, no more, may be visible beneath the surface, but you can sense the imposing presence of the whale. Perhaps the boat bobs a bit—or perhaps it is just your imagination—as the whale passes somewhere below. Suddenly, huffing like a steam engine as it blows, the whale surfaces some distance away. It looms out of the sea like an island being born and continues along its way.

The gray whale (*Eschrichtius robustus*) is seen by more people than any other large cetacean, for thousands of gray whales voyage twice yearly past the Pacific coast, close to shore, as they migrate between the warm, shallow lagoons of Baja California and the chill Arctic sea. The most primitive baleen whale in existence, the gray whale once ranged both the North Atlantic and the Pacific but the Atlantic gray has been extinct for several centuries. Over-exploitation almost led to the extinction of the Pacific gray as well, but conservation measures have allowed its population to rebuild to almost 20,000 individuals. Gray whales live on the Asian side of the Pacific as well as the American but those in American waters have been studied much more closely because the migratory route there is close to land.

California gray whales summer at the southern fringe of the Arctic ice pack, but as winter closes in they begin a 6,000-mile journey to Baja California, where they arrive in January to breed, have the young that were conceived the year before, and otherwise disport themselves. During this migration the grays plow past the southern California coast, sometimes cutting across bays and inlets from one headland to another, often only a mile or so from land. People swarm to the cliffs and

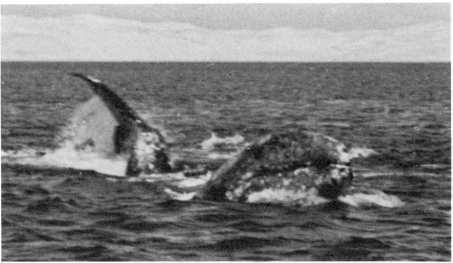

NATIONAL MARINE FISHERIES SERVICE

COURTING GIANTS: Two huge gray whales thrash the sea to froth as they mate in the warm waters of Scammon Lagoon off the desert coast of Baja, California.

beaches, and take to the sea in boats to glimpse the sea giants. Often the onlookers are rewarded by seeing one or more whales surfacing. As they surface the grays blow loudly; and when they sound, the last one sees of them is their mighty flukes, lifted high in the air as if waving farewell.

Their best-known winter home, a lagoon skirted by the wild desert of Baja California, is named for a 19th-century whaling captain and naturalist, Charles M. Scammon, one of the most resourceful men ever to ply his trade. While searching for new hunting grounds, Scammon chanced upon the 250-square-mile lagoon, which is behind a large triangular island that conceals it from the sea. The whales themselves told Scammon of its location, for as his vessel sailed down the Baja coast, a lookout sighted what appeared to be whale spouts coming from the desert. Knowing, obviously, that whales do

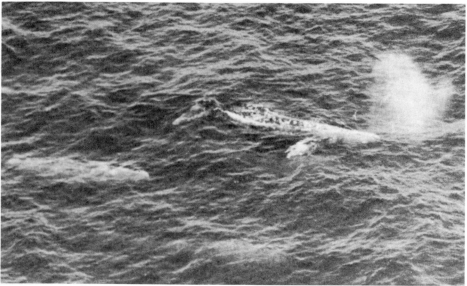

MARINELAND OF THE PACIFIC, BOB NOBLE

MIGRATING GIANTS: Gray whales pass the coast of southern California as they migrate between the Arctic and Baja, California. The lead whale is spouting.

not travel about on the land, Scammon reasoned that they must be in a hidden lagoon. His men set out in whale boats and shortly found the entrance to the lagoon and in it an astounding number of whales.

Doubtless rejoicing over the bounty they would receive from this unexpected windfall, the whalers began to slaughter the inhabitants of the lagoon. The whales fought back viciously, charging the boats when cornered. Scammon's whalers countered by firing explosive harpoons from boats in water too shallow for the whales to reach them.

Later other whaling captains, seeing Scammon's good fortune, tried desperately to find the source of his whales. Seldom was Scammon's ship without a shadow, but the crafty captain expertly confused his competitors. Eventually, however, because of a quirk of fate and a gust of breeze, the other whalers did find Scammon's Lagoon. One day, as a vessel belonging to one of Scammon's competitors was sailing in the area, those aboard smelled drying blubber. It came, strangely, from landward. By tracing the scent to its source, the competitors found Scammon's secret whaling ground. Other whalers flocked to

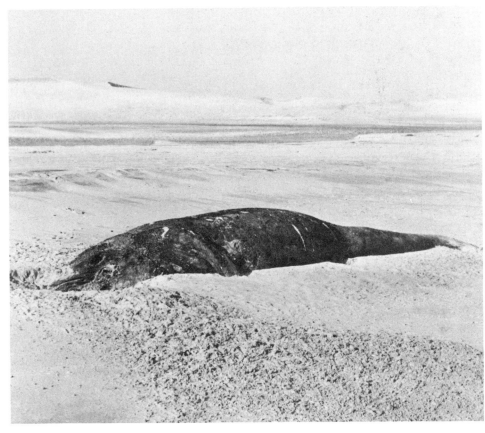

NATIONAL MARINE FISHERIES SERVICE

END OF A CALF: A dead gray whale calf lies in the sand of Scammon Lagoon, chief breeding and calving area for the California gray whale.

245

the lagoon, and a horrendous slaughter of the grays followed.

Whalers of the last century respected and feared the gray for its willingness to fight back. They referred to it as the devilfish. Old salts asserted that a gray whale that had been hunted for a few years learned to attack boats on sight.

More recently, a graduate student from the Scripps Institution of Oceanography had a shattering experience on meeting a gray whale underwater. As told by researcher and filmmaker Theodore J. Walker in the March 1971 *National Geographic,* the student was scuba diving when he came upon the whale. He reached out and touched the beast, whereupon the whale twitched and erupted into action. The student was knocked unconscious and had to be helped into his boat by a friend who had been in the water with him.

Dr. Walker also describes how the noted medical researcher Paul Dudley White was charged by a gray whale while trying to take the beast's heartbeat. Dr. White was implanting an electrocardiograph lead in the whale, when it slammed into his boat and knocked a hole in it.

When not disturbed, gray whales seem placid even when humans are quite nearby. John Prescott encountered a gray whale cow, 30 feet long and apparently pregnant, while diving off Catalina Island. The whale moved to within 6 feet of Prescott, who was diving on a rocky reef in 30 feet of water. The whale watched him and his diving companions closely, but departed when Marineland of the Pacific's collecting vessel, *Geronimo,* approached.

Encounters with Sea Lions and Other Pinnipeds

Cetaceans are considerably more aquatic than pinnipeds, the other large group of sea mammals. Including seals, walruses, and sea lions, the pinnipeds—the name means "wing-footed"—originated from the same root stock as the carnivores, and they generally remain true to their ancestry in their feeding habits. Essentially they are carnivores adapted for an aquatic existence, and they are the only large meat-eating animals that live in colonies. Pinniped colonies, especially during the breeding season, can be places of furious activity as the bulls defend their own little kingdoms against all comers. When the time to mate approaches, each bull takes possession of a particular piece of territory and tries to stock it with females. The resulting competition often causes violent battles among the bulls. At this time, the males of some pinniped species will charge a man who enters their domain; normally they would either pay no attention or flee to the water.

A few years ago a bull sea lion (*Zalopus californianus*) reportedly killed a man who had violated its territory. The sea lion is said to have sunk its teeth into the man's back, picked him up, and shaken him the way a terrier shakes a rat. David Hancock, who regularly visits pinniped colonies in the northwest, says he has been chased from the territories of bull sea lions many times. As with so many other animals, however, the bull sea lion directs aggression only against invaders of its territory. Each time he was chased, Hancock says, the bull gave up the chase when Hancock retreated beyond the border of the bull's personal realm.

During the breeding season, a sea lion colony is in constant hubbub, with the animals moving here and there and barking endlessly. Researchers believe that the continual barking of the males warns other bulls to keep their distance and thus helps avoid confrontations. The top weight for a California sea lion bull is about 600 pounds, but this is dwarfed by the size of the Steller's sea lion (*Eumetopias jubata*), which ranges the coast from California to the Arctic. A bull of this species may weigh close to a ton and is much more aggressive than the

247

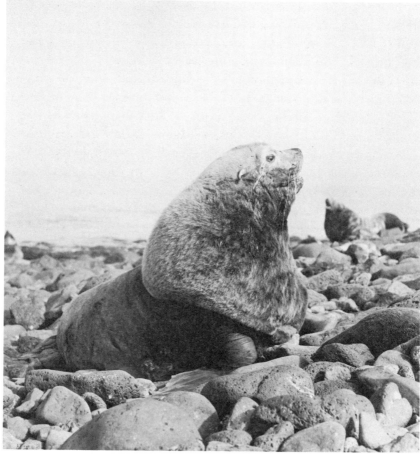

NATIONAL MARINE FISHERIES SERVICE, V.B. SCHEFFER

KING OF THE ROCK: A bull Steller sea lion, his huge neck scarred by battles with other bulls for a harem, surveys his territory on the shores of St. Paul Island, Alaska.

California sea lion. William Walker of Marineland of the Pacific told me how a huge bull Stellar's sea lion attacked him after he had beached his surfboard on a rock that was the site of a sea lion colony. The beast had been awakened by Walker and immediately charged him. Walker escaped by grabbing his

248

surf board and leaping into the water. The bull northern elephant seal (*Mirounga angustirostris*), a huge beast that can
reach a length of 16 feet, sometimes charges boats that come
too near during the breeding season. The reason may be that
at high tide the boats sailed over parts of a bull's territory that
would be dry at low water.

A big bull elephant seal once attacked a skiff carrying
John Prescott and four other men about 25 feet offshore. Prescott's party had been watching two bulls battling chest to
chest, shoving their ponderous forms against one another and
slashing with their huge canine teeth as they contested a piece
of territory. Another large elephant seal was in the water not
far away, but it disappeared under the surface. Suddenly it
made its presence known again by smashing into Prescott's
boat, knocking the small craft 3 feet into the air. The men
sped off before the seal could do further damage, but later,
Prescott reported, the brute had bitten through a layer of ply-
wood and chopped out chunks of the boat's keel.

When a bull elephant seal matures, its neck becomes
puffed and calloused. Competing bulls engage in highly ritualized battles in which the front of the neck of the opponent
seems to be the only target for the two antagonists. Sometimes
battling for as long as an hour, the two males slash downward
and across the front of one another's necks, spilling considerable blood from the puffy tissue but seldom inflicting a serious
wound. William Walker recounted for me an example of the
astonishingly ritualized nature of these contests. He once
watched a bull that remained upright, however, and withheld
its strike until the other male arose and again presented the
front of its neck. Walker believes that bachelor bulls that have
no harems and are kept at the edges of the colony have no pattern to their aggressiveness, but attack in erratic fashion, making them more dangerous than bulls with territories to defend.

When not breeding, elephant seals seem indifferent to a

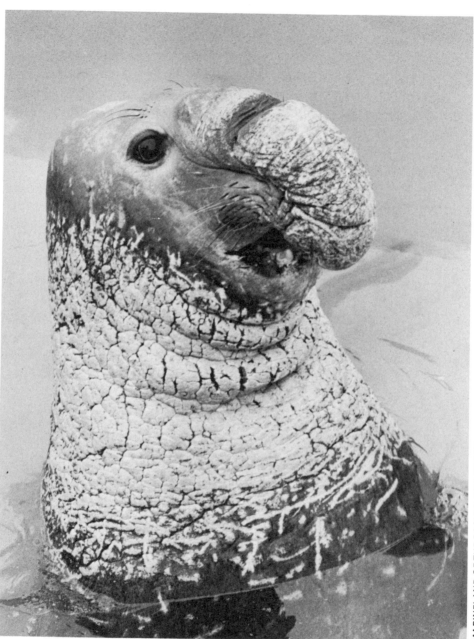

WARRIOR: When a bull sea elephant matures, callouses cover its neck. Sea elephant bulls strike at the front of one another's neck in their ritual battles over mates. The horizontal scars on this sea elephant are the reminders of past battles.

human who comes among them, especially if he keeps low and crawls between their mountainous forms. Biologists actually have crept among sleeping elephant seals and inserted thermometers into their rectums without arousing the ire of the beasts—an action prompted by what must be unquestionable curiosity. If a man suddenly stands up among a seal colony, however, he may be asking for trouble. He may look like another seal entering a bull's territory, or else he may frighten the seals and be run over as they stampede toward the water.

Nixon Griffis was charged by a Patagonian sea lion (*Otaria bryonia*) when he came between the bull and the water. But the bull stopped the charge when Griffis moved down the beach out of its line of sight.

The southern elephant seal (*M. leonina*) is larger than the northern species, reaching 20 feet in length and weighing as much as 8,000 pounds. Naturalist John Warham, writing in the January-February 1964 issue of *Animal Kingdom*, mentions that southern elephant seals will not attack a man unless he ventures among the cows. Cows of the species have bitten several scientists who came too close while studying them. Warham writes of one seal that charged him every time he passed the creature's particular stretch of beach.

Seals and sea lions sometimes act aggressively in captivity, but of course this behavior may not be normal. Peter Fennimore once told me how a large male crab-eater seal (*Lobodon carcinophagus*), just arrived at the New York Aquarium from the Antarctic, charged him after escaping from a crate. Fennimore had found the crate empty and had noticed traces of blood on the snow of the aquarium grounds. He followed the crimson droplets to discover that the seal was heading for the Coney Island boardwalk which runs between the aquarium and the beach. As Fennimore approached the seal, the animal whipped around and, snapping and snarling, lumbered toward him with frightening speed. Backing away quickly, Fennimore

251

summoned help, and other members of the aquarium staff arrived with a cargo net which they tossed over the seal. Fennimore, who had worked with other pinnipeds before but not the crab-eater, said the animal's reaction took him completely by surprise.

The Awesome Leopard Seal

Related to the crab-eater, and truly a terrifying creature, is the big leopard seal, which prowls the edge of the Antarctic ice, ready to rip unwary penguins to shreds. The leopard seal (*Hydrurga leotonyx*) sometimes ranges as far north as Australia, New Zealand, and Cape Horn. It reaches a length of 12 feet and weighs 1,000 pounds at its largest. The female exceeds the male in size, an unusual trait for a mammal.

The name *leopard seal* comes from the spots on the hide of this powerful animal, but it might just as well refer to its nature. Penguins, fish, squid, and other seals die under the fangs of the leopard seal, and recent evidence shows that it does not hesitate to attack man. Richard Penney, an expert on polar animals, described several encounters with leopard seals in an article he wrote for *Animal Kingdom*. Dr. Penney nearly became the victim of a leopard seal more than once. One time, he wrote, he fired four .38 caliber bullets into the head of a leopard seal without killing it. On another occasion, a leopard seal lunged at him through an ice fissure, snapping at his leg but missing. Another time a leopard seal erupted from a fissure and chased Dr. Penney and a companion for 100 yards across the ice.

Perhaps Dr. Penney's closest brush came as he was walking along the edge of the ice one time. He tossed a chunk of ice into the water where he had heard an odd sound a moment before, and suddenly a leopard seal raised its head above the surface. Possibly the seal appeared in response to the splashing ice which may have sounded like a penguin entering the water. The seal moved off, however, and Dr. Penney tossed in another chunk of ice. This time, 20 yards away, a leopard seal burst from the water, scrambled up onto the ice, and lunged at Dr. Penney, who jumped back, thrusting out a knife. The jaws of the seal clamped down on the knife blade, then the animal turned and made for the water.

Since leopard seals seldom are exhibited in zoos or aquariums, they are not too well known to the general public. Antarctic explorers long have been wary of them, however. Sir Ernest Shackleton, who led an Australian expedition to Antarctica in 1907, reported that a leopard seal had attacked one of his men on an ice floe. Another seal, according to Shackleton, was shot three times in the head and twice in the heart and remained alive.

It may be that leopard seals mistake men for large penguins, or other seals. But it is perhaps just as likely that these fierce predators view man as a desirable—if relatively new—food item in their frozen realm.

Beware the Walrus

For sheer ferocity and unbridled pugnacity, even the leopard seal must take second place among pinnipeds. The walrus (*Odobenus rosmarus*), so often pictured as a friendly, comical character, is a predator so powerful that it kills whales as large as belugas, as well as other pinnipeds. It can fight a polar bear to a stand-off with mighty slashes of its saber-like tusks. Men who have disturbed walruses have found that they respond in a horrifying fashion, seeking to tear their adversaries to pieces as if driven by a frenzied lust for vengeance—although vengefulness cannot be attributed to animals other than humans.

Walruses today seldom stray below the southern fringes of the Arctic, but in times past they ranged much farther south. Climatic changes and the pressures of hunting have driven them north. A bull walrus can weigh as much as a ton and can be a dozen feet long, with tusks a yard long. The tusks are canine teeth adapted for stabbing and for digging clams and crustaceans from the sea bottom.

British zoologist Gavin Maxwell, in his book *Seals of the World* describes certain rogue walruses, huge creatures with tusks that are smaller and sharper than those of normal walruses and that project sideways instead of straight down. These rogues, he says are excluded from the walrus herds and live almost exclusively on seals and other large prey.

Since medieval times, sea farers who have ranged northern waters have known that walruses are very protective of their young. They will assault a polar bear that threatens a young walrus and reportedly even have slaughtered killer whales that attempted to prey on their offspring.

Olaus Magnus, 16th-century archbishop of Uppsala, Sweden, wrote extensively on sea creatures. He stated that if walruses "see any man on the sea shore and can catch him, they come upon him suddenly, and rend him with their teeth, that they will kill him in a trice." Dutch navigator Willem Barents, in 1594, encountered walruses in the Orange Islands. He warned that if a female with young is threatened, "she will revenge herself upon the boats." An account from 1598 tells of a herd of walruses that were disturbed by men in small boats. They charged with an awful bellowing and shrieking, swimming directly at the boats, whose sails fortunately caught a breeze and whisked the terrified men away. "It was not wise of us," says the story teller, "to wake sleeping wolves."

Captain William Edward Parry, while searching the Arctic for a northwest passage in 1822, came across a walrus herd in the Fox Channel. About 200 walruses were scattered about on the ice in groups of 20 or 30 individuals. Parry's men harpooned one of the big beasts, which promptly smashed into their boat, plunging its tusks through the planking. On another occasion, after a walrus had been wounded, several of the beasts charged a boat, slashing at it with their tusks.

There are several accounts of entire herds of walruses charging boats in defense of themselves and their young. The full fury of such a mass attack was unleashed on a group of walrus hunters one day in July 1861 in Frobisher's Bay. As the hunters, in whale boats, approached a herd of walruses, the animals paid little attention until the men began to fire at one group. The beasts that were being fired upon dove for the bottom, but then they reappeared and charged the boats, shrieking wildly in unison. They uttered a sound described as "huk! huk! huk!" which echoed from ice floe to ice floe. At that sound, walruses that had been lying on other floes launched themselves into the water and headed for the hunters' boats. With walruses converging on them from all sides, and the air filled with fearful cries, the men battled back. They fought with lances, oars, and guns against the walruses, which slashed with their tusks, hooking them over the gunwales of the boats in an effort to upset them. Suddenly the herd parted as a monstrous walrus bore down upon the boats, his jaws open wide. As he reared up before one of the boats, a hunter shot him point blank in the mouth and killed him. With his death, the attack ended.

While not all pinnipeds are as dangerous as the walrus and the leopard seal, no animals of their size, and with their dental structure, should be treated lightly. Others among the pinnipeds may well endanger man at certain times. William G. Conway, general director of the New York Zoological Society, observed that Patagonian sea lions prey on penguins along the

Argentine coast. The sea lions swim under the penguins as they paddle through the water, grab the birds in their jaws, and wrench them apart.

Unquestionably, based on observations such as those above, pinnipeds under a wide range of circumstances can be highly dangerous creatures.

CHAPTER 6

The Hazards
of Reptiles

A huge reptile stalks its prey in the field waters of the brackish swamps that are common in much of the Indo-Pacific region. Lurking among the mangroves, sliding over the black mud, even competing with sharks for human prey off the beaches of some oceanic islands, this dread creature is the estuarine or salt-water crocodile (*Crocodylus porosus*). It is the largest and most ferocious of the order Crocodylia and is a man-eater that in many parts of its range is feared much more than the shark. Biologically it is but little removed from its ancestors, reptiles that survived when the last of the dinosaurs furnished carrion for little mammals that skittered through the night.

Estuarine crocodiles haunt the shores of small islands off the coast of New Guinea, and some of those who know these islands well believe an estuarine crocodile was responsible for the disappearance in 1961 of Michael Rockefeller, the son of New York's governor. Possibly no one will ever know if that adventurous young man was claimed by the estuarine crocodile, just as it is impossible to calculate the total number of the beast's victims. Certainly the number is high.

A grisly episode during World War II added considerably to the figure. During the winter of 1944-45, about 1,000 Japanese infantrymen were cornered by British troops in a dense mangrove swamp on the island of Ramree in the Bay of Bengal. The Japanese, battered and cut off from any possibility of help, fought on despite heavy pressure by the British. The fighting, and the presence of wounded men and corpses, drew a great number of estuarine crocodiles to the area. At night, the crocodiles thrashed about, devouring corpses, and then the men that still lived. The British troops outside the swamp could hear the gruesome sounds of screaming men within the dark tangle of the mangroves. By the end of the engagement, only 20 Japanese remained alive.

Dangerous and Endangered Crocodiles

Although the estuarine crocodile is better adapted to the marine environment than other members of its order, it is not the only crocodilian to enter salt water. The order Crocodylia includes alligators, caimans, and gavials as well as crocodiles. During the summer, American alligators (*Alligator mississippiensis*), living in coastal areas venture into salt water to feed on crabs, and the American crocodile (*C. acutus*) regularly inhabits brackish, and often salt, water.

More than a score of species exist today. With the exception of the American alligator and its smaller cousin, the Chinese alligator (*A. sinensis*), all are tropical or subtropical creatures. Even though some species, such as the estuarine crocodile, are extremely dangerous, crocodilians are feared more than is warranted. They are almost as maligned as snakes and are just as misunderstood. Man is actually more of a threat to them than they are to him, for destruction of habitat and uncontrolled hunting of crocodilians for their hides have placed almost every member of the order in danger of extinction.

Crocodilians are among the largest of reptiles, and no one wants to be eaten by one—but at the same time, it is possible

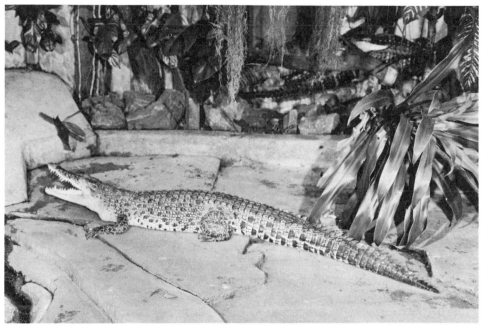

NEW YORK ZOOLOGICAL SOCIETY

KILLER CROC: The saltwater, or estuarine, crocodile is a proven man-killer. It lurks on the shores of many islands of the Indo-Pacific. This one, however, is in the Bronx Zoo.

to feel some sympathy for them because of their plight. They are the last of an ancient line that flourished during the Mesozoic Era, when reptiles were the dominant life form on earth. The order originated more than 180 million years ago, during the Triassic Period. As descendants of creatures that shared the earth with the dinosaurs, but, unlike the dinosaurs, managed to adapt to environmental changes, crocodilians are extremely interesting from an evolutionary point of view.

Crocodilians and dinosaurs both developed from creatures called thecodonts, from the Greek terms for *socket* and *tooth*. Their fossils show that thecodonts had teeth set in sockets of bone, a great advancement over animals that lived before

261

them. They were reptiles of large size, 15 to 20 feet long, and they walked mostly on powerful hind legs which enabled them to chase down smaller reptiles as prey.

The early crocodilians were not like those of today but instead lived largely on land, where they chased down their prey in much the same manner as their theocodont forebears. Some of the crocodilians, however, took to the water, possibly because of the pressure of competition from meat-eating dinosaurs. As aquatic forms developed, they reached immense size: one kind that lived in what today is Texas reached a length of 60 feet. It may have waited at the water's edge to prey on small dinosaurs. Although many dinosaurs were amphibious, few of the amphibious species were carnivorous, so the water was free of competition for crocodiles.

The climatic changes that altered the terrestrial habitat and helped remove the dinosaurs from the scene had less effect on the aquatic environment, so the crocodilians had felt less ecological stress than their dinosaur contemporaries. And few of the mammals, which succeeded reptiles as the earth's dominant life form, inhabited the same waters as the crocodilians, so these ancient reptiles remained free from competitive pressure.

For millennia the crocodilians thrived in their ponds, lakes, rivers, and swamps, with some venturing into the seas. Eventually the human species evolved but offered no serious threat to the crocodilians—until the past hundred years or so. Now, caught in a crunch between man's taking over their habitat, although it is wet and marshy, and his coveting their hides, the crocodilians have declined in numbers so seriously that many species will not survive without help.

Conservationists around the world are trying to preserve the various crocodilians. Some of these conservationists are outright preservationists, harboring the Utopian belief that with proper legislation all crocodilians can be perpetuated in a pristine state. Others want to maintain the creatures in the wild, but as a harvestable natural resource, free-ranging but managed, so their hides can be sold. Zoologists at many institutions are trying to breed crocodilians and have met with some success, although not on a scale that would permit farming the reptiles for their hides, and possibly their meat. To breed crocodilians, zoologists must not only mix the sexes in the right proportions, they must precisely duplicate environmental conditions that trigger the processes in crocodilian metabolism that are associated with reproduction. Those conditions include the right water level and photoperiod for the various species.

The state of crocodilian breeding programs was described succinctly in March 1971 at a meeting in New York of the crocodilian specialist group of the International Union for the Conservation of Nature. Rene E. Honegger of the Zurich Zoo asserted that ". . . breeding success with these reptiles is a rare and remarkable event." What the researchers have failed to accomplish, however, a Thai businessman, scientifically unschooled, has achieved. The zoologists at the meeting in New York listened with amazement as Utai Youngprapakorn told how, within 21 years, he had produced 11,000 crocodiles in Thailand from a breeding stock of 20 animals collected in the wild. The crocodiles—the estuarine species and the Siamese crocodile (*C. Siamensis*)—are native to Indochina and live in pools similar to those they might inhabit in the wild. Youngprapakorn, who began his crocodile farm in 1950 with an investment of $500, revealed his relatively simple formula to the scientists at the meeting.

Two ponds at the farm are reserved for breeding, and each contains 200 adult crocodiles, with a mix of three females to each male—a ratio designed to increase the chance that a male that is ready to mate will find a receptive female. Climatic conditions, of course, are no different on the farm than in the wild, which gives Youngprapakorn a decided advantage over someone trying to breed crocodiles in a temperate climate. Youngprapakorn feeds his crocodiles as much fish as they can eat, in the water where they naturally feed, and he provides them with roofless nesting stalls of vegetation similar to the type used by the animals to build nest mounds in the wild. The young are removed to nursery tanks after they hatch. Youngprapakorn harvests skin and meat from his stock, and he even makes curios out of young that happen to die. In addition, he helps pay the cost of the operation by charging an admission fee for visitors, who can see thousands more crocodiles on his farm than live in the wild in all of Thailand.

Crocodilians seem sluggish when they are basking in the sun, but these powerful creatures move surprisingly fast when in danger or when after prey. Sometimes they wait at the water's edge to seize animals that venture near to drink, but fish, turtles, and other aquatic animals, as well as carrion, constitute the major portion of the crocodilian diet. Rather than lunging forward at its prey, a crocodilian usually catches it with a sideways swipe of its jaws, which, if the prey is small, quickly crush it.

When a crocodilian seizes a large animal, it either rips it to pieces or, if it is a terrestrial animal, holds it under water until it drowns. Several crocodilians may home in on a large animal that one of their number has killed, ripping huge pieces of flesh from it, sometimes by gripping a limb in their jaws and spinning around until it tears loose. However, the familiar motion-picture scene of scores of crocodiles waiting by the river bank, ready to slither into the water and attack anyone who ventures near, seldom is enacted in the wild.

Nevertheless, conservationists who wish to protect crocodilians from extinction must face the fact that some species, and particularly certain individuals, readily prey on humans. Bernhard Grzimek, director of the Frankfurt Zoo and Europe's leading wildlife conservationist, told me of a woman who fell into the Nile River while viewing the scenery from an over-look, and was torn to pieces by crocodiles. The Nile crocodile (*C. niloticus*) and the Asian mugger crocodile (*C. Palustris*) have at times terrorized entire riverside communities. Often, however, it is only a few confirmed man-eating individuals that bring down wrath upon all members of their species.

C. Ralph De Sola, writing in the January-February 1933 issue of *Animal Kingdom,* says of the Orinoco crocodile (*C. intermedius*) of South America: "It does considerable damage to the natives, who retaliate by destroying its nests. Its presence has a decided effect on convicts quartered in the bush of French Guiana, whose attempts at freedom are inhibited or suddenly frustrated by the dreaded man-eater. Death from this crocodile is indeed terrible: a side-swipe of the powerful tail, a crackling report of closing jaws, a few bubbles rising from the river bottom—the prey is finished."

The only crocodile native to the United States is the American crocodile (*C. acutus*), whose range touches southern Florida. Some specimens are as much as 20 feet long. This crocodile is considered quite aggressive. A good comparison of the temperaments of the American crocodile and the more docile American alligator was made for me by Edwin Froehlich, who in conjunction with researchers from the University of Florida has maintained an alligator breeding farm in Lake Park, Florida. Froehlich keeps a 10-foot American crocodile on his farm and is much more wary of it than of alligators. An alligator, being inquisitive, will swim close to you if you pat your hand on the water. It makes no aggressive moves, and submerges and retreats at any sudden move on your part. With the crocodile, it is a different story. Froehlich says that when he pats the water with his hand the crocodile "stays offshore, submerges, and eases in toward your hand." When the crocodile is close enough, Froehlich, "it lunges out of the water, jaws open."

A closely related form, the Cuban crocodile (*C. rhombifer*), is particularly testy. An old Cuban crocodile has lived in the reptile house of the Bronx Zoo for many years, and despite its long captivity it occasionally lunges at a keeper. A few years ago, a blood sample was needed from this beast. The zoo's curator of herpetology, Dr. F. Wayne King, and his crew of keepers were preparing to hog-tie the crocodile when I happened by the reptile house. I changed into some work clothes and lent a hand in the operation, which proved to be quite strenuous, if not dangerous. The crocodile, hissing with toothy jaws wide open and thrashing its tail about, lunged here and there as we tried to get loops of rope over him and lash him to a board. It took a half-dozen of us almost an hour to tie the beast and tape its jaws closed.

The Cuban crocodile is one of the most endangered crocodilians. Many of the swamps that provided a habitat for the creature have been turned to farmland. A correspondent in Cuba wrote to me not long ago and described efforts that are under way to save the crocodile there. About 3,000 of the reptiles were rounded up from areas where their presence conflicted with agriculture and were placed in a fenced preserve in the Zapata Swamp of south-central Cuba. The Cubans hope the crocodile will breed in the swamp, but the project is complicated somewhat by the presence of the American crocodile within the preserve. American and Cuban crocodiles are interbreeding, a fact that has led to fears that the Cuban variety may disappear as a distinct species.

Caimans and Alligators

Caimans, which inhabit tropical America, are large crocodilians with an ugly disposition. Almost every time I have handled a caiman it has tried to bite me, although only one

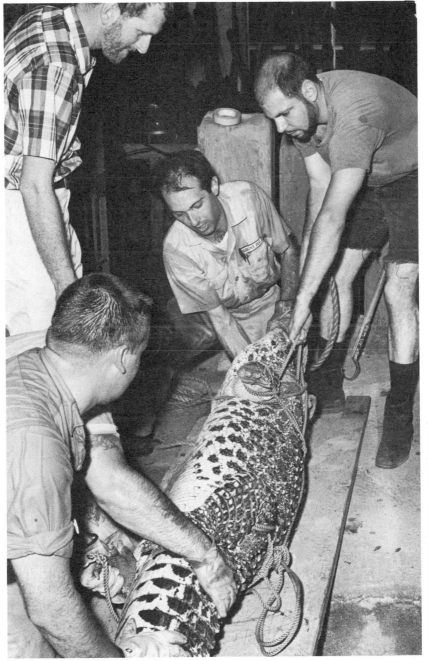

HOG-TIED CROC: *The author, at right, helps members of the Bronx Zoo's reptile department tie up a powerful Cuban crocodile so a blood sample can be taken.*

thus far has succeeded. This particular beast was a yard-long spectacled caiman (*Caiman crocodilus*) that managed to rip my hand, even though the animal was in a cloth sack. The same creature also urinated on me as I held it up before a group of squealing school children during a lecture.

Some species of caimans grow to more than a dozen feet long but even a caiman only a few feet long can inflict a serious bite. Another spectacled caiman of my acquaintance is one that arrived at my home from the Connecticut Audubon Society after it had bitten the hand of an attendant at the society's nature center. When just a hatchling, the caiman had been given as a gift to a family, which soon found that the creature was growing at an appalling rate. When it was almost 3 feet long, its owners brought it to the Connecticut Audubon nature center, and there it slashed the hand of a college student who worked there. The student was taken to a hospital, and the caiman was brought to my house. I kept it in a picnic cooler until I could take it to the Bronx Zoo, as a permanent home. A day or two passed before I could take the creature to the zoo, however, and each time I opened the cooler to feed it or check its condition, the caiman attempted to get at me.

Alligators are much less inclined to bite than caimans. Although the American alligator lives in the wild throughout the Southeastern United States—and only there, by the way—there is no record of a fatal attack on a human by one. This is not to say, however, that such an event never happened, unheralded, in some dank southern swamp. An alligator supposedly killed a member of a party headed by the French explorer La Salle in a Texas river, although this event is not documented to the satisfaction of scientists. More recently, the body of a nine-year-old boy was found in Florida, partially eaten by alligators. Some of the beasts seen near where the body was found were killed, and human remains were found in their stomachs, but it is uncertain whether they killed the youngster or found him after he had died.

Generally alligators flee from human approach, unless they have grown used to people. The most dangerous alligator is the one that has become accustomed to having humans about, and because people have fed it, associates them with food. Alligators in some parts of Florida station themselves in back-yard ponds and are taken for granted as part of the scenery. Every so often, an alligator of this type will make a pass at a person.

During the summer of 1972 two youngsters were attacked by alligators in Florida. One was an eleven-year-old boy who was swimming in a pond with a friend when the jaws of an alligator closed on his body. Bitten severely in the abdomen, the boy was taken to a hospital where he underwent surgery for five hours. The other victim was a six-year-old boy whose leg was grabbed by an alligator as he was scooping minnows from a pond. In 1973, a girl mangled by an alligator died in Florida.

Zoologist Wilfred T. Neil, in his key book on crocodilians, *The Last of the Ruling Reptiles*, suggests that the alligator's behavior toward man varies with time and place. He speculates that alligators might have been more aggressive before they became fearful of firearms. Of all the crocodilians, in Dr. Neil's opinion, only the estuarine crocodile regularly preys on humans. In Papua he witnessed two attacks on men by probably the same estuarine crocodile only two weeks apart. On the first occasion, the crocodile seized a man in the water, and vanished with its victim. The second instance occurred when a crocodile overturned a small boat with two turtle hunters in it. The crocodile managed to grab one of the men by the ankle, but let go when the other man speared the reptile.

Giant Snake: The Anaconda

There is one reptile that is so powerful that it occasionally makes a meal of a large caiman: the anaconda, or water boa (*Eunectes murinus*), reaches a truly enormous size, and is known to prey upon caimans, with some regularity. The anaconda, which may grow larger than 30 feet in length, belongs to the family Boidae, which includes the true giant snakes— anacondas, boas, and pythons. It is a larger relative of the familiar boa constrictor (*Constrictor constrictor*), but far more powerful and of a much more dangerous temperament. Like the boa constrictor, the anaconda loops its coils around its prey and squeezes it until it cannot breathe. With every breath the victim exhales, the anaconda tightens its coils, until the victim's heart and lungs are compressed to such an extent respiration is impossible. Constricting snakes do not, as often is believed, crush their prey.

Olive green, with dark markings, the anaconda spends most of its time in the waters of the South American rivers in which it lives. It sometimes drags its prey into the water to drown. While boa constrictors have a relatively docile temperament, anacondas, even small individuals, cannot be trusted. We have shared our home with a boa constrictor, 6 feet long, for several years, and I have handled many other boas of that size and larger. Never once has one attempted to bite me, although improperly handled, even our pet boa will bite. The anaconda is something else again and bites readily.

I never have handled an anaconda longer than 9 or 10 feet, and I hope never to undertake such a task. A boa constrictor is powerful, and when it tightens its coils it exerts a considerable pressure. But the coils of an anaconda are like loops of steel. The best comparison I can make between the two snakes is that the pressure that seems to be exerted around one's arm by a single loop of an anaconda's coils exceeds that of several coils of a boa constrictor when both snakes are of comparable size.

In all probability, a reasonably strong man could hold his

270

own with a 10-foot anaconda unless the snake was able to anchor its tail or managed to loop a few coils over his throat and face. But a 10-foot anaconda is a bantam; anacondas easily reach more than 25 feet in length. Although a 30-foot specimen never has been verified, a party of oilmen in the jungles of Columbia shot an anaconda that is said to have measured more than that. James A. Oliver, director of the New York Aquarium and one of the nation's foremost herpetologists, discusses the length of the giant snakes in his book, *Snakes in Fact and Fiction*. He accepts at least 37 feet as the maximum length of the anaconda.

For hundreds of years, tales of gargantuan anacondas, at least as large as the 60-foot constrictors that lived millions of years ago, have trickled out of the more remote regions of South America's vast tropical forests. I have heard stories myself, admittedly second or third hand, from herpetologists whose colleagues claim to have seen such snakes. In the early part of this century explorer Percy Fawcett, trekking through the wilderness where Peru, Brazil, and Bolivia meet, supposedly saw an anaconda more than 60 feet long swimming past his boat. A hunting party in the Brazilian rain forest once claimed to have seen a 75-foot anaconda. Considering that an anaconda 30 feet long weighs about 500 pounds, one twice that length would be an immense creature indeed. Do colossal anacondas prowl the backwoods of South America? I would like to believe the answer is affirmative, although the evidence is sparse.

Other dangerous snakes are at least as aquatic as the anaconda. Without question, the most dangerous creature in the fresh waters of the United States is the cottonmouth, or water moccasin (*Agkistrodon piscivorous*). This highly venomous and aggressive cousin of the copperhead ranges through much of the lower half of the country, lurking in swamps, rice fields, ditches, lakes, and streams, where it hunts fish, frogs, small mammals, and birds. The name *cottonmouth* derives from the

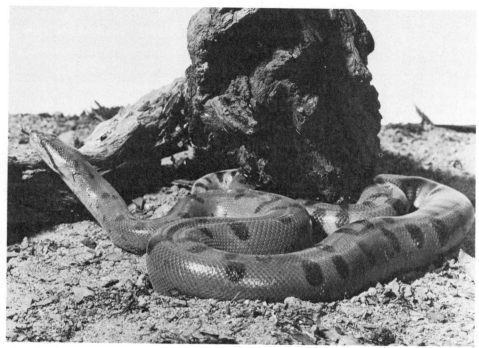

RIVER MONSTER: The anaconda, which lives in the rivers of South America, may grow to a length of more than 35 feet, making it probably the world's largest snake.

white color that is revealed when the snake opens its jaws to strike. The cottonmouth resembles a number of non-venomous water snakes because of its dark brown color. Some of them range much farther north than the cottonmouth and often are killed because of mistaken identity. The cottonmouth is generally larger than any of these "false mocassins," however. Big individuals can be more than 6 feet long and have a girth equal to that of a man's arm. Woodsmen who know the cottonmouth do not provoke it, for unlike many other venomous snakes it will stand and fight even if not cornered.

Sea Snakes: The Invading Horde

Although neither the cottonmouth nor the anaconda can be considered fully aquatic, there is one group of snakes that seldom, if ever, strays upon the land. These are the sea snakes of the family Hydrophiidae, which rove the seas of the Indo-

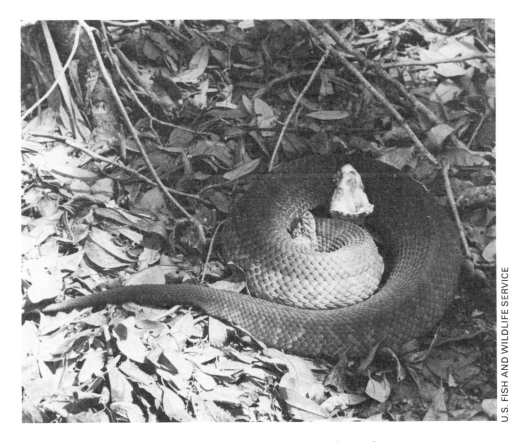

U.S. FISH AND WILDLIFE SERVICE

SOMETHING TO AVOID: The cottonmouth, the only venomous snake in the United States, is a creature to avoid. It leads its menacing life in the South.

Pacific region. Far more venomous than even the cobras, 50 species of sea snakes have adapted in form and physiology to a fully marine life. Their bodies are flattened laterally, particularly in the tail, which serves as an oar. They are extremely graceful in the water, but they barely can get about on land.

Although they breathe air, sea snakes can stay under the surface for hours at a time because of remarkable adaptations. The right lung of the sea snake (in all snakes the left lung has degenerated) reaches almost to its tail. Its windpipe has been modified into an auxiliary lung, which, like the true lung, takes oxygen into the blood. Thus the snake can use its air most efficiently.

Sea snakes generally range from Samoa to East Africa and from Japan to Australia. The far-rover of the group is the yellow-bellied sea snake (*Pelamis platurus*), a great traveler that drifts on the surface of the sea. This species is found from the Asian side of the Pacific to the Americas as far north as southern California. Sea snakes do not seem able to survive in waters colder than 68 degrees F. Therefore water temperature forms an invisible barrier, more effective than any material wall, that prevents them from entering the Atlantic Ocean around the Cape of Good Hope or Cape Horn.

Scientists believe that yellow-bellied sea snakes did not inhabit the eastern edge of the Pacific when the isthmus of Panama rose from the sea about 3 million years ago. Had that narrow neck of land not been there, the snakes probably would inhabit the Atlantic today. They cannot cross the isthmus through the Panama Canal because the freshwater lakes in the canals bar the passage of marine creatures from one ocean to another. If sea snakes should enter fresh water, they would lose critical amounts of body salts and die. Normally, salt from the marine environment replaces salt that is continuously eliminated by a special gland in the sea snake's lower jaw, so that the intake and elimination of salt in the snake's body balances out.

The freshwater barrier provided by the Panama Canal would be lacking in any sea-level canal across the isthmus, and a sea snake invasion of the Atlantic is one of the most feared consequences of such a project. Dire predictions of sea snakes swarming through the Caribbean, chasing tourists back to North America, follow any mention of a sea-level canal. There is more to fear from such an invasion, however, than a retreat of tourists from the West Indies. Introduction of sea snakes into the tropical Atlantic could have a serious effect on the ecological balance there.

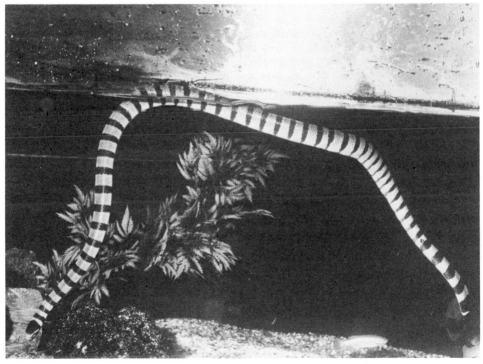

A REAL SEA SERPENT: The banded sea snake is an ocean-going serpent, living all of its life in the sea. This one swims in a tank at the New York Aquarium.

275

Fish of the Pacific habitually avoid sea snakes, even if the fish are large enough to make the snakes their prey. Scientists have placed sea snakes in aquariums with Pacific Ocean fish that were starving, but the fish refused to touch the snakes. One Pacific snapper that had been trained to gobble up live food the instant it hit the water went so far as to spit out a sea snake as soon as it realized the nature of its prey. Atlantic fish, on the other hand, seem to lack a fear of sea snakes and attempt to eat them. Several Atlantic fish have died from sea snake bites when snakes and fish were placed in the water together. Researchers suggest that fish living in the Pacific have evolved mechanisms that instinctively tell them to avoid sea snakes, but that their Atlantic counterparts lack such a safeguard.

Sea snakes have been known since very early times, but perhaps the first reference to them in literature was made in the first century. Spanish explorers who visited the Pacific coast of South America in the 16th century reported seeing vast numbers of yellow-bellied sea snakes close to shore. Although sea snakes generally remain near the shore, great armadas of these creatures, probably breeding or migrating, occasionally cover the surface of the open sea. One such horde, 10 feet wide and 60 miles long, was seen between the Malay Peninsula and Sumatra in 1932. Within that mass literally millions of serpentine bodies, undulating and stroking with their flat tails, surged forward toward some unknown destination.

Sea snakes may be the most numerous reptiles on earth. Many Asians value them for their skin and meat, and fishermen take thousands of them from the water yearly. Fifty thousand sea snakes are sold each year in Japan's Amami Islands, and twice that number are caught and sold annually on Gato Island in the Philippines. Vietnamese fishermen haul in hundreds of sea snakes with each cast of the net at certain seasons of the year. The fishermen work their nets with bare hands, so that many are bitten—and a goodly number reportedly die from the sea snakes' venom.

Once bitten by a sea snake, a person stands a good chance of dying, for paralysis develops a short time after the relatively painless nip of the reptile's fangs. A single ejection of the venom is powerful enough to kill one or two men. During October 1815, an unusual number of sea snakes ventured into a river near Madras, India, and several people died of their bites.

Not all sea snakes bite readily, however, so one man's experience with the creatures may differ from the next person's. I have seen banded sea snakes of the genus *Laticauda* picked up and handled with no apparent indication that they had any urge to use their fangs. Dr. Oliver, who has worked with sea snakes both in captivity and in the wild, summed up for me their unpredictability: "They vary from those that will bite anything to those you cannot *make* bite," he said.

John Prescott, who has captured sea snakes with hand nets, told me that never has he seen unprovoked aggression by one of these animals. But on two occasions sea snakes have given him a scare. While curator at Marineland of the Pacific, Prescott received a cardboard box, wrapped in plain brown paper, from a friend in the Caroline Islands. The box was labelled simply "Biological Specimens." Prescott removed the wrapper and began to open the box, when from beneath one of the flaps appeared a flat, oar-like tail which got longer and longer. Recognizing the nature of what was in the box, and remembering that his friend once had promised to send him some sea snakes, Prescott backed away. Just then the snake became wedged in the box, however, and Prescott was able to place it in a proper container.

On another occasion, this time in an undersea cave off Okinawa, Prescott narrowly missed a head-on collision with a sea snake about 5 feet long. He had entered the cave in search of fish, and as he approached the end of the cave he was looking at the bottom instead of ahead of him. Looking up, he saw the sea snake swimming directly at him. Inadvertantly he had cornered the animal in the cave, and it was trying to escape. Before Prescott could move, the snake flashed directly under him and shot out of the cave into the open sea.

Sea snakes seem more inclined toward pugnacity when on the surface than when underwater, according to the reports of some divers who have encountered them. David Hancock once followed one for an hour while scuba diving on the Great Barrier Reef. He first observed the snake at a depth of 90 feet, and closing in on it, he followed it at a perilously close distance. He even tried to grab the creature, but it easily evaded him. He continued to trail the snake as it headed for the surface, where its docile behavior changed and it approached Hancock menacingly. Once both of them submerged again, however, the snake, according to Hancock, ceased its aggressiveness.

Not-So-Tough Turtles

The most familiar aquatic reptiles are not snakes or crocodilians, but turtles. Among the species that inhabit North American ponds, lakes, and streams are some with disagreeable reputations. They are, of course, the snapping turtles—the common snapper (*Chelydra serpentina*) and the huge alligator snapper (*Macroclemys temminicki*), which is the world's largest freshwater turtle. Ranging from Florida to the southern Midwest, the alligator snapping turtle often weighs 100 pounds —and it has been recorded at twice that weight. With a huge head, wickedly hooked jaws, and dorsal keels that give its shell a sawback appearance, the alligator snapper looks like something created to frighten little children into being good. Few beasts look so forbidding, but while the alligator snapper could take a sizeable piece of meat out of anyone into whom it sank

278

its sharp-edged jaws, it is not particularly pugnacious nor does it seek large prey. Instead, this monstrous turtle prefers to spend most of its time waiting in ambush for fish on the bottom of whatever body of water that serves it as a home. With its rough-hewn shell, the turtle looks like a chunk of rock, a stump, or a piece of debris. Moreover, it has evolved a fishing lure that surpasses any device humans have invented to lure fish to a hook. On the floor of its mouth is a pinkish tab of flesh that not only resembles a worm in shape but wriggles with a motion so wormlike that it draws fish right into the snapper's jaws. Thus, rather than actively pursuing fish, the alligator snapper rests on the bottom, wriggles its lure, and waits for something to drop by for dinner.

The common snapping turtle is another case entirely. It prowls the water searching for ducklings, swimming mammals, fish, frogs, and anything else it can handle. But much of its diet consists of trash fish and carrion, so it serves an important function in maintaining the balance of nature in the waters it inhabits. Its range is wide extending from Canada to South America. At home in fresh water, it also ventures into the brackish waters of estuaries. Although not so large as the alligator snapping turtle, the common variety can weigh as much as 50 pounds. A specimen half that weight can be considered a big turtle, however. Personally, I never have seen a common snapping turtle that weighed more than about 30 pounds.

How dangerous is the common snapper? Not very, actually, especially when in the water, where it will flee from a human's approach. But on land, where the turtle cannot move as quickly as it can in water, it sometimes will do just what its name implies—snap at its adversary, to the accompaniment of some ferocious hissing noises. I have handled snapping turtles ranging in size from youngsters 2 inches long to adults too large to fit in the bottom of a standard-size trash can, and seldom has one tried to bite me. The ferocity of the common

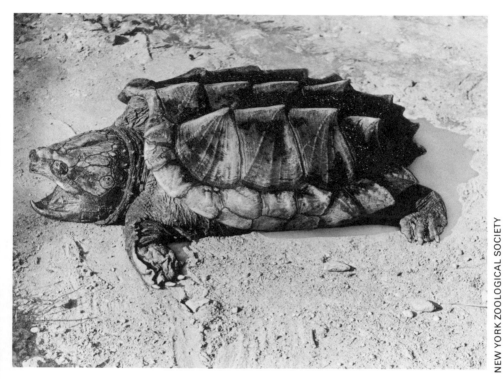

NEW YORK ZOOLOGICAL SOCIETY

HEAVYWEIGHT: The huge, 200-pound alligator snapping turtle, shown here out of the water, is not an active hunter. Instead it lies in wait on the bottom, wriggling a worm-like appendage near its tongue to lure fish to its jaws.

snapper is somewhat over-rated, as is the power of its bite. It is doubtful, for example, whether a fair-sized specimen could cleave off one's finger, much less, as often is claimed, chop a broom handle in two. There are many aquatic reptiles that truly endanger man, but the common snapping turtle is not one of them.

CHAPTER 7

Sea Monsters–
Past, Present,
and Future

Its form cloaked by the sea mist, its desolate cry masked by the rush of the storm surge, a creature passes close offshore, perhaps skirting the entrance to the bay, perhaps just beyond the rock-strewn base of the headland. Close though it is, weather and darkness conceal its presence as, driven perhaps by a dateless urging, it prowls through the sea and the night. So my imagination pictures the sea beast of legend, the shadowy creature that has been reported too often by rational, astute observers to lack substance, but whose existence nevertheless remains unproved. Somewhere, perhaps in a cove with waters black as pitch, or in a murky deep, lies a giant creature yet unknown to humankind, or at least that is what I prefer to believe. Sea serpents have had a place in lore and legend for countless centuries. The accounts telling of mysterious, unnamed sea creatures include too many substantive observations for anyone to deny that man has yet to identify all the large animals that inhabit the waters.

Many biologists, at least those whose scientific detachment is tempered with a touch of romance, privately confide their belief that not everyone who has seen a strange creature at the sea has been victimized by illusion. And certainly it stands to reason that if an unknown animal of large size exists on this planet, the chances are greatest that it lives in the water. Most, if not all, of the terrestrial creatures of reasonable size have long since been discovered, for the simple reason that we are far more likely to come in contact with them. It is estimated, for example, that we have identified 96 percent of all living birds—but still a vast number of the fishes that live in the sea remain without a name.

Assuming that an unknown creature exists, the question arises whether it is an aberrant form of an existing species, a creature that has kept pace with evolution, or a survivor from past ages, unchanged for millions of years. Plenty of precedent for all possibilities exists. In 1964 in the Bahamas, an oceanographer's net swept up an inch-long, pop-eyed fish previously unknown to science. Its discovery created a new family, genus, and species. And in the Indian ocean, a yard-wide deepwater jellyfish, also new to science, was collected during the 1950s.

Survivors From Past Ages

In 1888, scientists aboard the research vessel *Albatross* dredged up a surprisingly large fish from a depth of 6,000 feet off the coast of Chile. A photograph survives showing an elongate fish, somewhat primitive in appearance, with a double fin and a large, gaping mouth. It appears to have been at least 5 feet long, probably longer. Little else is known about it because a crewman, thinking to keep the deck neat, promptly heaved the creature overboard.

In 1959, a larval eel more than 6 feet long was brought up by the trawl of a research vessel west of the Cape of Good Hope. The normal counterpart of the creature would be an immature eel 2 or 3 inches long that, when adult, would grow to between 3 and 5 feet. How large is the adult stage of the 6-foot larva? Do huge eels 90 feet long snake through the depths?

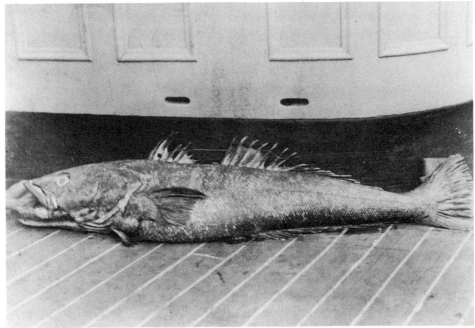

STRANGE FISH: This fish, about 5 feet long, was dredged from a depth of 6,000 feet by the research vessel Albatross *in 1888. Shortly after this photo was taken on deck, a crewman tossed the fish overboard, to the dismay of scientists who had never seen anything like it before.*

Perhaps the most startling discovery thus far of a sea creature new to science took place in 1938, when a large fish was captured in a trawl in 250 feet of water off an archipelago in the Indian Ocean. The creature weighed more than 125 pounds and was a lobe-finned fish much like those that first shed their aquatic existence during the Devonian Period of life on land. The fish was named the coelecanth (*Latimeria chalumnae*). Others have been collected since then, and scientists believe that large individuals may weigh as much as 180 pounds, possibly more. The species grows to a length of more

285

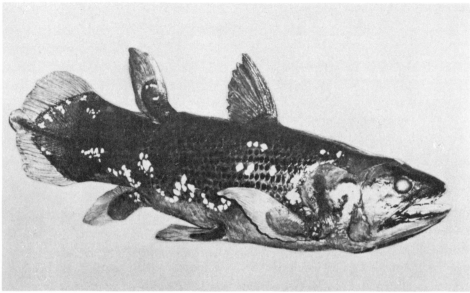

U.S. FISH AND WILDLIFE SERVICE. REX GARY SCHMIDT

SURVIVOR FROM THE PAST: The coelacanth, long thought to be extinct until its spectacular discovery in 1938, still roams the oceans. It is related to the fishes that gave rise to land-living vertebrates.

than 5 feet. Little changed from its ancestors of 300 million years ago, it is a chunky fish armed with very sharp cone-shaped teeth, and it is armored with heavy scales. The coelecanth is living proof that a creature of ancient lineage, of considerable size, and unknown to science, can turn up in the sea at almost any time.

Whether or not their species are unknown, some very sizeable animals must inhabit the deeper regions of the sea, perhaps where reefs meet deep water. Sportsmen fishing in deep waters off Bimimi often have had bait torn off large hooks by unidentifiable animals. About 20 years ago Robert Menzies, a well-known oceanographer, turned up a strong indication that something very large and very powerful roves the Milne Edwards Deep off the west coast of South America. Dr. Menzies baited a steel hook, 2 feet long, with a yard-long squid and lowered it into the depths. Something in those dark waters tugged at the bait, removed it, and left the hook badly bent.

Could the creature have been a giant squid? A huge shark? The monstrous parent of a 6-foot larval eel? Or something that should have vanished at the end of the Mesozoic Era?

Quite likely, if a sea monster is found, it will not be totally unfamiliar to biologists. The main lines of animal evolution have been quite thoroughly sketched, so there is little chance that whatever many have been seen and described as a sea serpent will be totally alien in biology. It may indeed be quite familiar in some respects, even closely related to a known form, but perhaps unpleasantly larger.

Six-Ton Octopus?

That possibility was raised by an incident that occurred in December 1896 on a beach near St. Augustine, Florida. Its full import was not made clear, however, until the magazine *Natural History* published an analysis of it in March 1971. The article described a sea creature of titanic bulk that was beached near St. Augustine and was identified, though not without dispute, as an octopus. But what an octopus. Its body was said to measure 25 feet in girth, to weigh an estimated 6 tons, and to trail tentacles at least 75 feet long. Before the article was published, the last specimens of tissue from the animal were examined in a laboratory and in fact proved to be octopus tissue. If 6-ton octopuses do exist, no legendary sea monster would be more terrible, for a cephalopod of that size could well account for many of the vessels that over the years have vanished at sea.

It would be appropriate if the creature was indeed a huge cephalopod, for these animals have contributed heavily to the lore of the sea monster. Scylla, the monster whose great arms reached for the seafarers of Homer's Odyssey, easily could have been a giant squid. And in Scandinavian waters, the giant squid and the kraken, or sea monster, virtually are indistinguishable from one another. The giant squid often is called a *kraken,* which also is a designation for sea monster. Olaus Magnus in 1555 described a "serpent of astonishing size in an island called Moos, in the diocese of Hammer." First seen in 1522, the creature was described as "raising itself high above the surface of the water and circling like a spire." The serpent, according to Olaus Magnus, was about 75 feet long. Was it really a serpent, or a giant squid reaching its tentacles high above the waves?

Olaus Magnus also described a serpent that lived in holes among the rocks at the shore near Bergen, Norway. Supposedly 200 feet long, it emerged from its caverns on summer nights to devour hogs, calves, and other livestock ashore. It was noted for its flaming, glaring eyes, an interesting observation in view of the fact that the eyes of a squid often are described in that manner. Olaus Magnus said that the serpent, in addition to raiding livestock, attacked boats, snatching men from the vessels as it towered over them.

Scandinavian clergymen seem to have had a near-monopoly on early sea serpent stories. Bishop Eric Pontoppidan of Bergen, in 1752, described a sea serpent of his day that was stranded by the tide in an inlet. Its remains were soft and slimy, a description that, with other characteristics mentioned by the Bishop make it appear to have been a large squid.

288

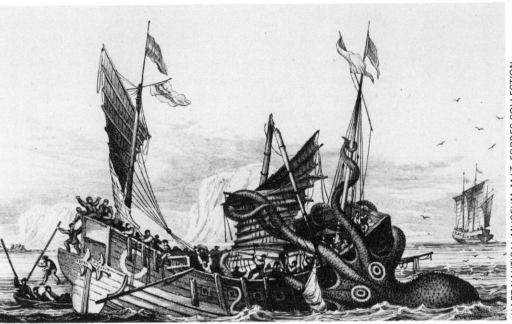

BASED ON FACT: The drawing shows a kraken, or giant squid, attacking a ship. Experts believe that giant squids have at times attacked, and possibly even sunk, ships at sea.

Myriad Monsters

Hans Egede, a Dane who wrote about sea serpents during the same period, told of seeing a monster in the Davis Straits near Greenland. It had a long snout and it spouted like a whale. The creature, which also had broad flippers, sounds very much like a whale, except that its body was serpentine. No modern whale has such a shape, but 40 million years ago whales with long snouts and snake-like bodies flourished in the seas.

Bishop Pontoppidan also wrote of a sighting by Captain Lorenz von Ferry, an official of Bergen known for his good sense, who chanced upon a sea serpent one day while sailing. The beast had a rather horselike head, with a long white mane streaming behind it. As the creature moved through the waves, von Ferry could see more than half a dozen coils about 6 feet apart. He fired a gun at the monster, which sank in a sea reddened with its blood.

Sea monster sightings became almost commonplace off Massachusetts during the early 19th century. A particularly colorful encounter, which some people branded a hoax, took

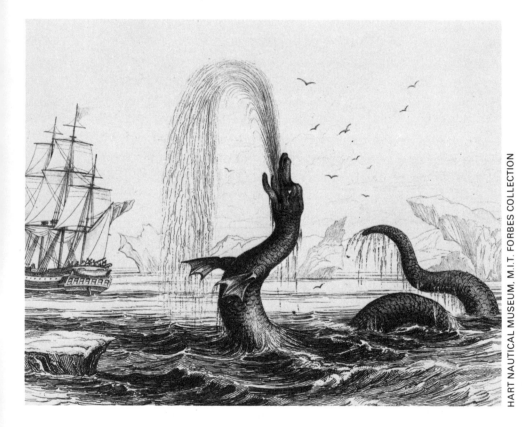

DAVIS STRAITS SERPENT: Hans Egede, a Dane, reported seeing the creature depicted above in the Davis Straits.

290

place on May 12, 1818, as the schooner *Adamant* was sailing from Penobscot to Hingham. According to the schooner's captain, Joseph Woodward, a large object was sighted in the water about two o'clock in the afternoon. Thinking he might be near the wreck of a ship, Woodward brought his vessel close by the form and found that it was "a monstrous serpent," coiling and uncoiling in a most unfriendly manner. When the serpent swam to a distance of some 60 feet from the schooner, the crew opened fire with a cannon and muskets. The missiles bounced off the beast like rain, and the serpent submerged, coming to the surface again with its head on one side of the boat and its tail on the other. The captain estimated the serpent to be 130 feet long and 6 feet in diameter. It remained near the boat for five hours but did not attempt to harm it.

In August 1848, the officers and crew of the British frigate *Daedalus* saw a creature about 60 feet long, with a snake-like head and a mane, and in May 1863, the Royal Mail steamship *Athenian* came across a snake 100 feet long in the water.

The link between the giant squid and sea serpent is strengthened by a report from the British barque *Pauline*, which in July 1875 was sailing for Zanzibar when it came across a sperm whale encircled by what those aboard the ship thought were the coils of a sea serpent. The serpent, according to those who saw it, had a huge head, a whitish belly, and a brown back. After a struggle of a quarter of an hour, the two vanished beneath the waves, with the whale diving, or being dragged down, head first. What the people aboard the *Pauline* probably witnessed was a battle between a sperm whale and a giant squid.

A most unusual type of sea monster, quite unlike the serpentine creatures usually reported, was seen by the captain and ship's surgeon of the British steamship *Nestor* in 1876. While steaming for Shanghai, the vessel drew near what appeared to be a shoal. Its presence surprised the captain, for his charts showed no such hazard. The "shoal" turned out to be moving, and on closer investigation it appeared to resemble a gigantic amphibian, like a frog or salamander. It had a yellow head about 20 feet long and a yellow and black tail, and its total length was more than 45 feet.

Most accounts of past sea serpent sightings are included in a classic book written in 1892 by A.C. Oudemans, a Dutch zoologist and botanist and director of the Royal Zoological and Botanical Society at The Hague. His book, *The Great Sea Serpent*, records 162 sightings from 1522 to 1890. He wrote it to support his conclusion that "the great sea serpent" was an unknown species of giant pinniped with large eyes and a mane that was as fearless as a walrus.

The giant-sea-mammal theory also has been proposed to explain sightings of strange objects in Scotland's lochs. Although today they hold fresh water, once the lochs were arms of the sea. The most famous of these creatures, of course, is the monster of Loch Ness, but other lochs have their own mysterious inhabitants. For centuries, in fact, the lochs of Scotland have spawned myriad legends of water monsters, and certainly no lakes could be better suited as the homes of strange and nameless animals. Cutting between rugged, misty hills, the lochs are incredibly deep: some go down more than 1,000 feet into the earth. They occupy deep valleys that were flooded by the sea when Ice Age glaciers retreated more than 12,000 years ago. The rise in sea level then ceased and the sea retreated slightly, cutting off the lochs from the ocean.

The Loch Ness monster has slithered in and out of the news regularly since the 1930s, when it first was heavily publicized. In most reports the monster has appeared in classic sea serpent style, with a long neck and a reptilian head raised above the water. Often witnesses describe it as having several humps on its back. In recent years, scientific teams have probed for the Loch Ness creature, using high-powered pho-

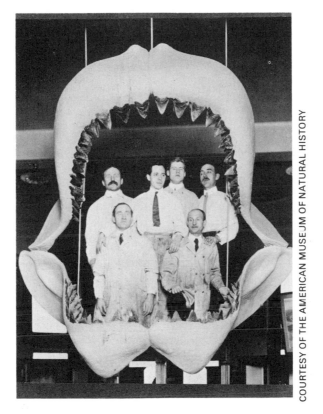

COURTESY OF THE AMERICAN MUSEUM OF NATURAL HISTORY

KILLER FROM THE PAST: The jaws of this fossil shark, a relative of today's great white shark, speak for themselves. The creature that owned them must have been at least the size of a sperm whale.

tographic equipment, sonar, and midget submarines. Film taken by these researchers shows images that look indeed like a humped, long-necked animal rising from the dark waters of the loch.

Perhaps the best evidence thus far for the existence of the Loch Ness monster is sonar echoes that have been picked up from moving objects deep in the loch. In 1972, searchers lowered sonar gear and a camera into the loch and recorded what appeared to be large objects chasing schools of salmon. The sonar echoes were such that they could have been produced by two large animals, 20 to 30 feet long, with long appendages and at least two humps each. The photographs showed what appeared to be a flipper as long as a man.

The creature of Loch Ness has a rival for publicity in a similar beast that haunts the waters of Loch Morar. From descriptions by those who have seen it, "Morag" resembles the Loch Ness monster in form and habit. Loch Morar, 11 miles long and more than a mile across at its widest point, is 30 feet above sea level, but only a quarter mile from the ocean's edge. The loch and its monster are discussed in *The Search for Morag*, a book by Elizabeth Montgomery Campbell and David Solomon. The authors are members of the Loch Morar Survey, a group that heads the search for the beast.

The survey began its work in 1970 by collecting legends and stories about Morag. Since then it has gathered accounts of sightings in recent years. One such sighting occurred in 1948, when a creature with an estimated length of 20 feet and five humps manifested itself before a boatload of tourists. Several other persons have seen a long neck, or a broad back, surface in the loch, whose waters, unlike the peat-stained waters of Loch Ness, are sparkling clear. The clarity of the water enabled a fisherman on the lake in July 1969 to see what looked like a giant lizard lying on the bottom 20 feet down. The beast, about 20 feet long, seemed to be peering up at him.

That same year two men who were voyaging across Loch Morar in a motor boat had a chilling encounter with whatever it is that hides in the loch. Shortly after 9 P. M. on August 16, Duncan McDonnell and William Simpson were motoring through the warm twilight when they saw a huge, humped animal with a rough, brown hide and what looked like a reptilian head. It surfaced behind their boat, swam alongside the craft, and bumped it. McDonell picked up an oar and tried to

294

beat the creature away, but the oar snapped. Simpson, meanwhile, picked up a rifle and fired a bullet into the creature. It promptly sank out of sight, although there was no evidence that it had been hurt.

In the two years following the McDonell-Simpson incident, thirteen more sightings were reported. Many of the observations were of large, hump-like objects moving through the water. The observers ranged from scientists to schoolchildren, both in boats and ashore.

Scotland is not the only land where people have seen strange creatures emerge from the waters of deep lakes. One of the large lakes in western Canada, Lake Okanagan in central British Columbia, has its own version of the monster of the lochs. Called *Ogopogo* by local Indians, the creature roves a body of water that is 2,000 feet deep and 80 miles long. Ogopogo is feared by the Indians who claim it will attack men on the water. Its appearance, according to those who have seen it, resembles that of the creatures of the lochs.

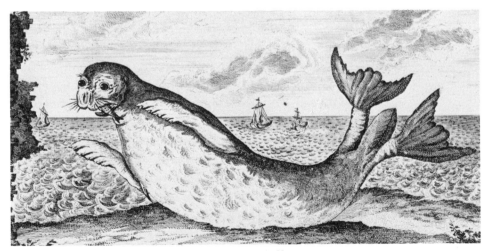

SEA MONSTER: This creature supposedly appeared on the shores of the Adriatic Sea in Italy some 200 years ago.

Certainly many sightings of "monsters" in lakes and at sea can be explained away as mistakes, as optical phenomena, or as already existing creatures viewed from a peculiar angle or under poor conditions of visibility. The fragile ribbonfishes (Trachipteridae), which are flat-bodied creatures about 30 feet long, but slight in build with a high-spined dorsal fin, undoubtedly can take credit for many sea serpent sightings. But when the entire question is considered, the possibility cannot be dismissed that there are indeed unknown creatures hidden by the waters, and that some may someday qualify as sea monsters.

Sea Monsters of Yesterday

Several aquatic creatures of the past, if they suddenly appeared today, would meet the qualification required for any good sea monster. An ancient crocodile, *Rhamposuchus*, which stalked its prey in India 10 million years ago, reached a length of 60 feet—larger even than the terrible tyrannosaur of 70 million years ago. A crocodile of Texas that was a contemporary of the tyrannosaur was as large as the great dinosaur, reaching a length of 45 feet.

Since early in geologic history, the sea has held monstrous creatures of one sort or another. During the Silurian Period, more than 400 million years ago, giant water scorpions, 6 feet long, boasting huge claws and vicious jaws, swam through the seas after primitive fish. The scorpions shared the waters with mollusks called nautiloids, which were 16 feet long and resembled large squid encased in cone-shaped shells.

Some of the amphibians that arose during the Denovian Period grew to considerable size. The British Museum of Natural History has on exhibit the reconstructed skeleton of a 7-foot amphibian, *Paracyclotosaurus davidi*, shaped like an alligator with a broad skull about 2 feet wide. *Eryops*, an amphibian whose fossilized remains were found in Texas, resembled a giant salamander 6 feet in length. Anyone who has seen a large frog or salamander eat its prey knows that a king-size amphibian would be a formidable beast.

During the Mesozoic Era, there were sharks in the sea as large as modern sperm whales. The reconstructed jaws of a fossil great white shark, on display in the American Museum of Natural History, gape wide enough to hold a half dozen men. It was during the Mesozoic that dinosaurs ruled the land, and at the same time other reptiles of great size evolved in the sea. The Mesozoic was a time when vast, shallow seas infringed on the continents, and in these seas flourished reptiles that were remarkably well adapted for an aquatic life. In form and habit, they mirrored fish and modern sea mammals.

Much of what scientists know about these ancient aquatic reptiles results from the curiosity of the daughter of an English carpenter, Mary Anning, who lived from 1799 to 1847. While a youngster she became intensely interested in fossils, and she pursued her avocation with such passion that by the time she was eleven years old she had discovered the first known complete skeleton of an ichthyosaur. Later she performed a similar feat by finding the first complete skeleton of a plesiosaur.

Ichthyosaurs and plesiosaurs were the two most important sea reptiles of the Jurassic Period, which lasted through the middle of the Mesozoic, from 180 million years ago to 135 million years ago. The plesiosaur, interestingly enough, resembles a seal with a long neck and a reptilian head. Its tail is relatively short, its body rounded, and its flippers long and broad. One line of plesiosaurs, known as the pliosaurs, evolved into a short-necked form with a body that was shaped rather like a torpedo.

297

The ichthyosaurs were totally adapted for the water and could not even get about on the shore, as could the plesiosaurs. In shape they resembled a modern dolphin, right down to the pointed snout, except for that fact that the tail was oriented vertically instead of horizontally. Among the largest of the ichthyosaurs was *Platyodon*, which reached a length of 30 feet. Ichthyosaurs bore living young, which entered the world tail-first as the female swam in the sea. An ichthyosaur fossil at the British Museum has a tiny embryo, barely visible, within it.

During the sunset of the age of reptiles, which ended about 70 million years ago, a huge lizard, related to the monitor lizards of today, roved the sea. It was the mosasaur, a creature with long jaws that were filled with huge teeth and which probably rivaled the giant sharks in ferocity. With a paddle-like tail and short flippers, the mosasaur probably inhabited inshore waters. The animals even may have hauled themselves up onto

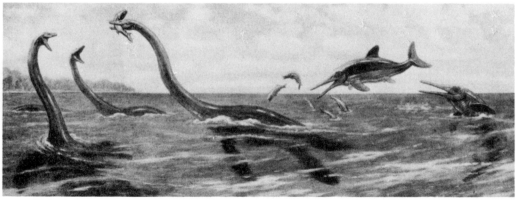

COURTESY OF THE

REAL MONSTERS: Long-necked pleisosaurs and leaping icthyosaurs, sea reptiles of the past, could well pass for sea monsters if they lived today. The question is—do creatures such as these survive somewhere in the vast depths?

298

the beach to lay their eggs. Without a doubt, the mosasaur ranks as one of the most frightening creatures ever to inhabit the ocean.

The mammals came into their own with the passing of the age of reptiles, and by 40 million years ago the sea was the home of the whale. Among the whales that flourished, but then vanished without leaving descendants, were the zeuglodons, the creatures whose description remarkably coincides with that given by Hans Egede of the animal he saw in the Davis Straits. Zeuglodons were at least 70 feet long, with tapering jaws, and then were only 8 feet in girth at the widest part of the body. Thus streamlined, they resembled a giant serpent. It would be ironic, indeed, if unknown to man such a primitive creature as the zeuglodon survived somewhere in the deeps while the blue whale, which has passed the test of natural selection but has fallen victim to man's greed, vanished from the sea.

Most Dangerous Creature of All

The sea, with its creatures large and small, awaits discovery. In coming decades man will unveil many of its inner mysteries—its treasures and its terrors. As man penetrates the hydrosphere, his view of this major portion of the earth's environment must adjust and change if he is to cope with it.

The posture that we must take toward water and its creatures was well summarized by my friend and former colleague, Robert Morris, in a letter he wrote when I asked him what animal in the sea is the most dangerous to man. "I feel," he wrote, "that the most dangerous creature in the sea is man himself. In venturing into the foreign environment of the sea he must be prepared to understand and meet it on its terms and not his. In diving and encountering many potentially dangerous creatures, my closest encounters with death have been

299

from human error. . . . From my more than 1,000 hours underwater with an Aqualung, I have come away with one profound idea—you must understand the ocean environment, the
creatures living there, and, more than that, your capabilities in
that environment."

The water world may hold terrors, but in itself it is not
terrifying. There are killers in the sea as there are elsewhere,
but the dangers they present, like other dangers, diminish in
the face of knowledge.

SUGGESTED READING

Bigelow, Henry B. and Schroeder, William C. *Fishes of the Gulf of Maine*. Washington: United States Government Printing Office, 1953.

Budker, Paul. *The Life of Sharks*. New York: Columbia University Press, 1971.

Campbell, Elizabeth Montgomery and Solomon, David. *The Search for Morag*. New York: Walker and Company, 1972.

Case, Gerard R. *Fossil Shark and Fish Remains of North America*. New York: Gerard R. Case, Jersey City, N.J.

Clare, Patricia. *The Struggle for the Great Barrier Reef*. New York: Walker and Company, 1972.

Cromie, William J. *The Living World of the Sea*. Englewood Cliffs, N.J.: Prentice-Hall, Inc., 1966.

Cromie, William J. *Secrets of the Seas*. Pleasantville: Reader's Digest Assoc., 1971.

Gilbert, Perry W. *Sharks and Survival*. Boston: D.C. Heath & Company, 1963.

SUGGESTED READING

Greenwood, P.H. and Norman, J.R. *A History of Fishes*. New York: Hill and Wang, 1963.

Lane, Frank W. *Kingdom of the Octopus*. New York: Pyramid Publications, 1962.

Lorenz, Konrad. *On Aggression*. New York: Harcourt Brace Jovanovich, 1966.

Neill, Wilfred T. *The Last of the Ruling Reptiles*. New York: Columbia University Press, 1971.

Oliver, James A. *Snakes in Fact and Fiction*. New York: The Macmillan Company, 1959.

Scheffer, Victor. *The Year of the Whale*. New York: Charles Scribner's Sons, 1969.

Thorson, Gunnar. *Life in the Sea*. New York: McGraw-Hill Boom Company, 1971.

Whipple, A.B.C. *Yankee Whalers in the South Seas*. Garden City: Doubleday Company, 1954.

INDEX

303

INDEX

INDEX